Histories of Health and Materiality in the Indian Ocean World

Histories of Health and Materiality in the Indian Ocean World

Medicine, Material Culture and Trade, 1600–2000

Edited by
Burton Cleetus and Anne Gerritsen

BLOOMSBURY ACADEMIC
LONDON • NEW YORK • OXFORD • NEW DELHI • SYDNEY

BLOOMSBURY ACADEMIC
Bloomsbury Publishing Plc
50 Bedford Square, London, WC1B 3DP, UK
1385 Broadway, New York, NY 10018, USA
29 Earlsfort Terrace, Dublin 2, Ireland

BLOOMSBURY, BLOOMSBURY ACADEMIC and the Diana logo are trademarks of Bloomsbury Publishing Plc

First published in Great Britain 2023
Paperback edition published 2024

Copyright © Burton Cleetus and Anne Gerritsen, 2023

Burton Cleetus and Anne Gerritsen have asserted their right under the Copyright, Designs and Patents Act, 1988, to be identified as Editors of this work.

Cover image © Delhi: selling rice in a bazaar. Watercolour by an Indian painter. Credit: Wellcome Collection. Attribution 4.0 International (CC BY 4.0)

All rights reserved. No part of this publication may be reproduced or transmitted in any form or by any means, electronic or mechanical, including photocopying, recording, or any information storage or retrieval system, without prior permission in writing from the publishers.

Bloomsbury Publishing Plc does not have any control over, or responsibility for, any third-party websites referred to or in this book. All internet addresses given in this book were correct at the time of going to press. The author and publisher regret any inconvenience caused if addresses have changed or sites have ceased to exist, but can accept no responsibility for any such changes.

A catalogue record for this book is available from the British Library.

A catalog record for this book is available from the Library of Congress.

ISBN: PB: 978-1-3501-9648-3
ePDF: 978-1-3501-9589-9
eBook: 978-1-3501-9590-5

Typeset by Deanta Global Publishing Services, Chennai, India

To find out more about our authors and books visit www.bloomsbury.com and sign up for our newsletters.

Contents

List of figures	vii
List of contributors	viii
List of abbreviations	xi
Acknowledgements	xii

1. Health, medicine and trade in the Indian Ocean world: A material culture approach *Anne Gerritsen and Burton Cleetus* — 1
2. 'Europe does not want you': Natural history, materia medica and the empire *Pratik Chakrabarti* — 25
3. *In pursuit of a healing Eden*: Exploring the medico-botanical networks of knowledge circulation in the Indian Ocean region with special reference to South India, 1600–1800 CE *Malavika Binny* — 41
4. Rhubarb in the Indian Ocean world: The entangled itinerary of a material complex *Anne Gerritsen* — 63
5. Perfumes in early modern India: Ephemeral materiality and aromatic mobility *Amrita Chattopadhyay* — 87
6. Letters to the Vaidyan: The circulation of Ayurvedic drugs and knowledge from Kottakkal Aryavaidyasala to South-east Asia *Burton Cleetus* — 111
7. Toxic trading: Poisons and medicines in British India *David Arnold* — 127
8. 'The all-cleansing soap'? History of soap in Keralam c. 1880–1950 *Greeshma Justin John* — 145
9. Chaulmoogra: Indian Ocean world leprosy remedies in the South Pacific *Jane Buckingham* — 171
10. Bodies in circulation: Determining age and regulating health of transported convicts to the Andamans, c.1860s–1920s *Suparna Sengupta* — 191
11. From tribal knowledge to Ayurvedic medicine: Transition of *Arogyapacha*, the wonder herb of Kerala *Girija KP* — 211

12 Of miracle drugs, Captain Hooks and Colonialism 2.0:
    Bioprospecting, biopiracy and the patenting of tribal bioresources
    and medicinal knowledge *Kaushiki Das*   231
13 Privileging the body: The bio-materialization of medicine and the
    asymmetrical production of pluralism *Harish Naraindas*   253

Select Bibliography   281
Index   297

Figures

1.1	Toothpaste pot, England, 1860–95	2
1.2	Ceramic pot for 'Oriental toothpaste', England, 1870–1910	3
1.3	Label for Areca nut tooth paste, 1900–10?	3
8.1	Malabar takes pride in hygiene	156
13.1	The bio-materialized world of medicine	258
13.2	Excluded esoteric circle	263
13.3	Fever, represented as a frenzied beast	265
13.4	Excluded exoteric circle	268

Contributors

David Arnold is a professor emeritus in the History department at the University of Warwick and a Fellow of the British Academy. He has written extensively on science, medicine, technology and environment in colonial and postcolonial India. Principal works include: *Colonizing the Body: State Medicine and Epidemic Disease in Nineteenth-Century India* (1993), *Science, Technology and Medicine in Colonial India* (2000), *Everyday Technology: Machines and the Making of India's Modernity* (2013), *Toxic Histories: Poison and Pollution in Modern India* (2016), *Burning the Dead: Hindu Nationhood and the Global Construction of Indian Tradition* (2021) and *Pandemic India: From Cholera to Covid-19* (2022).

Malavika Binny is an assistant professor in the Department of History at Kannur University, India. Her research interests include dalit studies, gender history, histories of medicine and science and South-Indian history. She has published on gender studies (2017), history of caste (2016) and on medieval Sanskrit poetry (2017) in international journals. She is currently engaged in the process of translating *Unnuneelisandesham*, a medieval champu kavyam from Manipravalam to English and is also working on the final draft of a book on the Mattancherry palace for Kerala Bhasha Institute.

Jane Buckingham is an associate professor of history at the University of Canterbury, Christchurch, New Zealand. She has researched extensively in India and the South Pacific and published in a range of areas including the history of medicine, law, health and disability. Her particular specialization is the history of leprosy in India and the Pacific. Her book *Leprosy in Colonial South India: Medicine and Confinement* (2002) remains current. More recent publications explore the link between leprosy, migration and indentured labour through colonial networks.

Pratik Chakrabarti is the NEH-Cullen Chair in History & Medicine at the University of Houston in the Department of History. He has contributed widely to the history of science, medicine, and imperial history. He is the author of several monographs including *Bacteriology in British India: Laboratory*

Medicine and the Tropics (2012) and *Medicine and Empire 1600–1960* (2014). His recent monograph is *Inscriptions of Nature: Geology and the Naturalization of Antiquity* (2020).

Amrita Chattopadhyay is a PhD research scholar at Jawaharlal Nehru University in the Centre for Historical Studies. Her research interests focus on Mughal history, material culture, perfume and sensory objects, maritime studies of medieval India and the early modern world. Her current PhD thesis looks at Mughal material culture with a special focus on sensory objects. Her forthcoming article is entitled 'A Study of Seventeenth-Century Aromatic-Woods' Dispatch in India: Circulation of Aloewood and Sandalwood through the Facilitating Port-cities and Trade Networks' (2022).

Burton Cleetus teaches modern history at the Centre for Historical Studies, Jawaharlal Nehru University, New Delhi. He specializes in the history of medicine and has worked on the institutionalization of indigenous medical traditions in India.

Kaushiki Das is a doctoral researcher at the Centre for the Study of Social Systems, Jawaharlal Nehru University. Her research interests lie in intellectual property rights and traditional medicine, decolonizing science and impact of technology on women. She has previously collaborated on projects, including the preparation of a position paper for the 32nd Session of Inter-Governmental Committee on Intellectual Property and Genetic Folklore at Geneva. Her most recent publication is entitled 'Digital Lakshman Rekhas: Understanding the Impact of Safety Apps on Women's Freedom of Movement in Urban Spaces' (*Global Perspectives*, 2021).

Anne Gerritsen is a professor in the history department at the University of Warwick and a Fellow of the British Academy. She has published on local religion in Jiangxi in *Ji'an Literati and the Local* (2007), on ceramics in *The City of Blue and White: Chinese Porcelain and the Early Modern World* (2020), and edited several collections on material culture with Giorgio Riello, including *The Global Lives of Things* (2015) and *Global Gifts: The Material Culture of Diplomacy in Early Modern Eurasia* (2017).

Greeshma Justin John is a doctoral candidate at the Centre for Regional Studies, University of Hyderabad, India. Her research focuses on the history of cleanliness in Kerala.

Harish Naraindas is a professor of sociology at Jawaharlal Nehru University and an honorary professor at Deakin University. His work wrestles with the epistemic premises of science and medicine, in an effort to arrive at a general theory of the emergence of medicine and alternative medicine in Europe and India. He has published on a range of themes, including tropical medicine, vaccination, childbirth, Ayurveda, the German Heilpraktiker (healer) and on the sacramental nature of anthropological explanation. His latest publication, *Psychedelic Therapy: Diplomatic Re-compositions of Life/Non-life, the Living and the Dead* (2021), is an ethnography of a psychosomatic department in a German Hospital.

Girija Kizhakke Pattathil is an independent scholar based out of Kerala. She is interested in gender studies, development practices, questions that explore the politics and history of knowledge formation, the liminal space of interaction among heterogeneous knowledge practices and their philosophical and psychological foundations. Her recent book is *Mapping the History of Ayurveda: Culture, Hegemony and the Rhetoric of Diversity* (2022).

Suparna Sengupta worked as a postdoctoral Junior Fellow at Nehru Memorial Museum and Library, New Delhi, on the project 'Occupying Islands and Controlling Sea: Andamans and Bay of Bengal' from a historical perspective to explore the relation of maritime jurisdiction and the process of Empire-building. She has been recently awarded the Charles Wallace India Trust Visiting Fellowship (2021–2) for research on imperial sovereignty and State Offenses in colonial India. Her research interests focus on issues of sovereignty, subjecthood, criminal law and jurisdiction and international law.

Abbreviations

BSM	Benefit-Sharing Model
GI	Geographical Indications of Goods
IPR	Intellectual Property Rights
ITDP	Integrated Tribal Development Project
JNTBGRI	Jawaharlal Nehru Tropical Botanical Garden and Research Institute
KIRTADS	Kerala Institute for Research, Training and Development of Scheduled Castes and Tribes
RRL	Regional Research Laboratory
TKDL	Traditional Knowledge Digital Library
WIPO	World Intellectual Property Organisation

Acknowledgements

The initial support for this project came from the Wellcome Trust. In December 2016, a project entitled 'Therapeutic Commodities: Trade, Transmission and the Material Culture of Global Medicine' was awarded with a Seed Award in Humanities and Social Science. The funding facilitated two international conferences, one in China, the other in India. The conference in China took place at Fudan University in Shanghai in March 2018 and was co-organized with Professor Gao Xi. The conference in India took place at the Centre for Historical Studies at Jawaharlal Nehru University (JNU) in New Delhi and was co-organized with Dr Burton Cleetus. Two smaller events were also organized under the aegis of this grant, in Johannesburg and at Warwick.

This volume comes from the workshop entitled 'Health and Materiality Histories of Health, Medicine and Trade across Cultures, 1600-2000', organized at JNU. Several people were instrumental in making this event possible, including Professor Radhika Singha and Professor Sucheta Mahajan, Chairperson at the Centre for Historical Studies. Dr Somak Biswas's contributions to the organization of the workshop were also fundamental to the success of the event. JNU and the Global History and Culture Centre at the University of Warwick were both very supportive in materializing the workshop, which led to the realization of this monograph. We are also very grateful for the support from the editorial team at Bloomsbury and the sage advice from the anonymous reviewers of this volume.

1

Health, medicine and trade in the Indian Ocean world

A material culture approach

Anne Gerritsen and Burton Cleetus

Introduction

In nineteenth-century Britain, chemists carried a range of products for oral hygiene. This included toothpaste marketed not only as an aid for 'preserving and beautifying the teeth' but also for 'perfuming the breath' and 'strengthening the gums' (Figure 1.1).

A key ingredient in many of these nineteenth-century toothpastes was the areca nut, the fruit of the areca palm, sometimes also referred to as the betelnut.[1] Of course, areca palms were not native to British soils, but a tropical crop imported from around the British empire. The areca palm was native to Southeast Asia but had long been dispersed throughout the Indian Ocean, including Kerala, Madagascar and Tanzania.[2] Popular in many parts of the tropics, betel or areca nuts were consumed in India by chewing them, sometimes in a preparation with betel leaf and slaked lime to release their stimulating properties, or used in Ayurvedic medicine. Early modern European visitors were less than impressed with the practice. John Henry Grose (*fl.* 1750–83) wrote in his *Voyage to the East-Indies*: 'They pretend that this use of Betel sweetens the breath, fortifies the stomach, though the juice is rarely swallowed, and preserves the teeth, tho' it reddens them; but, I am apt to believe, that there is more of vitious habit than any medicinal virtue in it, and that it is like tobacco, chiefly matter of pleasure.'[3] In the nineteenth century, visitors to India described the effect of betel on the teeth of the chewers as 'disgusting'; John Crawfurd (1783–1868) talked of the 'disgusting effects of the betel and areca preparation' on the gums,[4] while the young Prussian physician Werner Hoffmeister (1819–45) wrote, 'Would that

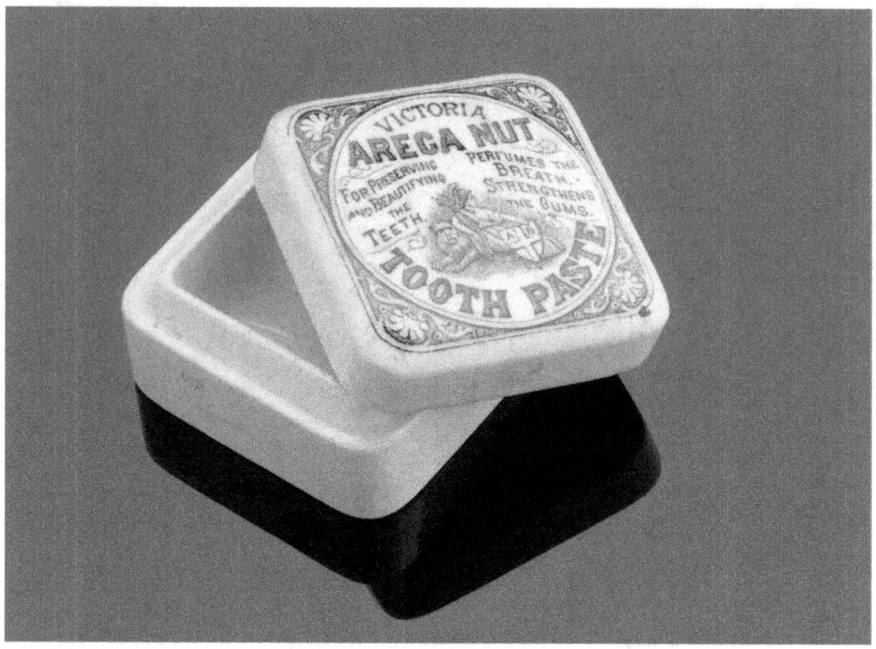

Figure 1.1 Toothpaste pot, England, 1860–95. Credit: Science Museum, London. Attribution 4.0 International (CC BY 4.0).

it were possible to win these people from the use of their betel-nut, which dyes their lips a vile yellowish red, and their teeth brown, and distorts their mouths with a perpetual grin! It is really impossible to imagine anything more disgusting than this unnatural custom.'[5]

It is perhaps somewhat surprising, then, that British manufacturers used areca nut as a key ingredient in toothpastes, which were marketed as 'oriental' products. In one case, a Lancashire-made toothpaste was branded 'Oriental toothpaste' (Figure 1.2), in another case, it was the image on the lid of the toothpaste, decorated with areca palm trees and onion-shaped dome, that revealed its 'oriental' associations (Figure 1.3). Yet another brand of toothpaste, produced in the Bedford laboratory in London by John Pepper and Company and known as 'Cracroft's areca nut tooth paste' was prepared, according to the label, 'from the Cingalese recipe' (i.e. Sri Lankan).[6]

These three toothpaste containers could form the start of several different discussions. They could be part of a study of the history of dental hygiene practices in general, or of toothpaste specifically, for example with a focus on nineteenth-century Britain, or indeed a history of tooth-cleaning

Health, Medicine, Trade in the Indian Ocean World 3

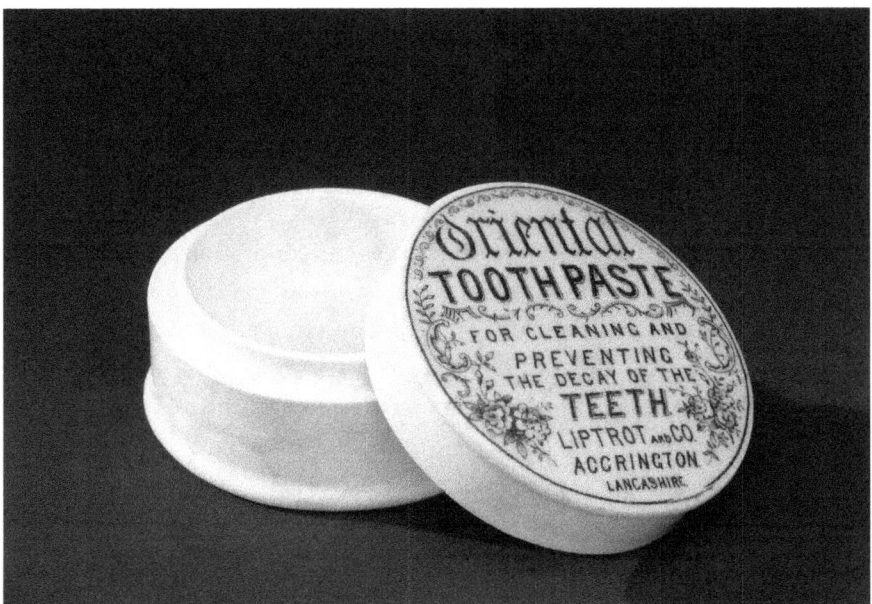

Figure 1.2 Ceramic pot for 'Oriental toothpaste', England, 1870–1910. Science Museum, London. Attribution 4.0 International (CC BY 4.0).

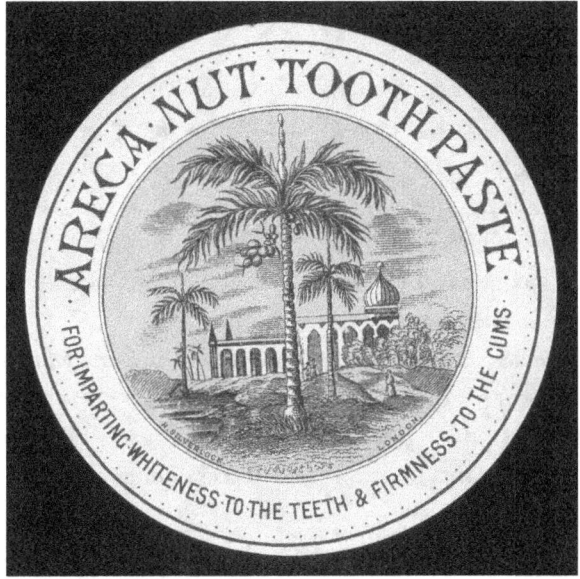

Figure 1.3 Label for Areca nut tooth paste, 1900–10? Credit: Wellcome Collection.

practices in different times and places. They could form part of a study of advertising or marketing, with these three examples revealing the ways in which goods and hygiene practices were made attractive for their potential consumers in nineteenth-century Britain. They might even form part of a discussion of collecting practices, considering the enduring appeal of such nineteenth-century pots and labels, as testified by their widespread availability online today. Interesting as such explorations might be, we propose to use these objects in a different way: as the starting point for a conversation about the history of trade in and circulation of health-related commodities in the wider Indian Ocean world between 1600 and 2000. In this volume, we are interested in approaching the history of medicine from an object-centred or material culture studies perspective. Before we consider the twelve studies that make up this volume and the contributions they seek to make individually, we need to explain in some detail what we mean by an object-centred perspective and discuss the ways in which we think a material culture studies approach can contribute to the histories of health in the Indian Ocean world.

The study of material culture

Material culture has long been a key feature of several very different disciplines, including archaeology, anthropology and the history of art. More recently, the historical sciences, including the histories of science, technology and medicine have also become more interested in objects and materiality. It might be useful to begin with a brief overview of what the concept of 'material culture' means in some of those contexts, before discussing the material culture approach we intend to follow in this volume.

For archaeologists, material culture refers very broadly to material remains that have been 'worked' in some way or another.[7] If a branch falls from a tree onto the ground, then that branch is a 'natural object' and does not form part of material culture unless that branch reveals traces of human interference, ranging from picking it up and placing it somewhere deliberate (when it becomes a so-called 'manuport'), and decorating it with notches or scraping off the bark, to planing it down to fashion it into a piece of furniture, which makes that natural object an artefact.[8] Material culture, in this sense, is the evidence of that human interaction. Across vast swathes of time and space, material culture can provide contemporary scholars access to the human hands that shaped it, as well as to the social worlds within which maker and user encountered, interacted with, shaped and were shaped by an object. Broadly speaking, archaeologists draw on the natural sciences (chemistry, biology, geology, engineering and so on) to extract meaning from objects as well as social sciences and humanities. While the former is more 'thing-centred', the latter is characterized by 'human-centredness', shifting the point of focus away from the object itself and towards the human relations within which the object is entangled.[9] The human-centred approach to things as it features in the work of social theorists and anthropologists is mostly concerned with the ways in which things are constructed in human minds. Things may well have material existence, but of greater interest is the ways in which those objects exist in human minds. The value of an object is not an intrinsic part of the object but established within the human mind, its meaning entirely dependent on the social context in which it exists. Arjun Appadurai's work on the ways in which value and meaning change over the lifespan of an object, suggesting the idea of an object with a social life, is perhaps the clearest example of this.[10] The field of material culture studies has benefited enormously from this work.

Art historians share many of the ideas about objects proposed by social scientists, but also bring a different set of analytical tools to the study of material culture. An older generation of art historians working in a Western disciplinary framework might impose a hierarchical difference between the fine arts, such as sculpture and painting, seen as the outcome of an individual creative genius, and the decorative arts, produced within a workshop context, without a single creator. While that Eurocentric way of distinguishing between art and material culture, which idolizes a particular form of art production has been broadly discredited, especially by those looking at art and material culture beyond Europe, the idea that material culture includes pieces made for use and enjoyment with or without an individual maker still holds. Being able to analyse the outward appearance of objects, the elements of design and the histories of use and meaning is important for object-centred approaches.

The work of scholars like Alfred Gell and Bruno Latour has added the element of object agency to the discussion.[11] Alfred Gell's work pointed to the ways in which an object can have a transformative impact on its environment. For Gell, this often means that humans delegate agency to things, rather than seeing the agency as initiating from within the object. Bruno Latour developed this idea much further in what he termed his actor-network theory (ANT). For Latour, 'actors' are a much broader category, which includes human as well as non-human actors, animals as well as actors from the material world such as tools, instruments and machines. To understand any technological change, according to Latour, we need to explore the entire assemblage of actors that is connected by that technology. So, to understand the change in energy provision, we need to focus not only on the human minds that made this possible but also on the actors from the material world, from vast oil rigs to tiny taps, from airplanes to bicycles, from intercontinental telegraph wires to WiFi boosters. For Latour, all actors, human and non-human, have agency, and all are entirely entangled in a complex network that cannot easily be disassembled.

For some historians, the written word continues to be the mainstay of their diet of sources, but for many other historians, sources have expanded beyond the written word: visual materials and the moving image, the worlds of fiction and fantasy, music and sound, food and drink as well as the world of things. This concerns studies of specific objects that have shaped our past, such as the pistol that shot President Abraham Lincoln or the three ships that came under attack in Boston Harbour in 1773.[12] Such objects were part of a significant change in the course of history and have come to be seen as representatives of that change. It also concerns a certain type of object, that again came to be associated with momentous changes in history: Ford's Model-T that exemplified conveyer-belt production, for example, or the gas chamber that made possible the extermination of millions of Jews during the Second World War. The objects, in such cases, are closely tied to technologies, which in turn facilitate a much wider social change.[13] For example, new technologies in creating lenses made the wearing of eyeglasses possible, which in turn facilitated reading beyond a certain age and those same technologies made it possible to create microscopes and star observation machines, which in turn transformed (parts of) the world.[14]

But objects are a much broader category than these objects that are associated with world-changing events and technologies. Objects are also part of the daily lived experiences of ordinary people, and the writing of material culture history has brought these ordinary objects more to the foreground than writing about special objects. Written histories now often take into account the material stories of ordinary people. The objects associated with slavery, for example, or the material culture of industrializing (and deindustrializing) urban spaces or the material culture of the world of work.[15] In such cases, the material world brings also the opportunity to expand the social classes about whom we write. Not all human experiences are recorded in written texts. Of course, equally, there are gaps in the material legacies of ordinary people.

The term 'materiality' is often mentioned in the context of material culture studies. Of course, in a common sense understanding of the term, materiality refers to the material aspects of an object. Such terms often appear more sharply defined when contrasted with their opposite, so materiality as opposed to visuality, in a similar contrast as textuality and orality. The terms point to the elements we are interested in analysing: the physical aspects of the object and the ways in which the material from which it was made shaped the object rather than its visual appearance. Textuality might refer to the ways in which words take meaning in the form of text appearing on a surface, as opposed to words that convey their meaning in spoken form. In literary criticism, however, textuality means far more than simply the textual form of communication: it includes analysis of such things as the status of a text, voicing in text (such as distinctions between monologues and dialogues), the organization of the text and the issue of power in and of text that allow for a far more nuanced reading of that text.[16] Similarly, materiality has come to mean far more than simply the material existence of an object: it aims for a better understanding of an object by asking questions about the agency of the material, its functionality, its relationship to space and spirituality and so on.[17] Not all are equally happy with this move away from the material existence of an object; Tim Ingold, for example, has proposed that we return to a meaning of materiality that focuses on the 'material and its properties':

> Thus the properties of materials, regarded as constituents of an environment, cannot be identified as fixed, essential attributes of things, but are rather processual and relational. They are neither objectively determined nor subjectively imagined but practically experienced. In that sense, every property is a condensed story. To describe the properties of materials is to tell the stories of what happens to them as they flow, mix and mutate.[18]

Here we arrive at the key meaning of materiality that we are interested in in this volume: objects made of materials that have properties, which in turn allow us to tell stories about their flows and mutations.

A key characteristic of the period covered in this volume, from 1600 to 2000, is the growth in volume and intensity of long-distance trade. Of course, in 1600, long-distance trade was far from new, and neither were periods of intensification in that global trade.[19] Several factors, however, made long-distance trade a more prominent feature of the period after 1600. Oceanic travel now happened along established routes with networks of ports for provisioning and knowledge-gathering. Such routes provided an attractive supplement to the long-standing land routes that criss-crossed the Afro-Eurasian landmass. Together, the land and sea routes had begun to create a regular exchange of people, things and ideas that connected the diverse parts of Afro-Eurasia, more intensely in some spaces, such as the Atlantic and Indian Oceans, and in more fragmented ways, such as on the Central Asian steppe or the Sahara. These maritime trade routes themselves, too, were nothing new in 1600; Chinese junks had sailed between the southern coast of China, the Southeast Asian islands and the Indian Ocean from at the least the ninth century, and Muslim traders had created an integrated sphere of trade in the region that connected the Red Sea area, the African coast, the Malabar and Coromandel coasts, to what is now Indonesia long before 1600. But it was the European trade companies, and their regular sorties between Europe and Asia, that intensified the movement of people, things and ideas. Building on bases established by the Portuguese from the late fifteenth century onwards, the Dutch and the English, and later the French and the Scandinavian companies, turned the maritime space to their advantage. They facilitated not only the arrival of large quantities of Asian goods in the European marketplace, and from there into commercial and domestic spaces, but also the introduction of European ideas about religion, politics and society in Asia. The increased availability of print technologies in Europe and Asia, too, increased the exchange of ideas and supported the mobility of goods and people significantly. Of course, other periods of intensification would follow, with the increasing presence of European imperialists in the non-European world, the growth of communication technologies with the arrival of the telegraph, and the establishment of multinational states.

The impact of the growth of trade and exchange on the worlds of consumption, technology and medicine has received ample attention in the scholarship and does not require further discussion here.[20] What does perhaps bear pointing out, however, is the impact this increase in the mobility of goods, people and ideas had on the material world, and especially on the ways in which things carry meaning. As established earlier, objects have their own material existence, but they are also constituted *as objects* within the human mind: they are constructed as objects within a particular knowledge framework that assigns a certain significance to that object. When objects move, however, those knowledge frameworks are displaced and objects gain new meanings, both *enroute* and within new contexts. Often, the result is a layering of meaning: the older meanings do not disappear, but those meanings may be transformed unrecognizably within the new context. The material culture of global connections takes seriously this layering of meaning that objects acquire as they move through time and space.[21] Aiming to understand the various contexts through which an object has moved and take account of how that movement shaped the multiple meanings of an individual object or object type should both be part of any material culture approach.

Histories of medicine in the Indian Ocean world: The state of the field

Historically, the Indian Ocean had been the centre of the spice trade. Arab and Chinese merchants traded in a variety of spices, including pepper, ginger, cinnamon, cardamom, cloves, nutmeg and mace.[22] However, as European powers began to replace Arabs in the sixteenth century in dominating the Indian Ocean trade, the nature and volume of the materials that were traded changed fundamentally. European mercantilism led to the wide circulation of information on the biological wealth of the tropics. Plants indigenous to the Americas such as maize, potatoes, tomatoes, peppers, okra, groundnuts, chillies, guavas, pineapples and tobacco were introduced by the Portuguese, and subsequently raised in colonial spaces in India and the Indian Ocean archipelago, demonstrating huge nutritional, commercial and medical value. As the metropole, European countries also became the collection houses of a variety of Asian and American plants, often marked as strange and exotic, which went on to have an important bearing on the medical market.

The task of collection, codification and circulation of plant matter was organized through a wide network, which involved sailors, soldiers, apothecaries, medical men, botanists, ethnographers and others. Yet at times such collection was undertaken under the direct patronage and supervision of the highest colonial officials themselves. The seventeenth-century Dutch Governor of Malabar, for example, a man named Hendrik Adriaan van Rheede tot Drakenstein (1631–91), or Hendrik van Rheede for short, compiled a compendium on the plants of Malabar. His *Hortus Indicus Malabaricus* was a multivolume text, produced in collaboration with local informants.[23] Similar medical/botanical texts were produced in different parts of the colonial world by men like Garcia Da Orta (1501?–68), Jan Huygen van Linschoten (1563–1611), Hans Sloane (1660–1753). Linschoten's text on the medicinal uses of nutmeg, edited by Linschoten's collaborator Bernardus Paludanus, mentions that it can be used for pain in the head, uterus or muscles.[24] The elaborate descriptions of plants produced a new abstraction, away from their epistemic and geo-cultural contexts, a process which is called 'bioprospecting' in modern times: the process of acquiring botanical and medical knowledge from local communities for commercial production. It has been argued that this process of abstraction was marked by different stages: in the initial stages of colonial knowledge production, ethnographers and botanists were more sympathetic towards local knowledge and cultures, while the centralization of knowledge and the advancements made in the botanical sciences that happened over time in Europe led to local knowledge being considered nothing more than barbaric and unscientific.[25]

The large-scale influx of botanical varieties from the colonial world in European markets and knowledge centres widened the medical market. Yet, as Schiebinger argues, culturally induced prejudices and preferences had a major role in shaping the nature of plant collecting and its uses, a process she calls 'agnotology', or culturally shaped ignorance.[26] Thus, the process of absorption of plants as medical material from the non-European world was marked by the working of power relations and culturally defined boundaries, which shaped the limits and possibilities of such interactions and transactions. Such cultural boundaries defined medicine in the non-European world as well.

A wide variety of new plants were introduced in the Indian subcontinent by the Portuguese and introduced into the diet, some of which also made their way into the local medicinal world. Along with plants and animals such as the turkey also came New World diseases. A sixteenth-century commentary on Ayurveda such as the *Bhavaprakasha* mentions the prevalence of Syphilis as *Phirangi roga* or 'disease brought by the Portuguese'.[27] Similarly, plants like *okra* or lady's finger, introduced to the subcontinent by the Portuguese, found their way into the Ayurvedic medical domain.[28]

The use of plants that were not indigenous to South Asia in the domestic kitchen increased substantially after the nature of colonialism changed with the arrival of the British. As the subcontinent was brought under the political authority of Britain, the relationship between plants and people underwent major changes, and consumption practices, dietary preferences and the medical domain in India all came to be fundamentally altered. In the last decades of the nineteenth century, locally planted and cultivated tea became the national beverage of the subcontinent. Coffee, which had been introduced a century earlier, had not gained the same popularity that tea enjoyed, yet from the mid-nineteenth century, at least among a sizeable section of the Indian educated elite, the consumption of coffee was gaining traction.[29] The commercial cultivation of tobacco also led to the creation of an internal market as people became increasingly addicted.[30] Thus, the new cultural taste, made familiar by British colonialism, backed by state power, both political and ideological, led to the rise of new consumption practices.

This process was marked by a concerted effort by people to abstain from prevailing cultural practices of the contemporary society. This was also because, unlike previous political regimes of the Indian subcontinent, the British administration in India was sustained by the use of science both as an ideological apparatus and as an everyday practice. The use of science under British colonialism challenged indigenous medical traditions and dismissed these as speculative and not adhering to scientific reason. In response, Indian social elites exposed to the cultural and political influence of Western science and medicine internalized the idea that Indian cultural and medical traditions lacked scientific reasoning. Indian elites strived to reposition local traditions in light of the epistemic challenges posed by Western reasoning.[31] Nationalist upsurge against colonial rule reflected a drive to revisit classical Sanskrit knowledge traditions in the light of Western science. The emergence of nationalist consciousness led to homogenization and centralization in Indian medicine, which often led to the marginalization of localized healing traditions and quackery. Thus, therapeutic objects were subjected to multiple layers of negotiations brought about both by colonial dominance as well as nationalist upsurge.

Under British colonial rule, Indian bodies came to be identified as the principal site of socio-cultural and religious backwardness. The colonial mind was thought to be speculative and unable to adhere to logical reason. A transition in the mind was deemed possible through an organized state-centred pedagogic process, including the forceful introduction of the disciplinary mechanisms of the state, such as prisons, lunatic asylums, state-centred vaccination programmes, law and education.[32]

Colonial ethnographers in India measured the bodies of their subjects, including the human skull, nose, hip and breasts, so as to form an 'objective' understanding of their colonial subjects.[33] European surgeons searched for marks on the body to understand bodily ailments, underlining human bodies as the primary material site for governance.[34] The extension of commercial cultivation forced the colonial administration to search for healthy bodies that could be used for labour.

As the introduction of Western medicine through the establishment of teaching hospitals and dissection of the human corpse as the entry point of enquiry into medical sciences continued, colonial authorities considered that touching the corpse and the internal gaze of the material body would enable Indians to transcend religiously bounded marks of purity and pollution associated with the corpse. It was for this reason that the 1836 dissection of a body by Madhusoodhan Gupta (1800–50), an upper caste medical student at

Calcutta Medical College, was seen as a major landmark not only in the history of the introduction of Western medicine in India but also in India's transition to modernity, signifying a radical deviation from the speculative world into a materially driven world.[35]

For colonial officials and ethnographers, diseases in the colonial contexts were culturally and socially defined. Diseases were understood in the context of birthing practices, sexual behaviours, religious rituals, life in domestic spaces and a host of other practices through which morbidity was defined in colonial India. People, places, environments and goods were marked as diseased spaces. At a wider societal level, hygiene and cleanliness were seen by the Christian missionaries as marks of progress, while dirt and disease symbolized sin.[36] In Asian and African societies, such questions of moral and physical hygiene spurred domestic movements towards internal reform, both social and individual. One of the major issues of central concern for both the colonial officials and the indigenous reformers was bodily constitutions of people in indigenous societies. The creation of a healthy Indian individual was thought to be possible only through a transition in the cultural and religious life of the subcontinent. Cultural backwardness was seen as a manifestation of physical morbidity, to be overcome only through altering the consumption patterns of the people. New dietary practices were familiarized by the colonial state, aimed at changing the body's internal and external constitution as a mark of transforming the social and therefore individual conditions of life.

By the late nineteenth century, the expansion of industrial capitalism in Europe led to the arrival of new goods in India for therapeutic and domestic consumption, which were gaining popularity among the emerging Indian educated elites. British colonialism also expanded patterns of domestic food consumption as new plants introduced within the subcontinent became popularized in the kitchen of the Indian household, through experiments with new dietary practices and the expansion of print and other communication networks. The introduction and the popularization of baking as a new mode of cooking in areas of British influence also introduced new consumption patterns, especially among those who benefited from the expansion of the colonial bureaucracy. The association of educated Indian elites with the colonial administration and the practice of transfers and postings increased familiarity with new recipes prevalent in different regions of the British presidencies. Kolladi Mootheri Kalyani Amma, for example, noted down the recipes she came across while her husband was posted in various parts of the Madras Presidency in South India as a civil servant. Her daughter, Kolladi Mootheri Parukutti

Amma, published the notes of her mother, which give an interesting account of the kind of cooking practices that reached her through her servants and became prevalent throughout South India.[37] The widening of print culture in turn led to the publication of cookery books; their circulation among the reading public brought about changes in taste, refreshments, food and dietary practices.

Individuals subjected to colonial modernization were fearful about their physical composition and bodily weaknesses, a concern central to the social reform movement in India. In tune with the concern for bodily weakness, a market for British consumption goods rolled out a variety of products aimed at addressing bodily weakness and increasing bodily vitality. Similar to the current enthusiasm for products like energy boosters, indigenous medical practitioners too ventured to produce new products that were aimed at regaining bodily and mental energy. Social reformers argued for new dietary practices, which included the consumption of new foodstuffs, while distancing from food that in earlier contexts had been seen as fundamentally responsible for physical and mental weakness. For instance, Narayana Guru, the leading social reform leader among the Ezhavas, a lower-caste community in Kerala, argued that the social backwardness of the community resulted from the consumption of fish, meat and toddy: a fermented alcohol, locally sourced from the sap of the unripe flowers of palm and coconut plants. He argued in favour of vegetarianism, advised to desist from the consumption of toddy and also urged community members to engage in new occupations in Ayurveda and industry. The new Ayurveda of the early twentieth century that Narayana desired was based on Sanskrit text and drugs with elaborate preparation methods.

Medicine in non-European contexts was often organized by an environmental ethic, where the body is constituted of the five elements of nature. Disease, therefore, was structured within a relationship between bodies and nature, a disturbance of which caused disease. It was this underlying theory of nature and bodies that maintained the balance or caused diseases.[38] It is into this environmentalist ethic that Western medicine introduced new theories of disease causation in the nineteenth century.

In the context of changing notions of diseases and cure, the non-European world was subjected to fundamental changes both in terms of epistemic premises as well as the integration of new drugs. The desire for new drugs was endowed with new meanings familiarized by British colonialism in India. Colonialism introduced a new ethic on bodies and disease. The body itself came to be seen as a material object that needs to be transformed through the integration with other objects. The identification and transition of material objects became a major concern of the colonial state.

The emergence of science was structured by the emergence of the material. As Harold Cook remarks, it was about the collection and examining of objects and artefacts, which he calls objectivity.[39] In the project of colonial knowledge production, plants, the environment and even the colonial subject came to be seen as material objects, which could be examined, understood and transformed. Colonialism set in motion a process by which the bodies of the people became the objects of study, defined primarily in terms of the morbid conditions. The tropics came to be seen as spaces of growth and fertility, of putrefaction, poisons and diseases.[40] The discourse on the tropics as miasmatic was the basic framework through which disease causation and the nature of bodies in the colonies were understood. The search for a materially grounded tradition in medicine led reformers in medicine to focus on drugs and their uses as has been depicted in ancient classical texts and their epistemic foundations. Plant-based materials came to be increasingly processed and marketed as symbol of ancient Indian medical practice. Indian nationalism, while being articulated in various streams of thought used Ayurveda, particularly the belief in its drugs and their efficacy, to prove its scientific strength.

The introduction of new plants in the colonial world changed the terms of reference for both medicine and food. New crops introduced by the Portuguese, Dutch and later the English had a lasting impact on consumption patterns. New plants changed the preferences of taste and came to be part of the ecological world. Though the transfer of biological wealth occurred from the sixteenth century, onwards the popularization and adaptation of new plants into the dietary practices occurred much later in the nineteenth century after the British emerged as a major political establishment in India. The British had a major impact on the kinds of plants that could be used both for medical and domestic food consumption in India. This was primarily for the fact that unlike its earlier counterparts the British administration created an educated elite exposed to new knowledge forms and social and cultural values that British administration in India. British administration also was guided by economic considerations, therefore was looking for a domestic market for processed drugs. Tea was introduced in the late nineteenth century and quickly gained popularity as a refreshing drink across the subcontinent, though its counterpart, coffee, introduced much earlier in the eighteenth century, failed to gain ground. Similar was the case of tapioca, a plant native to the Americas, which was introduced in the Indian subcontinent by the Portuguese. It was only in the 1860s that the consumption of its tuber gained popularity through the efforts of the princely ruler of Travancore Visakham Thirunal Rama Varma, introduced for the extension of tapioca cultivation to feed the state's marginalized sections, whose access to rice was limited. The Travancore State Manual notes: 'His name will ever be remembered for the introduction and extension of tapioca cultivation in Travancore; it is now the labourer's food *par excellence,* and "there is no poor man in the land who eats it without silently blessing the memory of *Vishakham* Rajah for it".[41]

Thus, the expansion of plants was guided by the expansion of the population, the rise of new state systems, the consolidation of British state power and the responses to it. The expansion of trade networks enforced migration of the people, and led to the expansion of commercial crops, widening the preference for new material goods. This was also possible due to the ideological changes that were emerging. The ideological contexts opened up by the colonial state were able to generate new cultural values and norms, which were highly valued and preferred at least by an emerging Indian educated elite. New cultural tastes meant new sartorial practices, new preferences for food and medicine. As the idea of the individual emerged, often in confrontation with traditional values and norms, the elites imagined building healthy bodies and therefore healthy nuclear families against the traditional joint family systems. As concerns over physical weakness as symptoms of socio-religious and political loss under colonialism emerged, plants that were deemed to have the potential to rejuvenate physical strength and vigour gained significance.

One of the major institutions that familiarized new moral values in India were the Christian missionaries. It was the missionaries who equated moral and physical weakness with sin and disease. Even when personal hygiene was stressed by the missionaries as a means to overcome dirt, disease and sin, missionaries considered the consumption of meat one of the ways of overcoming bodily weakness. Christian missionaries travelled across the non-European world armed with the Bible and the potato. The tuber was to adapt to all climates and therefore was considered to be an essential part of the missionary's proselytization efforts. Though religious conversion was not acceptable to the vast majority, the potato came to be widely popularized in colonial North India. British colonial intervention generated new cultural values and tastes, which created a new market for a variety of goods including soaps, clothes, food and drugs.

Health and hygiene were prime concerns in the familiarization and consumption of new kinds of food, plants and animal matter as well as in the use of new goods like soaps and clothes. This was reflected in the curriculum of the newly established schools and in the sermons of the social reformers, which identified the individual body as the site of India's transition to modernity. Health, then, was socially and culturally located through constantly changing perceptions of the body.

The chapters of the book

Some of the articles in this collection of histories of health and materiality focus on a single drug and recount the history of that medicinal commodity. In the chapter by Anne Gerritsen, for example, the drug at the heart of the story is rhubarb, and the chapter follows the itinerary of this commodity through time and space, starting with some of the earliest medical tracts in both the Chinese and Greek traditions and tracing the story through records of trade and knowledge transfer from rhubarb's roots in Central Asia to its use in China, India and Europe. The challenges become clear immediately: rhubarb is not a single plant but a plant complex, understood in very different ways across linguistic, chronological and cultural boundaries, hence the reference to rhubarb's 'entangled itinerary' in the chapter's title. The material culture approach in the study of rhubarb helps us to avoid essentializing rhubarb as a singular commodity, instead seeing the concept of rhubarb being reconstituted over and over again depending on the context.

Drugs like chaulmoogra and arogyapacha, too, have histories that can be traced through time and space, revealing the complexities in their constitution. Jane Buckingham's study of chaulmoogra focuses on the use of this therapeutic in the treatment of leprosy in the South Pacific. Here, too, we see chaulmoogra emerge out of different Indian Ocean world geographies, including South and Southeast Asia, and separate medical traditions, including Chinese, Buddhist, Ayurvedic and indigenous healing practices. Trade and migration brought both chaulmoogra itself and knowledge about its therapeutic value to new communities of users dispersed throughout the Indian Ocean world and the South Pacific. Once it had become part of the British colonial-medical system, chaulmoogra became the drug of choice for the treatment of those affected by leprosy and thereby implicated in colonial practices of control over imperial bodies. As Buckingham's chapter shows, in the Pacific world, especially New Zealand and Fiji, British colonial cultivation and application of chaulmoogra created landscapes or islands of isolation, with extended plantations of chaulmoogra-producing trees and settlements serving only the banished populations affected by leprosy. Cure and control are flipsides of the same colonial coin.

The story of arogyapacha, the subject of Girija Kizhakke Pattathil's chapter, is equally complex as it moves from being mostly known as a rejuvenating substance in the indigenous medical context of the Western Ghats region in Kerala in South-western India to being formally legitimized in Ayurvedic medical texts and eventually commercially exploited on a global scale. The chronology is more contemporary here, dealing with the last decades of the twentieth century and the first of the twenty-first, and the agents involved are not the colonial powers but organizations such as the Kerala Kani Community Welfare Trust or the government of India. While many profited financially from the appropriation of knowledge about arogyapacha and from its exploitation as a health-giving substance, the inhabitants of the hills where this plant was harvested and other members of the Kani tribe were generally excluded from such profits.

The importance of material culture studies in this research is that they bring to the fore the ways in which values and meanings of material objects change over time. Rather than stable or essentialized, goods and materials are unstable and only gain meaning and value in context. In other words, the values and meanings assigned to materials can serve as a way of highlighting important historical changes in context. In the chapter by Amrita Chattopadhyay, we see that perfumes perform this role of revealing patterns of socio-cultural change in early modern India. Perfumes are ephemeral, perhaps suggesting their materiality is harder to study. Yet, Chattopadhyay shows that perfumes have not only complex material histories but also material agency. Perfumes were of great interest to those writing about health and well-being within both the Ayurvedic and Unani medical contexts, but their often-complex combinations of ingredients also had aesthetic and emotional associations. Such ingredients had to be sourced in distant locations, their remoteness often enhancing their value; their procurement connected the culture of aromatics within India to global networks of circulation and mobility. Chattopadhyay assigns agency not only to the traders who move the aromatics and manufacturers who created the perfumes but also to the perfumes themselves, which connected remote parts of the world and combined the bodies of emperors, princes, courtiers and servants into single regimes of fragrance and olfactory well-being. Greeshma Justin John's chapter on Keralam's history between 1880 and 1950 reveals how soap can also perform this role of revealing historical transformations. The meaning of soap depended not only on its ingredients – did it or did it not contain animal fats? Was it pure or adulterated? – but also on its manufacturing methods, its marketing strategies, its uses, its associations with social class, caste and gender and so on. By tracing the complex changes in the meaning of soap over time, Greeshma Justin John is able to tell a highly nuanced history of a region that was transforming into a society with modern ideas about health and hygiene but also undergoing major social transformations. The materiality of soap brings those to the fore in ways that are both striking and revealing.

The concept of materiality, which explores the ways in which material meanings are culturally constructed stretches well beyond commodities like rhubarb, chaulmoogra, perfume and soap. It even includes bodies, in this case the bodies of convicts, as the chapter by Suparna Sengupta shows. The physical health of convicts determined their ability to perform labour duties, and thus was of great interest to the colonial state. The colonial administration saw it as its duty to diagnose the signs of both age and health of a convicted criminal that had been judicially sentenced to transportation. Under the colonial criminal justice system, the bodies of the convicts were seen as material objects, to be deported and used for the transformation of putrid geographies of the Andaman Islands. The bodies of the convicts were deemed to undergo transition when subjected to hard labour in an alien space. For the colonial state, the bodies of convicts served the objectives of the colonial state just as state initiatives on health, hygiene and medicine did.

The poisons that form the subject of David Arnold's chapter equally change in meaning depending on their context. His chapter features three commodities: nux vomica, arsenic and kerosene, each of which brought both benefits to (public) health and potential harm. As these goods travelled across the oceans and entered into new social contexts, their meanings changed. Their trajectories were different, but all three commodities were part of the networks of mobility that connected Europe and Asia generally, and Britain and India specifically. Rather than seeing this as a story of individual substances moving in single directions, Arnold shows that medical substances like nux vomica and arsenic travelled in both raw and compound form in both directions along with other goods and people, transforming medical and botanical knowledge along the way. The story of kerosene, a by-product of the petroleum industry, reveals something slightly different: while it could be used as an effective disinfectant and as an agent to incinerate disease-spreading animals and objects, its high flammability also led to the accidental or intentional death of large numbers of the population. By focusing on the materiality of the three substances, more nuanced stories are revealed that challenge both the idea that new therapeutic substances always lead to improvements in health and society and the idea that they increasingly damage bodies and environments. These three commodities show that they do both.

While individual commodities feature at the core of many of the chapters in this volume, other chapters explore the material in the Indian Ocean world through the lens of empire. The chapters by Malavika Binny and Pratik Chakrabarti are examples of this approach, while of course empire and the colonial state feature in the background in almost all of these studies. The study by Binny explores the formation between 1600 and 1800 of medico-botanical networks of knowledge, especially in southern India. With the arrival of the European proto-colonists in India, attempts to take stock of the indigenous knowledge of the natural world led to the creation of new textual traditions. These include both the European medico-botanical texts about the natural world in India and new Ayurvedic texts that integrate European techniques and medical practices. And as we saw in the chapter by Arnold about a much later period, even in this early modern period, we are seeing flows in both directions, transforming not only knowledge about the natural world but also the natural world itself.

Chakrabarti's chapter similarly focuses on the transformations of *materia medica* that occurred not in Europe but beyond Europe, thereby bringing different spaces of empire within our field of vision. In these spaces beyond the boundaries of Europe, transformations that created hybrid knowledge worlds emerged. As Chakrabarti's study shows, a variety of agents were involved in these transformations, including the European botanists, imperial agents and local intermediaries that were based in the far-flung corners of the empire. In the central spaces of empire, at the European capitals and centres of learning, there was less interest in what the imperial agents had to say about the varied contexts in which *materia medica* were understood in India, hence the title 'Europe does not want you', but as the chapter shows, the transformations of *materia medica* in India were more hybrid and interactive than those occurring at the centre.

Several of the chapters included in this volume feature indigenous actors of different kinds. The chapter by Burton Cleetus focuses on the ways in which Ayurvedic practices changed under the colonial regime. He does this by exploring the history of an indigenous medical institution, the Kottakkal Aryavaidyasala clinic in Kerala, through its rich record of letters patients sent to the clinic demanding medical help. In the context of intense demand for labour in different parts of the colonial state, such as on the tea plantations in the northern provinces, displaced peoples suffered ongoing health problems.

Located far from home, Keralan migrants wrote to the clinic to ask for remedies and dietary regimes. Cleetus shows the instability that characterized this transforming world, as everything was in flux: the displaced bodies of indigenous migrants, the ailments they suffered, the treatments and dietary instructions they received, indigeneity, in fact, the entire constitution of Ayurvedic medicine. The focus on the material brings the constancy of this flux to the fore.

The indigenous actors that feature in the chapter by Kaushiki Das play quite a different role. Like Girija K. P. in her study of arogyapacha, Kaushiki Das focuses on the exploitation of 'miracle drugs' but shifts her attention away from the colonial state and its bioprospecting tendencies towards the role played by domestic pharmaceutical firms. Her chapter challenges the idea that the competition over natural resources simply pits the Global North against the Global South; those who compete over resources like indigenous medicinal plant substances and their accompanying plant knowledge include also the profit-driven domestic pharmaceutical companies, the so-called collaborative governmental institutions that seek to catalogue, codify and regulate that indigenous knowledge and even certain indigenous organizations. The landscape Das reveals is not simply 'neo-colonial', nor is it shaped by global north-global south divisions; it is a landscape that can only be viewed fully by seeing its material forms through the lens of indigenous knowledge.

In more ways than one, the chapter by Harish Naraindas poses a challenge to the emphasis on materiality that forms the key feature of the volume. Naraindas takes a series of ethnographic vignettes as the starting point for his study of South Asian therapeutic practice, which ultimately allows him to make a claim about all alternative therapeutic practices and the ways in which they relate to biomedicine, namely, that this relationship is fundamentally asymmetrical. By privileging *materia medica*, and specifically privileging the active ingredients that have been identified as the cure for a disease, all other aspects of therapeutic practice are excluded: incantations and other tantric practices, the role played by ghosts, planets and deities, or, in short, the role of the non-human and the incorporeal as both the cause and cure of diseases. The privileging of the material over the immaterial is not only a characteristic of the East/West divide but also of the past/present and mind/body divides, as much as it is of the institutionalized versus the 'folk' versions of Ayurvedic practice. Privileging the material has a long history, and, as Naraindas shows, turns fundamentally on recasting the meaning of the Eucharist and what follows in its wake. The premise of materiality, on which this volume rests, is thus used as a wedge to both problematize it and to offer a general theory of the asymmetrical relationship within biomedicine, and between biomedicine and alternative medicine worldwide.

Together, the chapters in this book offer a wide spectrum of views on what it means to focus on histories of health through the lens of materiality. For some, it means that a material, usually a substance with healing properties, features as the main character in the narrative. Aided by a cast of other actors, including healers and botanists, colonial administrators and bioprospectors, therapeutic substances reveal stories about the transformation, codification and commercialization of medical knowledge and practice as well as stories of global trade, imperial expansion and environmental exploitation. For others, the focus on the material world means more than stories of substances that can heal; it includes also substances that harm, and material worlds and regimes of healing that are harmed by the expansion of imperial, colonial and postcolonial power. Yet others see material culture studies as a way of problematizing what something 'means', destabilizing essentialized understandings of substances, and using the shift in meanings that can only be known by their contexts as a way of grasping larger patterns of change. The wide range of meanings assigned to the areca nut with which we started this chapter illustrates this: chewing the nut could work as a stimulant for some and an abhorrent for others; a substance that discoloured teeth in one part of the world was sold as an attractively 'oriental' tooth-cleaning additive in another. The Indian Ocean world was undergoing major and complex processes of change during the period encompassed by this volume (1600–2000), and we hope the chapters in this volume help to reveal the potential of the material culture approach for understanding those changes.

Notes

1. On the terminology and its associations, see Jaclyn Rohel, 'Empire and the Reordering of Edibility: Deconstructing Betel Quid through Metropolitan Discourses of Intoxication', *Global Food History* 3, no. 2 (2017), 153.
2. Nicole Boivin et al., 'East Africa and Madagascar in the Indian Ocean World', *Journal of World Prehistory* 26, no. 3 (2013), 215.
3. John Henry Grose, *A Voyage to the East-Indies* (London: S. Hooper and A. Morley, 1757), 376.
4. John Crawfurd, *History of the Indian Archipelago: Containing an Account of the Manners, Art, Languages, Religions, Institutions, and Commerce of Its Inhabitants*, vol. 1 (Edinburgh: Constable, 1820), 105.

5 Werner Hoffmeister, *Travels in Ceylon and Continental India: Including Nepal and Other Parts of the Himalayas, to the Borders of Thibet, with Some Notices of the Overland Route* (Edinburgh: W. P. Kennedy, 1848), 148.
6 Such lidded pots appear regularly for sale in antique markets. An example was listed in Ben Z. Swanson, *The Ben Z. Swanson, Jr. Collection of Antique Pot Lids: A Premier Absentee Auction in Two Sessions* (New York: Harmer Rooke Galleries, 1990), 16.
7 Laura Hurcombe, *Archaeological Artefacts as Material Culture* (London and New York: Routledge, 2007), 11.
8 Ibid., 4–5.
9 Ian Hodder, *Entangled: An Archaeology of the Relationships between Humans and Things* (Malden, MA [etc.]: Wiley-Blackwell, 2012), 41.
10 Arjun Appadurai, ed., *The Social Life of Things: Commodities in Cultural Perspective* (Cambridge: Cambridge University Press, 1986).
11 Alfred Gell, *Art and Agency: An Anthropological Theory* (Oxford: Clarendon Press, 2013); Bruno Latour, 'On Actor-Network Theory: A Few Clarifications', *Soziale Welt* 47, no. 4 (1996): 369–81.
12 Anne Gerritsen and Giorgio Riello, 'Material Culture History: Methods, Practices and Disciplines', in *Writing Material Culture History*, ed. Anne Gerritsen and Giorgio Riello, 2nd ed. (London: Bloomsbury Academic, 2021), 1–4.
13 Lorraine Daston, *Things That Talk: Object Lessons from Art and Science* (New York: Zone Books, 2004).
14 Anne Gerritsen and Giorgio Riello, eds, *Writing Material Culture History*, 2nd ed. (London: Bloomsbury Academic, 2021); Karen Harvey, *History and Material Culture: A Student's Guide to Approaching Alternative Sources* (London: Routledge, 2010).
15 See, for example, the chapter by Manuel Charpy in Giorgio Riello and Anne Gerritsen, eds, *Writing Material Culture History* (London: Bloomsbury, 2015).
16 W. F. Hanks, 'Text and Textuality', *Annual Review of Anthropology* 18 (1989): 95–127.
17 Tim Ingold, 'Materials against Materiality', *Archaeological Dialogues* 14, no. 1 (2007): 2.
18 Ibid., 14.
19 See, for example, the work on the late medieval world by Janet L. Abu-Lughod, *Before European Hegemony: The World System A.D. 1250-1350* (New York: Oxford University Press, 1989); the Silk Road has a history of global exchange that goes back to antiquity: Christopher I. Beckwith, *Empires of the Silk Road: A History of Central Eurasia from the Bronze Age to the Present* (Princeton: Princeton University Press, 2011); the trade in ceramics in the Indian Ocean is a good example of this early global trade: Zhao Bing, 'Global Trade and Swahili Cosmopolitan Material Culture: Chinese-Style Ceramic Shards from Sanje Ya Kati and Songo Mnara

(Kilwa, Tanzania)', *Journal of World History* 23, no. 1 (2012): 41–85; Zhao Bing, 'Chinese-Style Ceramics in East Africa from the 9th to 16th Century: A Case of Changing Value and Symbols in the Multi-Partner Global Trade', *Afriques. Débats, Méthodes et Terrains d'histoire*, no. 6 (2015); finally, cotton, too, has a very long and global history: Giorgio Riello and Prasannan Parthasarathi, eds, *The Spinning World: A Global History of Cotton Textiles, 1200-1850* (Oxford: Oxford University Press, 2009).

20 Harold John Cook, *Matters of Exchange: Commerce, Medicine, and Science in the Dutch Golden Age* (New Haven, Conn.; London: Yale University Press, 2008).

21 Anne Gerritsen and Giorgio Riello, eds, *The Global Lives of Things: The Material Culture of Connections in the Early Modern World* (London: Routledge, 2016).

22 Kapil Raj, *Relocating Modern Science: Circulation and the Construction of Knowledge in South Asia and Europe, 1650-1900* (Basingstoke: Palgrave Macmillan, 2007).

23 Hendrik Adriaan van Rheede tot Drakenstein, *Hortus Indicus Malabaricus: continens regni Malabarici apud Indos celeberrimi omnis generis plantas rariores* (Amstelodami: Joannis van Someren et Joannis van Dyck, 1678).

24 Cook, *Matters of Exchange*, 126.

25 Londa Schiebinger, *Plants and Empire: Colonial Bioprospecting in the Atlantic World* (Cambridge, MA [etc.]: Harvard University Press, 2004).

26 Schiebinger, *Plants and Empire*, 3; on agnotology, see also Robert Proctor and Londa Schiebinger, eds, *Agnotology: The Making and Unmaking of Ignorance* (Stanford: Stanford University Press, 2008).

27 K. R. Srikanthamurthy, trans., *Bhāvaprakāśa of Bhāvamiśra: Text, English Translation, Notes, Appendeces [Sic] and Index* (Varanasi: Krishnadas Academy, 1998); Tarun Kumar Dutta, Subhash Chandra Parija and Jamini Kanta Dutta, *Emerging and Re-Emerging Infectious Diseases* (New Delhi: Jaypee Brothers Medical Pub., 2013).

28 Colleen Taylor Sen, *Feasts and Fasts: A History of Food in India* (London: Reaktion Books, 2014), 212.

29 A. R. Venkatacalapati, *In Those Days There Was No Coffee: Writing in Cultural History* (New Delhi: Yoda Press, 2008).

30 Kathinka Sinha-Kerkhoff, *Colonising Plants in Bihar (1760-1950): Tobacco Betwixt Indigo and Sugarcane* (India: Partridge Publishing, 2014).

31 K. N. Panikkar, *Colonialism, Culture, and Resistance* (New Delhi: Oxford University Press, 2007).

32 Uday Singh Mehta, *Liberalism and Empire: India in British Liberal Thought* (New Delhi: Oxford University Press, 1999).

33 James Poskett, *Materials of the Mind: Phrenology, Race, and the Global History of Science, 1815-1920* (Chicago: University of Chicago Press, 2019).

34 Gyan Prakash, *Another Reason: Science and the Imagination of Modern India* (Princeton: Princeton University Press, 1999).
35 David Arnold, *Colonizing the Body: State Medicine and Epidemic Disease in Nineteenth-Century India* (Berkeley: University of California Press, 1993).
36 David Hardiman, *Missionaries and Their Medicine: A Christian Modernity for Tribal India* (Manchester: Manchester University Press, 2008).
37 *Paachayogangal* (recipes) written by Kolladi Mootheri Kalyani Amma published by Kolladi Mootheri Parukutti Amma Basel mission press. Mangalore, 1917.
38 Dominik Wujastyk, *The Roots of Ayurveda: Selections from Sanskrit Medical Writings* (New Delhi: Penguin, 1998).
39 Cook, *Matters of Exchange*, 2007.
40 Harish Naraindas, 'Poisons, Putrescence and the Weather: A Genealogy of the Advent of Tropical Medicine', *Contributions to Indian Sociology* 30, no. 1 (1996): 1–35.
41 V. Nagam Aiya, *The Travancore State Manual* (Trivandrum: Travancore Government Press, 1989), 589.

2

'Europe does not want you'
Natural history, materia medica and the empire
Pratik Chakrabarti

In recent years, scholars have extensively explored the history of early modern natural history and materia medica. There are fascinating histories of how European naturalists collected exotic plants and other curiosities from remote places, named and sketched them, or placed them inside their field diaries and shipped them across the oceans.[1] There is also a growing trend of juxtaposing various texts of early modern natural history, determining the intricate classificatory differences between them.[2] We have also learnt the various pluralistic forms of the history of nature in Europe in the early modern period.[3] At the same time, historians have shown that this world of *naturalia* had a relatively 'coherent' vision, based on experimental, observational and empirical methods that appeared in Europe from the seventeenth century.[4] Therefore, despite the plurality of collection and classifications, a distinct vision of natural history, based on secular observation, objectivity and empiricism defined European natural history from the seventeenth century.[5]

At the same time, the vibrant literature on the emergence of the global history of materia medica has rendered some of these European histories of natural history and materia medica relatively provincial. Historians have established that non-European princes, physicians, traders and scholars played significant roles in channelling these plants, herbs and animals through complex geographical and epistemological routes in the making of the global natural historical heritage.[6]

How do we frame the materiality of materia medica that emerged beyond Europe? The global history of materia medica poses specific questions to the materiality of nature and natural history based on European intellectual traditions of observation and empiricism. The European frames of natural history, based on the objective and empirical knowledge of nature, are inadequate here, as these objects were often ephemeral and belonged simultaneously to different historical and empirical contexts, where they enjoyed diverse meanings and were often used simultaneously by diverse intellectual traditions. While the distinctiveness of the new world of nature that appeared in Europe from the seventeenth century was based on experimental, observational and empirical methods, in Asia, America and the Caribbean, these objects were often seen through frames which are not themselves always empirical in the conventional sense of the term. The need is to appreciate the complex genealogies of these items, their pluralistic epistemologies and their hybrid medical lineages.

The empiricism of natural history has a particular colonial legacy as the rise of European commerce and colonial extraction facilitated the collection and transfer of plants and other material objects of nature. Materiality is also at the heart of the colonial history of drugs, plants and bodies. From the seventeenth century, Europeans were engaging with a complex world of nature in the colonies in Asia, Africa and America. They were simultaneously imposing their own spiritual and empirical ideas on them. That particular history of nature is often lost in the conventional narratives of natural history. This history was not only based on the observation, collection and relocation of nature, but also diverse conceptions of nature. This is also not just a case for appreciating the vernacular or the indigenous traditions of knowledge, as the vernacular did not remain distinct from the 'European'. European knowledge systems themselves in the colonies, as this chapter will show, were not a singular category. The need is to understand the contexts of the moral, physical and mystical encounters out of which materia medica emerged, away from Europe. An important part of this alternative world of nature in Asia was in the pursuit of spirituality. For example, an integral part of the expansion of the Portuguese empire in Asia and America from the seventeenth century was the expansion of Catholicism. The Portuguese collected plants and other Oriental exotics in Asia through the Catholic 'information order'.[7] These traditions were continued by the Protestant missionaries who came to Asia at the start of the eighteenth century. These missionaries collected, used, codified and defined a new world of materia medica in Asia. In doing so, they defined a material culture of nature that was deeply imbued with spirituality. The pursuits, due to their divergent trends, were not always compatible with the emergent trends in Europe. Often rejected in the metropolis of natural history, these worlds of plants, drugs and their uses framed the materia medica of Asia.

Spiritual pursuits: *Materia medica* and the missionaries in the Coromandel coast

The British and the Danish traders had built some of their early colonial settlements on the Coromandel coast of India from the seventeenth century. Madras was the base of the English East India Company (EEIC) and further south (around 300 km) at Tranquebar, the Danish set up their settlement, where the German-Danish Pietist missionaries started their first mission. These missionaries belonged to the Halle Orphanage or the Francke Foundation, started by the German Lutheran, August Hermann Francke. They were formally known as the Lutheran missionaries of the Royal Danish-Halle Mission, also as the Tranquebar Mission. In 1759, the Moravians arrived at Tranquebar, as the Danish king permitted them to propagate the gospel in the region as well.[8] While in Madras, British surgeons and naturalists studied the plants, drugs and therapeutic traditions of southern India and the Indian Ocean from perspectives of commerce and profit, at Tranquebar, the missionaries explored the world of nature and medicine as part of their interest in Tamil culture, history and spirituality. These two distinct encounters with nature coexisted on the Coromandel coast of the Indian Ocean.

The German missionaries who settled in the Danish settlement in Tranquebar collected and codified local plants and medical traditions of southern India extensively. As Kelly Whitmore has shown, their collection of the *naturalia* of southern India was accompanied by their engagement with local knowledge systems and social norms.[9] As they collected local plants, the Pietists also read Tamil texts, deliberated on Tamil religious traditions and nomenclatures of plants and medicines. One of the reasons why the Pietists and the Moravians on the Coromandel coast engaged extensively with local traditions, along with the local natural world, was because they were religious dissenters; their work was shaped by a rejection of certain forms of modern materialistic life. The spirituality and natural world they encountered in southern India confirmed that renunciation. The preoccupation of the missionary works with Indian culture, religion and plants was in search of an alternative moral repository in the East. Their texts about Indian religion, plants and customs appeared in Europe as advertisements of Eastern culture, in which the reference points remained the East.

Among the early missionaries was Johann Ernst Gründler (1677–1720), a Pietist who came to the Tranquebar Mission in 1709 and spent his entire life on the Coromandel coast studying Tamil medical texts and culture. To understand these more closely, he left the mission and settled in Poreiar, a nearby village, in 1710. There, he practised local habits and dressed like the locals. As part of this, he acquired several medical palm leaf bundles from the local scholars, which had information on various diseases, medicines and herbs, all of which were compiled in his *Malabar Medicus*.[10]

Other early Protestant missionaries such as Bartholomäus Ziegenbalg (1683–1719) and Heinrich Plütschau (1678–1747) similarly developed cultural links with the local population as part of their religious duties and in their curiosity for local spiritual instructions. They maintained diaries, which they sent home periodically. These diaries, along with the station registers, letters, private papers and so on, described Tamil life: festivals, temples, arts and crafts, music and dance, legends, fables, rituals and religious practices, ceremonies and customs. The diaries also detailed the diseases prevalent among the Tamil population and the medicines used, forming a major repository of Tamil culture and materia medica of the eighteenth century. He compiled these into the *Genealogy of the Malabarian Gods*, which he sent to Europe, along with extensive notes on the plants collected near Tranquebar.[11] At the same time, these early Danish missionaries introduced printing in southern India in 1712.[12] Ziegenbalg, who was instrumental in setting up the press, published texts in Tamil and on Indian religion and culture, among which were his *Genealogy of the South-Indian gods* and a text on Tamil grammar, *Grammatica Damulica*.[13] His translation of the New Testament into Tamil was printed in 1715. They also set up a paper mill at Poreiar where Gründler was based around the same time.[14] These led to a distinct print culture around plants, religion and drugs along the eighteenth-century Coromandel coast. While compiling these, Ziegenbalg came to question the predominant idea among missionaries in Europe that 'Malabarians are barbarians'. He conveyed this to his pastor Francke in Halle:

> they are a People of a great deal of Wit and Understanding, and will not be convinced but with Wisdom and Discretion. They have an exact *Analogy* and Coherence in all the fabulous Principles of their Faith. As for a *Future Life*, they have stronger Impressions, than our Atheistical Christians. They have many Books, which they pretend to have been deliver'd to them by their Gods, as we believe the Scriptures to be delivered to us by our God. Their books are stuffed with abundance of pleasant Fables and witty Inventions concerning the Lives of their Gods. They afford plenty of pretty Stories, about the World to come. And at this rate the Word of God, which we propose, seems to them to contain nothing but dry and insipid Notions.[15]

Plütschau, a contemporary of Ziegenbalg, wrote about local Tamil medical practitioners who took the 'greatest pain imaginable to search into the secrets of nature', and how they would amaze the European physicians back home, 'our Physicians in *Europe* would wonder at the Performance of our *Malabar* Doctors here'.[16] He added that since European drugs were not efficacious in Indian climates, the missionaries often depended on medicine prepared by the 'black doctors'. While discussing the Tamil texts like *Kalpastanum*, the Moravian Benjamin Heyne showed a similar appreciation of local medical traditions. He argued that their knowledge was not altogether false, 'The medical works of the Hindoos are neither to be regarded as miraculous productions of wisdom, nor as repositories of nonsense. Their practical principles, as far as I can judge, are very similar to our own; and even their theories may be reconciled with ours.'[17]

The Moravians, who settled along with the Pietists, followed a distinct lifestyle with a particular focus on being self-sufficient. They maintained common housekeeping and tried to earn their livelihood by 'work of their hands'. They purchased and cultivated lands for their subsistence.[18] As part of their close knowledge of the land, the Moravians of southern India sent carefully prepared botanical specimens to Joseph Banks and others in Britain as well as to the United States in the eighteenth and nineteenth centuries.[19] Due to their distinct lifestyles, the Moravians soon became popular among the local population as well as other Europeans.[20] Oluf Maderup (1711–76), a Lutheran missionary who came to Tranquebar in 1742, commented:

> I cannot describe how the Moravians have insinuated themselves in so short a time into the good will of the Danes, French and even Hindus by their voluntary humility and angel-like conduct as they consider it . . . The Natives therefore call them the 'Saints' or the 'Nyanigol' which means 'the wise men' that being the name which they gave here to some of their own holy men.[21]

By 1803 the Moravians had almost disappeared from Tranquebar, the last two having left for Europe after selling their land and garden. Despite their brief stay, they left an important impression, as we shall see, on the study of both plants and medicines of the Coromandel. Most importantly, they set the pattern of Protestant missionary engagements with indigenous plants and people. Christopher Samuel John (1747–1813) was a German missionary based in the Danish settlement of Tranquebar. In his account of the missionary contribution to the Indian school education system, John wrote, 'It is well known what good service the united brethren or Moravians at Tranquebar and Nicobar have rendered with respect to natural history, and knowledge of mechanics. The public on the coast continue to lament the loss of these advantages from their return to Europe.'[22]

Protestant missionaries, like the Dutch missionary Abraham Rogerius (1609–49), who worked with Tamil scholars at Pulicat, the Dutch settlement on the

Coromandel coast, had collected and studied Indian religious and mythological texts from the seventeenth century.[23] In his *Open Door to the Hidden Heathen Religion* (published in 1651), Rogerius had referred to the Puranic traditions of avatars. The Dutch missionaries had simultaneously interacted with Portuguese Catholic missionaries.[24] John inherited this vast intellectual tradition, primarily through his mission library. When he arrived at Tranquebar in 1771, John found the mission library filled with Tamil and Sanskrit medical and scientific texts collected by missionaries before him.[25] His study of Tamil materia medica was informed both by the exploration of the local flora as well as the reading of local texts.

John complemented his textual studies with the cultivation of plants in the mission garden. He collected plants with the help of his fellow missionaries such as the lexicographer Johan Peter Rottler (1749–1836), another Lutheran missionary and the Moravian Johan Gottfried Klein (1766–1821). In their mission garden, they kept local and exotic plants, both as a source of food and also for teaching the locals about God's work.[26] John wrote on natural history and the missionary schools drawing inspiration from his spirituality: 'The usefulness, beauty, and fertility of nature, leads us to admire the immense goodness, power, and wisdom of our great Creator, and the paternal love of our heavenly Father.'[27] His work on the materia medica of the Indian Ocean was defined by his Christian faith:

> Our Lord Jesus Christ, by his parables, directs our attention to surrounding objects, which we daily see before us, and teaches us by them to take up a due attention to our moral character and its consequences, exciting us to look up to our Creator with filial confidence as our best Father, and to submit ourselves entirely to his holy will and providence.[28]

These led to a distinct tradition of the *naturalia* in Tranquebar in the eighteenth century; combining the study of Tamil materia medica and religious practices with missionary observation of local plants, their Christian sentiments and European natural history.

Material pursuits: spices, plants and materia medica in the Coromandel

Adjacent to these spiritual-natural explorations on the Coromandel coast, there was another pursuit of natural history, undertaken primarily by the British employees of the East India Company. Company naturalists such as William Roxburgh (1751–1815) had different motivations for collecting Indian plants. These were either for the commercial benefit of the company or for recognition from the intellectual circles in Europe. Roxburgh conducted experiments in growing cinnamon, clove, tobacco, indigo and teak in his garden in Samulcottah, north of Madras. He also wrote extensive treatises on the medical plants of the coast seeking to publish these in the publications of the Royal Society in London. While the missionaries sought to attain their fulfilment in the study of Indian materia medica at the spatial-cultural site of the Orient itself, for Roxburgh Europe remained the site of his intellectual recognition.

Such commercial pursuit of Oriental spices and medicinal plants was started by the Portuguese. The Portuguese explorer Vasco da Gama arrived in India in 1498 in search of spices, which would go on to transform European maritime and commercial history from the sixteenth century. Since most spices were also used as medicines, interest in spices led Europeans to study the medical botany of south-east Asia. Spices enticed the European taste for exotic tropical flora, an attraction that remained with them for several centuries. Italian physicians and botanists like Caspar Bauhine, Prosper Alpinus and Dutch botanists like Willem Piso and Jacobus Breynius were the first Europeans to study the plants of Malabar.[29]

The other aspect of this was the search for alternative medical specimens, shaped by the global search for alternatives in commercial products. Monopolies of trade required the availability and cultivability of similar species within areas of control. This search figured prominently in drugs as it was closely linked to the procurement of and control over natural resources. James Petiver, the London apothecary, who collected plants from all over the world was a pioneer in this, and asserted that herbs of same nature and class tend to have 'like Vertue and Tendency to work the same effects'.[30]

Alongside this study of spices and materia medica in Asia, European naturalists were engrossed with objects of scientific interest arriving from different parts of the world. A major part of the Royal Society's scientific work from 1660 was in conducting global correspondences started by its first Secretary Henry Oldenburg. The urge was to collect and order natural historical specimens throughout the extent of the expanding empire. The Royal Society was captivated by the exotic and curative virtues of southern Indian plants: 'Providence seems admirably kind to those hot Countrys in providing them with such rare coolings and Cordial profitable against Feavours, Calentures, and such like distempers as may probably arise . . . for corroborating and exhilarating the Bodies and Spirits of men.'[31] Whitelaw Ainslie (1767–1837), the British Superintendent

Surgeon at the EEIC's establishment in Madras in the early nineteenth century, similarly marvelled at the exotic vegetation and materia medica he found along the coastlines. The medicinal plants were 'to be met with in the jungles, amongst the woods of Malabar, and mountains of the lower tracts of the peninsula, and more especially, in Travancore, that country so beautiful, so rich, I may say, in vegetable productions.'[32]

Although by the eighteenth century, spices had ceased to be the crucial commodity of Asian trade of the European East Indian companies, interest in Asian materia medica had emerged as a distinct intellectual tradition. British surgeons such as Roxburgh studied Indian medical plants and spices and reared them in their gardens for both scientific and commercial interests. The Malabar and the Coromandel coastlines were looked upon as a region of exotic plants valued both for medicine and spices; sometimes for both at the same time, the spices being often acknowledged for their medicinal values.

These practices transformed European drug markets. During the seventeenth century, the importation of drugs from the Orient and the New World increased twenty-fivefold.[33] New drugs from Asia and the Americas changed European materia medica fundamentally with the expansion of its medical catalogues and dispensatories, incorporating plants and herbs from different parts of the world. The history of the importation of Asian and American drugs and spices into European drug markets and how these transformed European drug markets, materia medica and natural history is relatively familiar. What is less obvious are the complex intellectual and material traditions from which these plants and therapeutics emerged and the consequences of these global transits at those sites.

'Europe does not want you'

The association between the East India Company surgeons and naturalists and the Danish–German missionaries along the coast of the Coromandel took various forms. On the one hand, the missionaries assisted British surgeons in their search for botanical and medicinal knowledge of the Indian Ocean region. Rottler, a Lutheran missionary with the Danish settlement, was responsible for looking after the garden at the Danish settlement in Tranquebar. Between 1799 and 1800, Rottler made several trips from Tranquebar to Madras collecting botanical specimens.[34] His collection was distributed in Kew, Liverpool and Madras. The English surgeons of Madras also appreciated Rottler's knowledge of local medical botany. In 1788, when the surgeons of the Madras Hospital Board insisted that Rottler should be put in charge of looking after the local medicines there as he had 'great proficiency in the Knowledge of Botany' of the region.[35] The government, however, was not too enthusiastic in appointing someone from outside the English establishment and appointed Mr Ponton (a surgeon from the Guntoor) in the post.[36] Ainslie dedicated his *Materia Medica* to Rottler, 'as a token of respect for his scientific celebrity . . . and the kind and liberal aid which has been received from him'.[37] In several parts of the book, he drew from Rottler's deep knowledge of indigenous plants, and their names and therapeutic uses. In 1795, Rottler accompanied Lord North, the first British Governor of Ceylon, who wanted a botanist to accompany him on a trip to the island.

Johann Gerhard Koenig (1728–85) was the surgeon-botanist who initiated the Linnaean study of Indian botany. A Baltic German and a student of Carl Linnaeus, Koenig came to India in 1768 as a surgeon and member of the Danish medical missionary in Tranquebar. He gave up his missionary duties to serve as a naturalist at the court of the Nawab of Arcot between 1773 and 1785. During this period, he studied the study of the flora of the Madras region and travelled to Ceylon.[38] In 1778, Koenig joined the EEIC, undertaking several scientific journeys for them.[39] His work is significant since it, along with introducing the new taxonomical methodology of Linnaeus in southern India, also drew from the earlier natural historical studies by Rheede and D'Orta.

Chronicling of the natural and cultural history of the region formed the primary link between the English surgeons in the Madras establishment and the German missionaries of Tranquebar. To the missionaries, the English settlement promised a larger site for missionary preaching than the relatively small Danish settlement. From the very beginning of the missionary settlement, Ziegenbalg and his fellow missionaries maintained close contact with the English neighbours. Their letters were sent to Europe by the EEIC ships, first to the Anglican Society for the Promotion of Christian Knowledge (SPCK) and then to Germany; some went to Copenhagen.[40] The British, who did not have any missionary representatives from home in these parts, invited the Lutherans to serve their troops. In 1751, the Court of Directors ordered the Madras government to 'Encourage the Danish missionaries to be active in their duty'.[41] Throughout the British rivalry with the French in southern India, the Danes maintained their neutrality. When Benjamin Schwartz visited Trichinopoly in 1762, in the middle of the war with the French, the EEIC's garrison commander, Major A. Preston requested him to assist them following the deaths of many soldiers and *sepoys* in an explosion at the fort's powder magazine. In return, Preston promised to build a prayer school for Tamil Christians. In 1764, when troops were ordered to march and besiege Madurai against the local rulers of Mysore, Preston again urged Schwartz to act as his military chaplain.[42] Through these encounters, the missionaries were drafted into the military, materialist and commercial world of the EEIC.

John and Roxburgh formed a close friendship while being at the two ends of the study of natural history in the Indian Ocean. Roxburgh familiarized John with the new cultures of collecting and growing exotic plants. He helped John to publish his paper on a Tamil philosopher called Avyar in the *Asiatick Researches*.[43] John also became an honorary member of the Asiatic Society in 1797.[44] Roxburgh also wrote to Charles Taylor, the Secretary to the Society for the Encouragement of Arts in London about John 'a most worthy Dane, at Tranquebar near Madras, an able friend & zealous philosopher'.[45] In doing so, Roxburgh ignited John's interest in natural philosophy and medicine. In 1790, Reverend John wrote to Roxburgh: 'You have almost made [me] a Malabar Doctor. '[46] In 1793, he wrote again about his desire to become a botanist, even at the expense of his missionary activities: 'I would wish to have or make myself wings like Dœdulus to fly to you to see your large tract of country & to have a share in the superintendence of it. I would forget my chief employment but teach the inhabitants at the same time how to plant & rear Coconut.'[47] In the mission headquarters in Halle, John was regarded as someone unduly in love with Indian natural history and secular studies.[48]

In return, John helped Roxburgh to collect plants through his missionary network based in the Indian Ocean. He inspired Roxburgh to continue his work in India with a missionary zeal: 'Go on in your zeal in studying the beauties & wonders in the works of our Glorious God & in promoting this excellent knowledge for the benefit of your fellow creatures.'[49] He also offered to procure books on botany for Roxburgh from Europe through his missionary networks.[50] John also regularly shared his research on snakes and snake poison with Roxburgh.[51] While doing so, John suggested to Roxburgh the need to develop informal networks in intellectual explorations away from Europe, similar to the way missionaries had functioned in this region. They had, as John elaborated, played an important part in collecting the curiosities of distant lands, and thus were a great ally to naturalists of Europe:

> Those who cultivate this study in Europe of whom very few can travel into foreign countries must depend upon their friends who have better opportunities for gratifying their desires by sending them their observation and collections. Amongst these Missionaries and Mission servants, and those who correspond with them, their native pupils and itinerant catechists have often been of great

service on their journey by procuring curiosities from distant countries and islands.[52]

John contacted his missionary friends in Ceylon who helped Roxburgh in his botanical collections.[53] He employed the Danish Lutheran Engelhard in Ceylon to collect cinnamon plants for Roxburgh.[54] John's Dutch friends also helped with his collection of plants.[55] From Tranquebar, John sent him lists of medicinal plants found in the surrounding regions as well as from where his missionary friends were posted.[56] He also sent a list of plants and information of their medical uses collected from 'Malabar Physicians', with their names written in Tamil.[57] Revd John also appointed a 'black Natural Philosopher' (his local assistant) to collect plants, shells, seeds, insects and fishes from Nicobar for Roxburgh.[58] John described the virtues of several medicinal plants in the surrounding areas and sent Roxburgh a list of the exotic plants in the mission garden along with a list of medical plants used by the local physicians.[59]

Despite their close friendship and the shared pursuit of the natural history of the Indian Ocean, there were important divergences. For Reverend John, serving in a mission in India and working among the locals and close to the natural world was an experience in salvation and fulfilment. The contentment of such a project was in the East itself. The missionary texts about Indian religion, plants and customs appeared in Europe as advertisements of Eastern culture, in which the reference points remained the East. As Roxburgh searched for recognition from Europe for his scientific pursuits and became restive with the delay in and often the loss of plants in transit to Europe, Reverend John sought to comfort him. He urged Roxburgh to find similar meaning in his work in studying local plants and to continue to serve the cause of humanity through his research:

> Europe does not want you so much as India. . . . Can you make so many discoveries for the benefit of the world in England . . . than you have done and will do here. You will be torn in pieces with all your plants, manuscripts and Drawings and you shall never have my blessings in such a degree as you have and shall have as long as you remain in India.[60]

The liminal, peripheral existences away from Europe, geographically and culturally, provided significant creative space for the development of diverse formulations about nature, morality, history and spirituality. These, however, did not gain recognition and acknowledgement from those undertaking those pursuits from Europe. Colonial botanists and missionaries who collected plants and local knowledge through their multifarious networks received little recognition from the scientific world of the eighteenth century John's words to Roxburgh also highlight a tension between the worlds of John and Roxburgh although they participated in the same networks of collection; while the missionaries could attain fulfilment in their study of nature at the spatial-cultural site of the Orient, the mainstream pursuit of eighteenth-century natural history, which Roxburgh had sought, was more firmly attached to Europe.

John's sense of fulfilment in the East too had its limits. The missionaries were sent to India with an obligation to write about their work and activities in India to their superiors in Europe. They were supposed to spread the words of the gospel to the locals, not collect the spiritual and intellectual wisdom of the East. Ziegenbalg, Plutsau, Rottler and John's collection of Tamil materia medica and religious insights were received with indifference among the missionaries in Europe. When Ziegenbalg requested his superior Francke in Halle to publish his letters so that the biased notions about Asian religions could be dispelled in Europe, the latter dismissed it emphatically, 'the missionaries were sent out to exterminate heathenism in India, not to spread heathen nonsense all over Europe'.[61]

The estrangement from Europe, as evident in John's words, 'Europe does not want you', was therefore twofold. At one level, Roxburgh and other naturalists based in Asia did not receive the metropolitan recognition that they craved, nor did the missionaries, who studied Tamil religion, culture and materia medica, from their superiors in Halle. The rejection was more fundamental; it was of the essential spiritual, commercial and material world which both John and Roxburgh inhabited on the coast of Coromandel. Both appeared redundant to the empirical and secular traditions of natural history and materia medica of Europe, which placed these distant and dried plants, seeds and barks within their order of things. In doing so, the European scholarship rejected the materiality of that world. It is therefore not surprising that John's premonition about the materiality of Roxburgh's work being 'torn in pieces' in Europe, came true.[62] Roxburgh's botanical collections and his manuscripts are now scattered in different places, in the British Library, Natural History Museum Library, in the Botanical Garden Library in India. The tapestry of that world remains dispersed in these fragments.

Notes

1 Ken Arnold, *Cabinets for the Curious: Looking Back at Early English Museums* (Aldershot: Ashgate, 2006); Susan Scott Parrish, *American Curiosity: Cultures of Natural History in the Colonial British Atlantic World* (Chapel Hill, NC: University

of North Carolina Press, 2006); James Delbourgo, 'Divers Things: Collecting the World under Water', *History of Science* 49, no. 2 (2011): 149–85; Pamela H. Smith and Paula Findlen, eds, *Merchants & Marvels; Commerce, Science, and Art in Early Modern Europe* (New York; London: Routledge, 2002). Also see Kay Dian Kriz, 'Curiosities, Commodities, and Transplanted Bodies in Hans Sloane's "Natural History of Jamaica"', *The William and Mary Quarterly* 57, no. 1 (2000): 35–78.

2 Matthew Cobb, 'Malpighi, Swammerdam and the Colourful Silkworm: Replication and Visual Representation in Early Modern Science', *Annals of Science* 59, no. 2 (2002): 111–47.

3 Gianna Pomata and Nancy Siraisi, eds, *Historia: Empiricism and Erudition in Early Modern Europe* (Cambridge, MA: MIT Press, 2005).

4 Nicholas Jardine and Emma Spary, 'Introduction: Worlds of Natural History', in *Worlds of Natural History*, ed Helen A. Curry, Nicholas Jardine, James A. Secord, and Emma Spary (Cambridge: Cambridge University Press, 2018), 3–16.

5 Harold John Cook, *Matters of Exchange: Commerce, Medicine, and Science in the Dutch Golden Age* (New Haven: Yale University Press, 2007).

6 Anna Winterbottom, *Hybrid Knowledge in the Early East India Company World*, Cambridge Imperial and Post-colonial Studies Series (Basingstoke, Hampshire: Palgrave Macmillan, 2016); Kapil Raj, *Relocating Modern Science: Circulation and the Construction of Scientific Knowledge in South Asia and Europe, 17th-19th Centuries* (Delhi: Permanent Black, 2006); Preetha Nair, *Raja Serfoji II: Science, Medicine and Enlightenment in Tanjore* (New Delhi: Routledge India, 2014); Simon Schaffer, Lissa Roberts, Kapil Raj, and James Delbourgo, eds, *The Brokered World: Go-Betweens and Global Intelligence, 1770–1820*, Uppsala Studies in History of Science 35 (Sagamore Beach, MA: Watson Publishing International, 2009).

7 Ângela Barreto Xavier and Ines G. Županov, *Catholic Orientalism: Portuguese Empire, Indian Knowledge (16th-18th Centuries)* (New Delhi: Oxford University Press, 2015).

8 C. S. Mohanavelu, *German Tamilology: German Contribution to Tamil Language, Literature and Culture during the Period 1706–1945* (Madras: Saiva Siddhanta, 1993), 35–7.

9 Kelly Joan Whitmer, 'What's in a Name? Place, Peoples and Plants in the Danish-Halle Mission, c. 1710–1740', *Annals of Science: In Kind: Species of Exchange in Early Modern Science* 70, no. 3 (2013): 337–56.

10 Mohanavelu, *German Tamilology*, 43–5.

11 The text was published much later in 1869: Bartholomaeus Ziegenbalg, *Genealogy of the South-Indian Gods, A Manual of the Mythology and Religion of the People of Southern India. Including a Description of Popular Hinduism* (Madras: Higginbotham, 1869).

12 Arno Lehmann, *It Began at Tranquebar: The Story of the Tranquebar Mission and the Beginnings of Protestant Christianity in India: Published to Celebrate the 250th*

Anniversary of the Landing of the First Protestant Missionaries at Tranquebar in 1706 (Madras: Christian Literature Society on behalf of the Federation of Evangelical Lutheran Churches in India, 1956), 101.

13 Ziegenbalg, *Genealogy of the South-Indian Gods*; Bartholomaeus Ziegenbalg, *Grammatica Damulica* (Halle an der Saale: Litteris et impensis Orphanotrophei, 1716).

14 P. Maria Lazar, 'Making a Mission of Understanding Tamil', *Indian Express – Tamil Nadu Notes* (1994), www.trankebar.net/article/indian-express/1994-12-12_mission-(lazar)/making.htm (accessed 21 February 2004).

15 Bartholomaeus Ziegenbalg, Heinrich Plütscho, and Johann Ernst Gründler, *Propagation of the Gospel in the East: Being an Account of the Success of Two Danish Missionaries, Lately Sent to the East-Indies, for the Conversion of the Heathens in Malabar. In Several Letters to Their Correspondents in Europe. . . . Rendered into English from the High-Dutch:* . . . (London: printed and sold by Joseph Downing, 1718), 55–6.

16 Bartholomaeus Ziegenbalg, 'Extract of another Letter, Relating to Some Diseases Incident to the Malabarians: Likewise of Some Remedies they Commonly Use Against Them', in *An Account Of The Religion, and Government, Learning, and Oeconomy, etc. Of The Malabarians: Sent by the Danish Missionaries to Their Correspondents in Europe* (London: Downing, 1717), 61–2.

17 Benjamin Heyne, *Tracts, Historical and Statistical, on India with Journals of Several Tours. Also an Account of Sumatra in a Series of Letters* (London: Baldwin, 1814), 124.

18 August Gottlieb Spangenberg, *An Account of the Manner in Which the Protestant Church of the Unitas Fratrum, or United Brethren, Preach the Gospel, and carry on their Mission Among the Heathen, Translated from German* (London: H. Trapp, 1788), 58, 83–4.

19 J. L. Reveal and J. S. Pringle, 'Taxonomic Botany and Floristics', in *Flora of North America North of Mexico. Volume I: Introduction*, ed. Flora of North America Editorial Committee (New York: Oxford University Press, 1993), 157–92.

20 Mohanavelu, *German Tamilology*, 12–27.

21 J. Ferdinand Fenger, *History of the Tranquebar Mission: Worked out from Original Papers, published in Danish and translated in English from the German of Emil Francke* (Tranquebar: Evangelical Lutheran Mission Press, 1863), 268.

22 Christopher S. John, *On Indian Civilization, or Report of a successful Experiment, Made during Two Years on That Subject, In Fifteen Tamul, and Five English native Schools; With Proposals for Establishing a Separate Liberal Native School Society* (London: Printed for F. C. and J. Rivington, 1813), 39.

23 Abraham Rogerius, *De open-deure tot het verborgen heydendom ofte Waerachtigh vertoogh van het Leven ende Zeden; mitsgaders de Religie, ende Gods-dienst der Bramines, op de Cust Chormandel, ende de Landen daar ontrent* [Open Door to the Hidden Heathen Religion]. (Leyden: Françoys Hackes, 1651).

24 Ângela Barreto Xavier and Ines G. Županov, *Catholic Orientalism: Portuguese Empire, Indian Knowledge (16th-18th Centuries)* (New Delhi: Oxford University Press, 2015).
25 John, *On Indian Civilization*, 39.
26 Ibid., 40-2.
27 Ibid., 36.
28 Ibid., 37.
29 'An Account of Some Books', *Philosophical Transactions (1683-1775)* 13 (1683):100.
30 James Petiver, 'Some Attempts Made to Prove That Herbs of the Same Make or Class for the Generallity, have the Like Vertue and Tendency to Work the Same Effects', *Philosophical Transactions (1683-1775)* 21 (1699): 289-94.
31 'An Account of Some Books', 104.
32 Whitelaw Ainslie, *Materia Indica, Or, Some Account of Those Articles which Are Employed by the Hindoos, and Other Eastern Nations, in their Medicine, Arts, and Agricultural* (London: Printed for Longman, Rees, Orme, Brown, and Green, Paternoster-Row, 1826), xxxvii.
33 Roy Porter and Dorothy Porter, 'The Rise of the English Drugs Industry: The Role of Thomas Corbyn', *Medical History* 33, no. 3 (1989): 277-95.
34 K. M. Matthew, 'Notes on an Important Botanical Trip (1799-1800) of J. P. Rottler on the Coromandel Coast (India) with a Translation of his Original Text, Explanatory Notes and a Map', *Botanical Journal of the Linnean Society* 113, no. 4 (1993): 351-88.
35 Surgeon General's Records (Tamil Nadu State Archive), vol. 3, Hospital Board, 10 October 1788, 200-1.
36 Surgeon General's Records (Tamil Nadu State Archive), vol. 5, Hospital Board, 22 May 1789, 17.
37 Whitelaw Ainslie, *Materia Medica of Hindoostan* (Madras: Government Press, 1813), front page.
38 Ray Desmond, *The European Discovery of the Indian Flora* (Kew: Royal Botanical Gardens, Oxford: Oxford University Press, 1992), 39.
39 See Niklas T. Jensen, 'The Medical Skills of the Malabar Doctors in Tranquebar, India, as Recorded by Surgeon T L F Folly, 1798', *Medical History* 49, no. 4 (2005): 497.
40 Ernst Benz, 'Pietist and Puritan Sources of Early Protestant World Missions (Cotton Mather and A. H. Francke)', *Church History* 20, no. 2 (1951): 29.
41 Asia Pacific and Africa Collections (hereafter APAC), E/4/856, Court of Directors to Madras council, 23 August 1751, paragraph 63.
42 Schwartz to Mission College, 10 July 1766, in Fenger, *History of the Tranquebar Mission*, 219.
43 Christopher S. John, 'A Summary Account of the Life and Writings of Avyar, a Tamul Female Philosopher', *Asiatick Researches* 7 (1803): 343-61.

44 Sibadas Chaudhuri, *Proceedings of the Asiatic Society. Vol. 1, 1784–1800* (Calcutta: The Asiatic Society, 1980), 275.
45 Botany Library, Natural History Museum (hereafter NHM) MSS. ROX, 1789, Roxburgh to Charles Taylor, undated.
46 APAC, European Manuscript D809, John to Roxburgh, 9 December 1790.
47 NHM, MSS. ROX, 1793, John to Roxburgh, 17 August 1793.
48 Indira V. Peterson, 'The Cabinet of King Serfoji of Tanjore: A European collection in early nineteenth-century India', *Journal of the History of Collections* 11, no. 1 (1999): 75.
49 APAC, European Manuscript D809, John to Roxburgh, 24 November 1789.
50 Ibid.
51 Ibid.
52 John, *On Indian Civilization*, 38.
53 NHM, MSS. ROX, 1793, John to Roxburgh, 17 August 1793.
54 Ibid.
55 APAC, European Manuscript D809, John to Roxburgh, 29 September 1789.
56 John sent a list of medicinal plants collected by him to Roxburgh with details of their uses by Indian practitioners. APAC, European Manuscript D 809, John to Roxburgh, 13 October 1790.
57 APAC, European Manuscript D809, John to Roxburgh, 20 June 1791.
58 APAC, European Manuscript D809, John to Roxburgh, 9 December 1790.
59 Ibid., John to Roxburgh, 13 October 1790. Also, see John to Roxburgh, 20 June 1791 and 24 November 1789.
60 APAC, European Manuscript D809, John to Roxburgh, 26 November 1792.
61 Quoted in Lehmann, *It Began at Tranquebar*, 32. Also see Ziegenbalg, *Genealogy of the South-Indian Gods*, xv.
62 APAC, European Manuscript D809, John to Roxburgh, 26 November 1792.

3

In pursuit of a healing Eden

Exploring the medico-botanical networks of knowledge circulation in the Indian Ocean region with special reference to South India, 1600–1800 CE

Malavika Binny

The confluence of the diverse yet deeply entangled fields of the history of science, materiality studies and Indian Ocean studies have opened up a terrain of questions into the nature and constitution of circulatory flows of early modern knowledge and imperial networks. It has also unravelled deep and unparalleled epistemological inquiries into the worlds of the trade, religion and medicine particularly in South India. These questions become particularly fascinating in the Indian Ocean littoral regions as they were deeply entwined with the regional politics of state formation, courtly culture and the reconstitution of elite and non-elite domains of cultural knowledge. They were often marked with a deep sense of materiality attached to the climatological significance of the ocean, manifest in the many readings of traditional medicine such as Ayurveda on the one hand and the inflow of new commodities which had to be made intelligible to native healing discourses on the other. The emergence of botany in Europe as a major avenue of academic interest as well as the pursuit for profits using botanical and medical knowledge and the quest to recreate the gardens of Eden in European cities led to what we will refer to as bioprospecting endeavours by European officials.[1] This led to a profusion of cultural encounters between South Asian and European medical traditions, which paved way for changes with both. The primary argument of the chapter will be that the exchange of information was mutual albeit asymmetrical. While medico-botanical knowledge about the Indian Ocean region moved to European shores, European *materia medica*, botanical products and therapeutic techniques also impacted the medical systems of the Indian subcontinent. Ayurveda proves to be a prime example of the exchange with Sanskritic texts produced after the sixteenth century CE including detailed information on the 'new' therapeutics.

One of the main aims of this chapter is to argue that while we do have plentiful evidence of a dynamic European and local exchange of knowledge from the south-western coast of India from the fifteenth century onwards, the knowledge that was extracted and transferred from south-west India to Europe was stripped of its cultural attachments and divorced from the local epistemological framework and reformulated according to European interests and 'scientific' traditions. This chapter will question the idea of Ayurveda as a crystallized and static form of knowledge associated only with Hinduism, with the aim of showing that even those traditions of medicine which existed prior to the arrival of the European mercantilism on the coasts of South India were not homogenous. They were the results of the inter-mixing and convergence of multiple knowledge systems, whose roots can be traced to widely divergent backgrounds including Buddhism, Jainism and tribal and folk medicine.[2]

In the early modern period, medical knowledge was vital not only in terms of nursing the injured and the sick of the trading companies, but also to gain access to imperial circuits of power. Interwoven into the global web of knowledge transfers are the histories of botanical science and state systems often couched in the language of both power and religion, which this chapter will be analysing in the context of the Indo–Portuguese–Dutch engagements on the Malabar Coast.[3] The relevance of botanical transfers in Empire-building has become clear from studies on the role of agents, actors, micro- and macro-networks and the analyses of the emergence of botanical gardens and botanic departments in European universities in the early modern period.[4]

In the case of diplomacy with countries such as China in the early modern period, it was medico-botanical knowledge that created opportunities for European trading companies and their missions to the Chinese courts which otherwise were deemed impenetrable.[5] Medical knowledge was essential for the survival of the personnel of the European trading companies in the tropical regions. Injury and disease represented a more serious, constant and certain threat than any rival nation's military challenge; no other factor constituted a greater drain on resources and source of anxiety for both soldiers and sailors. Walker and Cook have suggested that in the case of the colonization of the Atlantic Coast, especially during the initial phase, 'European commanders, dismayed at the ineffectiveness of their own home remedies against previously unknown tropical diseases and desperate to preserve the military effectiveness of their forces, looked to native healing practices for the alleviation of their ills.'[6]

The same process seems to also have been at work on the Indian Ocean coast where, faced with an immensely different geographical locale, dietary patterns and new types of flora and fauna, engagement with native medical knowledge was unavoidable. Hendrik Van Rheede (*c.* 1636–*c.* 1691), for instance, mentions the efficacy of medicine from Malabar as well as the expense of transporting medicine from Europe that might be avoided.[7]

The whole idea of the portrayal of the Indian Ocean as a tropical miasmic region of disease should also be factored into the narrative here.[8] A resilient and long-standing narrative in the history of science has envisioned the flowering of modern botany as the rise of taxonomy, nomenclature, and 'pure' systems of classification during this phase. One might say that one of the defining schisms of the eighteenth century, one that has shaped the history of the discipline and determined the limits of what may be termed as scientific rationality, was the struggle between the ancient and modern. This European contest between the ancient and the modern reappears in the history of science of the non-Western world as a dichotomy that distinguishes tradition and modernity.[9] Historians who have internalized this distinction have more often than not assumed a static view of both culture and knowledge, wherein the traditional is typically depicted as unchanging, threatened by and fighting against a modernity that would like to see it buried.[10] This image is true not only for the history of science but also for the history of knowledge production and the approach has been criticized and challenged by stressing the multi-vocality and fluidity of both knowledge systems.

Early modern bioprospecting ventures: Reconstituting the epistemological worlds

The verdant geographical space of modern-day Kerala, which is referred to in European and Mediterranean sources as Malabar or *Keraladésa*, has been of historical interest for about two millennia. The trade connections between the Malabar Coast and Europe have been effectively traced to Greco-Roman antiquity by historians on both sides of the Indian Ocean.[11] The modalities of the trade involved the exchange of materials, ideas and ideologies both ways. The mechanism that enabled the socio-economic intercourse up to the fifteenth century was facilitated and mediated by middlemen from the north-eastern coast of Africa and the Arabian Peninsula.[12] The source of interest which brought ships from Europe, Africa, Arabia and East Asia to the ancient coast was its fame as a garden of spices, prompting some authors to call it 'the pepper coast', but the land was equally famous as a treasure trove of potent medical herbs. Some of the most notable bioprospecting attempts in the early modern period were those by European physicians and administrative scholars such as Garcia Da Orta (*c*.1501–*c*.68), Christobal Acosta (*c*.1525–*c*.95), Nicolas L'Empereur (1660–1742) and Van Rheede.

The period from the fifteenth to the seventeenth centuries witnessed the composition of major botanical works on the flora of the Malabar and to a lesser extent of the Konkan coast. Richard Grove suggests that 'the number of available or relevant texts involved is very small, while, correspondingly, each has a life of extraordinary influence and longevity, far more than is the case with, for example, narrative histories'.[13] The first attempt at what can be termed as 'bioprospecting' specifically in the realm of medicine was by Garcia Da Orta who has been referred to as a pioneer of tropical medicine, especially with regard to the *materia medica* of the tropics. His work, the *Colóquios dos Simples e Drogas da India*, in many ways influenced later works such as that of Carolus Clusius (1526–1609), Jacobus Bontius (1592–1631) and Herman Boerhaave (1668–1738), and played a crucial role in expanding the horizons of disciplines such as botany, medicine, pharmacology and ethnology. Da Orta is also credited as the first physician to have systematically introduced South Asian drugs and healing methods to a European audience in the format of a printed book. The significance of the work can also be inferred from the fact that his book on medicine in general, and on tropical drugs in particular, was only the second book to be published from Goa under the Portuguese. Written in Portuguese, the work was first published by a certain João de Endem at Saint Paul's College in Goa in 1563.[14] It contains 59 *colloquies* in the form of conversations between the author and other characters, some historical and some fictional. In it, Da Orta discusses in detail 75 botanical and non-botanical drugs and 200 other floral and faunal elements. Having inherited the best of Renaissance teaching from Iberian universities, he was extremely familiar with the Greco-Roman traditions of medicine. There are several references to Galen and Hippocrates, and his work is interspersed with quotes from Dioscorides and Pliny, while he is also respectful of the Arabic-Persian medical scholarship by Avicenna and Mesué; on several occasions, he claims that they are more credible on tropical herbs than the Greco-Roman texts. Suffice to say that Da Orta was a polyglot and maintained close contact with merchants from China, the Malay Islands and the Malabar Coast which helped him cross-compare the various types of the same herbs from different parts of the globe.

Colóquios dos Simples e Drogas da India was translated into Latin by Clusius, who was by then an acclaimed botanist, under the title: *Aromatum et Simplicium Aliquot Medicamentorum apud Indios Nascentium Historia*.[15] Christobal Acosta also borrowed heavily from Da Orta's *Colóquios* in his *Tractado de las drogas y medicinas de las Indias Orientales*, which published in Spanish and became even more popular than Da Orta's original work.[16] While Orta was a physician, and his work an individual initiative pursued during the years he spent on the Indian peninsula collecting, analysing and studying indigenous herbs and healing practices, Van Rheede's monumental work, the *Hortus Malabaricus*, was in many ways an initiative pursued within the framework of the Dutch VOC apparatus. His position as the Dutch Governor of Malabar greatly helped him in the endeavour. A variety of exhaustive accounts by scholars like Heniger, Manilal and Fournier now enable us to chart the ideological and practical history of the compilation of the *Hortus Malabaricus*.[17]

The epistemological worlds of *Colóquios* and *Hortus Malabaricus* are quite different from one another. While *Colóquios* is dialogic and interested in understanding the semantic world of medicine, *Hortus* is pedantic about the drugs without exploring their cultural milieu. Da Orta's world is inhabited by spirits, demons and myths, in which medicine is not yet separated from its socio-cultural and ritual contexts. It is a world of competitive healing traditions, without a monolithic notion of medical or botanical science. That world is still new to European eyes, viewed using European perceptions, though not necessarily a European world view. On the other hand, *Hortus Malabaricus* was the product of the combined efforts of persons hailing from multiple traditions, yet it seems to follow a single and clear perception of 'botanical science'. This unified vision can be seen through all twelve volumes, in its clear-cut and precise schemata, its systematic elucidation of the nomenclature (in Latin, Malayalam, Arabic and Sanskrit), plant anatomy and its characteristics followed by utilities. The text suggests a well-planned structure and strategy according to the newfound interest in botany of the period in Europe, a phenomenon sometimes termed 'Renaissance botany'.[18]

Asymmetries of knowledge extraction: The social world of medicine in South India

Hortus Malabaricus was published over fifteen years, from 1678 to 1693 CE. It contains detailed information on 725 plants and has 791 illustrations of the flora of Malabar. Van Rheede had the support of the king of Cochin and organized teams of local experts and herb collectors to collect and compile botanical specimens on the Malabar Coast and beyond. In the foreword to the third volume of *Hortus*, Van Rheede claims that he would organize and send teams of people numbering up to 200 people to collect herbs and shrubs on plant-collecting missions on visiting new places.[19] He gives high praise to the contributions of Brahmin priests who are referred to as having a 'high born' social status.[20] He also mentions that the panel of 'experts' constituted by him with the help of the ruler of Cochin also had people belonging to different social backgrounds.[21]

The third and the fourth certificates in the first volume of *Hortus Malabricus* mention the contributions of an Ezhava physician, Itti Achuden, who is referred to as 'Doctor Malabaricus' in the Latin translation in Roman script in the fourth certificate and as 'Kōlāṭṭu Vaidyan' in the third certificate in Malayalam in *kōlezhethu* script. This certificate states that the document is drafted by a Malayali physician born in Kodakarapally in the land of Karapuram (in present-day Alappuzha district in Kerala) who according to caste rites belongs to the Ezhava caste.[22] The Ezhavas, who were initially a toddy-tapping caste, had by the sixteenth and seventeenth centuries also become middlemen in the spice trade and physicians. Their familiarity with trees owing to their caste-based profession of tree climbing and toddy extraction also led them to have knowledge about a large number of botanical products. The Ezhavas were referred to as *Chegos* in the Portuguese and Dutch sources and the Latin translation of the certificate mentions Itti Achuden as a *Chego* physician. The fifth certificate also points to the involvement of three Konkani Gowda Saraswath Brahmins: Appu Bhatt, Vinayaka Pandit and Ranga Bhatt. According to the *Skanda Purāṇa,* an eighth-century Sanskrit text, Gowda Saraswath Brahmins were a community of Brahmins who had migrated to the Konkan coast and Kerala from northern India.[23]

The preface to the third volume of *Hortus Malabaricus* states clearly that Van Rheede lacked any kind of botanical expertise.[24] Thus, he formed a panel of physicians and experts from diverse traditions, including *Brahmana* such as Vinayaka Pandit, Ranga and Appu Bhatt, *Ezhava* physicians such as Itti Achuden, *Konkani* experts and a Carmelite priest (Father Matthew), to help with collecting and identifying plants. Several other figures were involved, such as Johannes Casearius (1642–77), who was in charge of the church in Cochin, several princes from other royal houses as well as a number of Dutch botanists.[25] These included Johan van Someren (1622–76) and Joannes van Dyck (1678–1703), both professors in botany at Leiden University, who had played instrumental roles in the identification and precise illustration of plants, and Johannes Munniks (1652–1711), a renowned botanist at Utrecht University, who helped with finding the correct Latin translation of the botanical specimens.[26]

This was no small feat even with the royal sanction of the Cochin Maharajah in the case of Kerala, because of the caste composition of the experts involved. Of course, the discourse on caste and its complex processes and impact on the history of medical traditions on the Indian subcontinent is a much under-represented topic to date. The practice of caste as graded social inequality which extended to non-commensality, endogamy and untouchability necessitated the existence of multiple object worlds of therapeutic knowledge which were both insular and porous to various degrees. Both early Ayurvedic treatises and native codes of conduct (*dharma-sastric* texts) such as the sixteenth-century Sanskrit treatise *Vyavahāramāla* refer to the distinct practices of medicine followed by people belonging to different castes.[27] In fact, the practice of untouchability made it almost impossible for upper caste physicians to treat lower-caste patients. This in turn led to the evolution of separate medical traditions for the different castes. Yet, as the inclusion of Itti Achuden, who belonged to a lower caste, shows, scholars from multiple castes belonging to different schools of medical traditions worked together. This points to an important moment of confluence in the history of South Asian botany and medicine, in which several traditions of medicine present on the Malabar Coast, until then without much exposure to each other, collaborated. Van Rheede himself expressed his apprehension about this, claiming that he had devised strategies and assigned specific tasks to different groups, and frustration that the experts from different traditions would not see eye to eye in the identification and use of herbs.[28] He also explicitly mentions that the physicians and experts 'did not know each other though they were from different parts of Malabar'.[29] They were suspicious of each other and very eager to receive praise, but not admit their lack of information about some plants.[30]

The impact of both Da Orta's and Van Rheede's works on the development of botany has been the subject of intense academic scrutiny.[31] While scholars more or less agree on the relevance of Da Orta ad Van Rheede for the perception of botany as 'big science' in the early modern period, the question of the provenance of the indigenous knowledge still remains unanswered.[32] Da Orta seems to have amassed the information from his many interactions with native physicians, including those in the court of Burdan Nizam Shah I of the Nizam Shahi dynasty of Ahmadnagar (to whom he was physician) and other local healers and merchants.³³ For instance, in the tenth Colloquy, Garcia Da Orta takes a detour from narrating the qualities of pharmacological products to recount the history of the Ahmadnagar and the Deccan.³⁴ He does the same in the sections on the use of mercury as medicine for leprosy,³⁵ the use of lemon, and in the medical uses of *acoro* (Acorus Calamus)³⁶ and *galanga* (Alpinia officinarum).³⁷

Van Rheede very specifically mentions the involvement of 'high caste' Brahmins and the use of Brahmin language as the functional language in which most ancient texts were composed.³⁸ It can be argued that no other texts than 'Ayurvedic texts' could be the source of their information. Yet, the Malayalam certificate in *kōlezhethu* script given by Itti Achuden also points towards a Malayali or an Ezhava component at work. Itti Achuden mentions a text called *Cholkettapustakam*. It is not clear whether this is a reference to a particular text or to the oral tradition of healing which was prevalent among the lower caste; the literal translation title of the text would be 'a book based on listening to recitals'.

Moreover, the certificates provided in the text by Ranga, Vinayaka and Appu Bhatt mention 'they referred to ancient works and have been engaging plant collection teams who would collect the flowers, fruits, seeds, trees and creepers of medical and other herbs for them according to the seasons in which the plants bloom'.³⁹ They mention an ancient text called *Manhaningattanam*, which could be a corrupted reference to *Maha-niganṭu*, one of the Sanskrit Ayurvedic herbal compendia. Curiously, the reference to this particular text is only present in the Latin translation of the certificate and not mentioned in the original certificate, which only refers to texts of medicine and other *niganṭus* (medical encyclopaedia). The language of the original certificate is Konkani (referred to as the *lingua Brahmana* in the text), which was written in the Devanagari script.

At this point, it is important for us to look at Ayurveda and its knowledge structure to understand the flow of information from South Asia to the global context. Some of the issues we deal with in the second section of the chapter involve the epistemic structure of the evolution of Ayurveda as one of the prominent systems of knowledge that the European networks tapped into. It is important to remember that the Ayurvedic system of medicine is not only a 'Hindu or Brahmanic' form of medicine, as it has been projected in recent times, but also a system of healing drawing its roots from multiple traditions. So, the movement of information flows between knowledge systems were not merely contingent on the European exercise of knowledge collection but goes back to the ancient and the early medieval period, the European enterprise being the more recent and systematic one.

The peripatetic world of medico-botanical materialities

It can be suggested that the evidence provided by texts such as that of Garcia Da Orta and Van Rheede informs us of a period of close interaction of divergent and often contradicting knowledge systems. Da Orta, in the case of most of the botanical herbs discussed in his *Colóquios,* mentions the Arabic, Portuguese, Greek/Roman, Malay, Canarese and, in some cases, Malayalam, Bengali, Gujarati and Sanskrit names for the same plant. For instance, in the case of the coconut, Da Orta mentions that it is called *coco* in Portuguese, *jauzalindi* in Arabic (as mentioned by Avicenna), *nihor* in Malay and referred to as *narel* by the Persians and Arabs. *Narel* could be a corrupted version of *Narikela,* the Sanskrit term for coconut. There is also a similar elaboration of the other products of the coconut tree such as the leaf, coconut milk, water, sugar and so on in various languages. In the case of *Hortus Malabaricus,* it seems that the work presents the information in more organized and systematic way. In the case of the coconut tree, the *Hortus* mentions the name of the tree and not just the major product as Da Orta does, and that it is called *tenga* in Latin, *mado* in the language of the Brahmanas, *tengu* in Malayalam and *narajil* in Arabic. Da Orta presents whatever information he has to hand about the botanical element under study, so he mentions the name of a plant in all the languages he knows, leaving out the name in the languages for which he does not have the information. *Hortus* Malabaricus, on the other hand, consistently mentions the titles of all the plants throughout the twelve volumes in four specific languages: Latin, Malayalam, Arabic and 'brahmin language' (*lingua brahmana antiqua*), that is, either Sanskrit or Konkani. This led to a standardization of the botanical method of description and illustration and enabled a very precise identification of the plants and their cultivation techniques. It also shows that the information from different cultural contexts was being woven together and formatted according to a new Western pattern.

In *Colóquios,* the emphasis is on procuring drugs and grading the efficacy of the same herbs/drugs from various places; hence it is clearly a book which narrates the story of mercantile and apothecary networks. In his second Colloquy, for instance, Da Orta mentions the various regions in which aloe is cultivated, pointing out that even though it grows in great abundance in Cambay and Bengal, the aloe from Socotra has the highest value. *Hortus Malabaricus,* on the other hand, describes not only the techniques of cultivation of the plants but also the ways and means to effectively commercialize their products, suggesting an urge towards territorial expansion and the arrival of European settlements marked by botanical gardens in the colonies. Using the same example of the coconut, it describes the plant in great detail and the various stages of the development of the fruit, the cultivation of the plant and the preparation of arrack from the fruit.[40] The detailed description of the plants and their utilities also reveals the close ties with multiple communities in Malabar, especially the ways in which information that may have been exclusive to particular communities was reformatted and subsequently disseminated.

Ayurvedic materia medica on the move

Historians in the recent past have focused on the explosion of knowledge associated with the scientific revolution and global expansion, and the large-scale transfer of trade goods and plants between Europe and its colonies. In particular, historians of science and medicine have explored the influx in Europe of botanical knowledge from Asia and the Atlantic world as well as the movement of medical knowledge from Europe to the rest of the world as part of Christian and so-called 'civilizing' missions. Until the last couple of decades, most of the work dealt with themes such 'the march of progress against barbarism' or the triumph of modern medicine against 'savage diseases' whose origins were traced back to the colonies.[41] It is only recently that such a framework has been intensively questioned and dismantled by interlinking the influx of botanical knowledge and the growth of modern medicine, thereby contextualizing the role of indigenous knowledge in the growth of science and medicine in Europe. For instance, in *Matters of Exchange*, Harold Cook traced out the networks of the Dutch East India Company, including the apothecary networks, in the transfer of *materia medica*, commerce and science in the early modern period.[42] Others, including Richard Grove, Kapil Raj, Richard Drayton and Donald Lach have conclusively shown that knowledge itself was a vital commodity transferred along the sprawling trade networks of the Portuguese, Dutch, English and French.[43] Few scholars other than Londa Schiebinger have tried to use native sources, particularly those in the vernacular native languages, to understand the interplay and deep discursivity of the complex processes at work in the extraction and circulation of knowledge. While the colonial archival record offers us one side of the story, it is the rich and extensive sources in Sanskrit, Tamil and *Manipravalam*,[44] which continued to be produced well into the nineteenth century, that can provide the other. This will also widen our understanding of the reception of early modern European medical traditions in culturally distinct areas such as South India.

The Ayurvedic texts, be it the early texts such as *Suśruta Samhitā*, *Caraka Samhitā* or *Aṣṭāngahṛdaya* or *Aṣṭāgasamhitā* of the Vāgbhaṭṭa tradition, medieval texts such as the fourth-century *Bhela Samhitā* and the seventh-eighth-century *Śārangadhāra Samhitā*, or the *Yōgaratnākara* of the mid-seventeenth century, do not deal with the description of the herb. Instead, the herb would be described in connection with its use-value in treating the disease. *Suśruta Samhitā* and *Caraka Samhitā* are considered to be the early foundational texts of the healing tradition known as Ayurveda. These texts written in Sanskrit in the period between the second century BCE and the fifth century CE are detailed medical compendia detailing diseases and cures, medical treatments, dietary regulations and pharmacopoeia and were used by medical practitioners well into the eighteenth century. They continue to have a considerable influence on Ayurvedic medical practice. The *Aṣṭāngahṛdaya* and *Aṣṭāgasamhitā* of the Vāgbhaṭṭa tradition were composed in the seventh century CE and it is the Vāgbhaṭṭa tradition which continues to have a lasting influence on the Ayurveda practised on the Malabar Coast. All of the Ayurvedic texts follow a style of classifying diseases into types and then elucidating the herbal remedies for them. While the diseases and their symptoms are elucidated in great detail, plant description is not found in these texts: the herbs are discussed in association with the remedies. Nigaṇṭus such as the tenth-century *Dhanvantari Nigaṇṭu* and the seventeenth-century *Bāvaprakaśa Nigaṇṭu* which were later additions to the Ayurvedic literature, on the other hand were compendia on drugs and *materia medica* used for Ayurvedic remedies.

The second chapter of the first volume of *Caraka Samhitā* begins with a typology of root herbs, but both the classification and the identification of the herbs are in connection with specific diseases.[45] So, in the treatment of conjunctivitis of the eye, *Caraka Samhitā* advises to apply breast milk, coconut water or a paste made of *halaga* (*Alpinia Galanga*), a root herb and the leaves of the *neem* tree (*Azadirachta indica*) to the eye, but there is no description of either the coconut or *neem* or *halaga*. While the disease, its symptoms, its treatment, the therapeutic herbs, the diet to be followed during the period of treatment, exercise, contact and patient care are all discussed in great detail, there is no description of the plant or its cultivation, nor do any of the Ayurvedic texts provide an illustration of the plant. In fact, illustrations of plants are very rare in general in early Ayurvedic material and there are only a few references to the cultivation techniques of the herbs. Contrary to this, *Hortus Malabaricus* provides an illustrated index of South-Indian flora, with elaborate drawings of the plants, trees, fruits and flowers, with detail on the cultivation techniques and seasonality of the plants.

A comparison of the Ayurvedic text with Da Orta reveals that *Colóquios* does borrow from these texts; what he describes as medicine from Malabar and, in some cases, Gujarat and Deccan, are in fact Ayurvedic medicines and practices.[46] *Suśruta Samhitā* and *Caraka Samhitā* classify herbs according to heat, dryness, unctuosity, fieriness, brittleness and bitterness. Da Orta uses the classification given by these texts, replacing unctuosity with 'moisture', and fieriness with 'heat'. At times, when the classification given by Galen or Dioscorides is contrary to that given by South Asian traditions, Da Orta gives more credence to the South Asian medical traditions. Da Orta is also clever in adapting the local knowledge which seems to have been borrowed, as mentioned earlier, from Ayurvedic traditions as well as from several other traditions including folk remedies. One of the characters in Da Orta's work is a 'slave girl' called Antonia who provides him with herbs and information about 'home remedies' from her native place.[47]

While *Hortus Malabaricus* was certainly used by later botanists such as Clusius and Carl Linneaus who challenged Dioscoridian and Greco-Roman classifications and pioneered modern botany, the text itself followed the patterns of European botanical texts based on Galenic medicine even though the botanical elements presented in them were from a totally different climate, culture and topography. The texts move from an attempt to 'make sense of a foreign or exotic land' as seen in Da Orta, thereby creating a picture of the other, the exotic and the Oriental, to addressing the objects of the natural world through modern eyes, attempting to 'represent objects as they are' to bring out categorizations and classifications of these specific South Asian flora in an attempt to 'universalize' botanical science.

Forbidden circulations: Towards a history of non-circulation?

As we engage with the theme of circulation, let us also try to refract the logic of circulation through the idea of the non-circulation of certain types of medico-botanical elements. It might seem ironic that the logic or the politics of circulation is most effectively brought out if we discuss what is being not circulated. Londa Schiebinger, in her work on the botanical transfers from the Atlantic coast to Europe, uses the theme of non-circulation effectively to bring out the nature of knowledge transfers between the native community and the Europeans; the non-circulation of abortificents in any of the *materia medica* compiled by either the missionaries, travellers or the officials is suggestive of the practices of inclusion and exclusion by both sides with meticulous methods of checks and controls which characterize the information flow. We shall be using Schiebinger's methodology to understand the South-Indian situation, but with slight modifications. Knowledge, especially related to non-technical and non-crafts-based learning such as Vedic learning, was a highly valued commodity; such learning was also highly esoteric with numerous checks and guards to restrict outsiders from gaining it. In the case of Vedic learning, only the *dvijas,* the higher castes, were permitted to access Vedic learning. This had grown to amazing heights in South India. The *Vyavahāramāla,* a sixteenth-century *Sastraic* text, says that molten lead should be poured into the ear of a low-caste person who listens to the *Vedas.* On the other hand, technical knowledge such as *Ayurveda* and *taccuśāstra* (carpentry) was more or less caste (*jāti*) and family based. Knowledge was thus not only exclusionary but also formed the basis of social structuring mechanisms.

Ayurveda was practised by certain Brahmin families, but a similar healing system which is referred to as *Ezhavavaidyom* was also practised by some Ezhava families especially from the medieval period (*c.* 1300–1600) onwards.[48] The mode of transmission was by word of mouth from generation to generation. There were *śālas* and *vidyāpīṭhams* where skill- and craft-based education in addition to textual knowledge was taught; admission to these schools was strictly on the basis of *jāti* and family networks. It is in this context that the efforts of those such as Da Orta, Van Rheede and L'Empereur become all the more relevant as gaining access to information, either medical or botanical, would have meant gaining the trust of those who traditionally held control over the knowledge. Da Orta, in fact, laments the fact that the *Gentoo* physicians are very reluctant in sharing their knowledge and often use confusing and ambiguous terms.[49] He also points out that South Asian physicians, except what he calls *Moorish* physicians, do not divulge details about the preparation methods or the ingredients of their medical concoctions.[50] It is often seen in Ayurvedic and Ezhava medicine that the preparation of medicine or the mixing of ingredients to prepare medicine is highly individual, and depends on season, place of birth, occupation and humoral nature of the patient. Also, it is seen that the practitioners were more open to giving details pertaining to botanical elements, rather than about medicines as the latter would mean a loss of monopoly over their healing practice.

The early modern world of medical encounters on the Malabar Coast – new understandings of the Ayurvedic schemata

By the beginning of the early modern period, new political patterns had emerged in South India with the South-Indian vernacular texts registering several indications of the European presence in India. These can be found in terms of the introduction of non-indigenous plant products into the Ayurvedic pharmacopoeia such as the use of tobacco, guava, onions, papaya and cashew nuts as therapeutic commodities in the post-sixteenth-century texts,[51] the inclusion of new diseases such as *Śitalā* (a variety of pox), *phirangaroga* (syphilis) and *parangipuṇṇu* (a venereal disease similar to syphilis),[52] and the introduction of new techniques such as bloodletting and smoking.[53] The case of *phirangaroga*, for instance, is mentioned in the sixteenth-century text of Bāva Misra, the *Bhāvaprakāśa*, considered to be one among the three later venerated classical texts of Ayurveda. Though the prognosis of the disease is not elucidated in the text, it can be inferred that the disease had already been studied, categorized under *pāṇḍurōga* (skin disease), and matched with a remedy at the time of inclusion.[54] In other cases, such as the use of tobacco in the pharmacopoeia, the absorption took longer as it is only mentioned in great detail in later texts such as the *Yōgaratnākara*, though there are references to it in *Bāvaprakaśa*.[55] The practice of bloodletting, prevalent in early modern Europe until the advent of germ theory, was also adopted by some physicians though it did not gain much popularity.[56] In the Ayurvedic tradition, the claim is not that these additions revolutionized the field of Ayurveda, but these were significant additions to an already existing corpus of medical knowledge. Some of these Western elements were incorporated gradually while others made their way into the native practices quite swiftly.

The *Bāvaprakaśa*, the first text to mention tobacco, does not refer to the qualities of the plant, though the uses of the plant are also mentioned in the *Bāvaprakaśa Nigaṇṭu*.[57] The eighteenth-century *Yōgaratnākara* has an entire chapter dedicated to the introduction of tobacco into the therapeutics of Ayurveda. It begins with introducing the plant and its ten synonyms – *dhūmākhya, dhūmavṛkṣa, bṛhatpatra, dhūsara, tamākhu, guccaphalaka, dhūmayantraprakāśaka, bahubīja, bahuphala, sūkṣmabīja* and *dīrghaka*.[58] By the sixteenth century, *Bāvaprakaśa* references papaya (*madhukarkati/karkati*),[59] and the *Yōgaratnākara* has detailed descriptions of 'new' botanical products such as the orange (*nāranja*) and guava (*bījapuraphalam*). By the seventeenth century, one can see that the products have been integrated into the Ayurvedic *materia medica*. The *Yōgaratnākara* discusses the therapeutic uses of the fruit, leaves and even the peel of the guava.[60] The botanical products are placed into the typology according to the Ayurvedic format. The effects of medicine extracted from specific parts of the plant is also mentioned along with predominant 'qualities' of the plant according to the *doṣa* (bodily humour) it activates on consumption.

Such incursions into the *materia medica* were nothing new to Ayurveda, which routinely accommodated pharmacopoeia and techniques from other native medical systems such as Siddha and tribal medicine. It can also be argued that Unani medicine, which made its way to the South-Indian coast through Arab intermediaries, influenced the *materia medica* of the Ayurvedic texts, albeit in an indirect way. Epistemologically, Ayurvedic sources like other Sanskritic texts have a penchant for classification to the minutest of details. Unlike other Brahmanic texts, however, Ayurveda had a garb of being empirico-rational, which meant that the classificatory schemes had to be based on empirical observation and a certain level of understanding of the samples while also being based on intricate mythologies. For instance, the *jaṅgāla*, *anūpa* and *sādharana* classification,[61] which Zimmerman in his *Jungle and the Aroma of Meats* points out, is one among the many typologies of classification of Ayurveda.[62] The parameters of classification included that of *tridoṣa* (bodily humours), *kāla* (season), *deśa* (place), *jāti* (caste/profession) and *guṇa* (temperament). The division of all land into *jaṅgāla*, *anūpa* and *sādharana* is one among the multiple classifications that Ayurveda employs.

The types and patterns of classification range from those which encompass sets of environment-nature characteristics, the order of things according to the *tridoṣa (humoral)* aspects, to a hierarchy of beings and on seasonality or even distance from the ocean or forest terrains. Most of the materials mentioned within the texts not only figure under multiple categories but are also sifted through these layers of classification to make them comprehensible under the Ayurvedic schemata. So, when a new entity is introduced into the Ayurveda knowledge system, its properties have to be analysed 'empirically' by the authors of the Ayurvedic texts, while having to be placed at a particular position within the classificatory hierarchies of Ayurveda.

In certain cases, like in the introduction of metallic compounds into the Ayurvedic medical pantheon, the incorporation occurred by placing them in the Sanskritic mythological universe through mythmaking and the creation of sub-stories within larger pre-existing narratives. The incorporation of new *materia medica* involved multiple processes and conscious layering within the particular system of medicine. So, at one level, the introduction of new *materia medica* indicates a new wave of therapeutics entering the lexicon, its interaction with European systems and on the other, it also indicates the process of adaptation and accommodation strategies employed. Of particular interest are the introduction of new botanical elements such as that of tobacco, papaya, orange, guava, China root and cashew nuts, all of which by the seventeenth century were well shaped into native herbal compendia and of the appearance of new kinds of diseases and treatments discussed in the later texts. The bioprospecting ventures by the European scholars such as by De Orta and Van Rheede, aided by the native physicians, experts, royal officials and herb collectors, paved the way for South Asian therapeutics to enter into European networks. Their not-so-equal counterparts in South India forged new epistemic and semiological networks to accommodate the new medical materialities.

Conclusion

In the very recent past, scholars have suggested that early modern science was a one-way process of plant transfers to suit the interests of mercantile colonialism; while there can be no refutation of the use and abuse of botany to serve imperialist purposes, the working of the evolution of both botany and medicine was a much more nuanced process and needs to be addressed in all its complexities. While bioprospecting was indeed the keyword in the initial phases of proto-colonial expansion, the relationship and the interaction between knowledge systems as well as people who engaged with the diverse forms of knowledge changed over time – a change that is reflected through the texts that were produced on both sides. While attention has been paid to the mechanisms and agents engaged in the knowledge transfer who were in many ways crucial to the continued existence of the European empires in non-European contexts, there is very little work that has been done on the knowledge actually transferred and produced, and how the interactions played out on both sides. The knowledge transfer as this article argues was more of an exchange than a transfer, even though it was an asymmetrical exchange. In no way can it be claimed that both sides benefited favourably, if we are to analyse the situation through the eyes of knowledge production and as a dialogue between diverse knowledge systems, a more vibrant discourse emerges. Certainly, a tendency to over-indulge in the idea of collaborative efforts will not be welcome, as imperial and political power opened up portals to specific types of knowledge to European eyes which were not even accessible to a large section of the South Asian masses. However, a certain sort of genuine engagement, accommodation and appreciation need to be acknowledged as the texts themselves clearly reveal.

Notes

1. For a detailed analysis, see Ângela Barreto Xavier and Ines G. Županov, *Catholic Orientalism: Portuguese Empire, Indian Knowledge (16th-18th Centuries)* (Oxford: Oxford University Press, 2015), particularly Part 1, Chapters 1, 2 and 3; Richard H. Drayton, *Nature's Government: Science, Imperial Britain and the 'Improvement' of the World* (New Haven: Yale University Press, 2000).
2. Scholars like Jan Breman and David Hardiman have argued that the tribal population of India and their practices must be considered as a separate category rather than conflating them with the peasant and lower-caste population of India. (See David Hardiman, 'Healing, Medical Power and the Poor: Contests in Tribal India', *Economic and Political Weekly* 42, no. 16 (2007): 1404–8.) Though the term folk medicine is used to refer to both the traditional practices of the non-dominant castes as well as the tribes of India, it is useful to identify both of these as separate categories particularly owing to the presence of forest-based tribal healers called 'lādavaidyans' in South India.
3. Various historians have argued on the significance of the Malabar Coast in Indian Ocean trade and cultural contacts including Ashin Das Gupta, *Malabar in Asian Trade: 1740–1800* (Cambridge: Cambridge University Press, 1967); M. N. Pearson, *The Portuguese in India* (Cambridge: Cambridge University Press, 2006); and Pius Malekandathil, *Portuguese Cochin and the Maritime Trade of India, 1500–1663* (New Delhi: Manohar, 2001); and Jonathan Israel, *Dutch Primacy in World Trade, 1585–1740* (New York: Oxford University Press, 1989), to name just a few.
4. For detailed analyses on the theme of imperial knowledge networks, see Kapil Raj, *Relocating Modern Science: Circulation and the Construction of Knowledge in South Asia and Europe, 1650–1900* (Basingstoke: Palgrave Macmillan, 2007); Drayton, *Nature's Government*; Ray McLeod, *Nature and Empire: Science and the Colonial Enterprise* (Chicago: University of Chicago Press, 2000); David Arnold, *Science, Technology and Medicine in Colonial India* (Cambridge: Cambridge University Press, 2000); Londa Schiebinger, *Plants and Empire: Colonial Bioprospecting in the Atlantic World* (Cambridge, MA: Harvard University Press, 2004); Pratik Chakrabarti, *Materials and Medicine: Trade, Conquest and Therapeutics in the Eighteenth Century* (Manchester: Manchester University Press, 2015).
5. See Shu-Jyuan Deiwiks, Bernhard Führer, and Therese Geulen, eds, *Europe Meets China, China Meets Europe; The Beginnings of European-Chinese Scientific Exchange in the 17th Century* (Sankt Augustin: Institut Monumenta Serica, 2014).
6. Harold Cook and Timothy D. Walker, "Circulation of Medicine in the Early Modern Atlantic 'World', *Social History of Medicine* 26, no. 3 (2013): 338.
7. Hendrik Adriaan van Rheede, *Hortus Malabaricus*, trans. K. S. Manilal (Thiruvananthapuram: University of Kerala Press, 2008), xii.

8 David Arnold, 'The Indian Ocean as a Disease zone; 1500–1950', *South Asia* 14, no. 2 (1991): 1–21; Burton Cleetus, 'Tropics of Disease; Epidemics in Colonial India', *Economic and Political Weekly* 55, no. 21 (2020).

9 S. Irfan Habib and Dhruv Raina, "Reinventing Traditional Medicine: Method, Institutional Change and the Manufacture of Drugs and Medication in Late Colonial India', in *Asian Medicine and Globalization*, ed. Joseph S. Alter (Philadelphia: University of Pennsylvania Press, 2005), 67.

10 Ibid.

11 See A. Sreedhara Menon, *A Survey of Kerala History* (Kottayam: DC Books, 2007); Ranabir Chakravarti, *The Pull towards the Coast and Other Essays: The Indian Ocean History and the Subcontinent Before 1500 CE* (Delhi: Primus Books, 2020); Rajan Gurukkal, *Rethinking Classical Indo-Roman Trade; Political Economy of Eastern Mediterranean Exchange Relations* (Oxford: Oxford University Press, 2016). Also see Raoul McLaughlin, *The Roman Empire and the Indian Ocean: The Ancient World Economy and the Kingdoms of Africa, Arabia and India* (Barnsley: Pen and Sword Books, 2014), and Matthew Adam Cobb, ed., *The Indian Ocean Trade in Antiquity Political, Cultural and Economic Impacts* (London: Taylor and Francis, 2018) among many other works.

12 African records such as the *Geniza* records from Cairo (ninth to the nineteenth centuries CE) have several references to the role played by Jewish, Middle Eastern and African middlemen in the vibrant trade between South-Indian and African ports. See for instance, S. D. Goitein, 'Portrait of a Medieval India Trader: Three Letters from the Cairo Geniza', *Bulletin of the School of Oriental and African Studies* 48 (1987): 449–64.

13 Richard Grove, *Green Imperialism: Colonial Expansion, Tropical Island Edens and the Origins of Environmentalism, 1600–1860* (Cambridge: Cambridge University Press, 1995), 79–80.

14 João de Endem was one of the first printers at the Catholic Press at Goa. Not much is known about him other than his name being mentioned in Da Orta's work and an earlier book titled *Compendio spritual da vida Christãa* by Gaspar de Leão published from the same press in 1561. Garcia Da Orta, *Colóquios dos simples e drogas he cousas medicinais da Índia e assi dalgũas frutas achadas nella onde se tratam algũas cousas tocantes a medicina, pratica, e outras cousas boas pera saber* (Goa: João de Endem, 1563).

15 Garcia Da Orta, *Aromatum, et simplicium aliquot medicamentorum apud Indos nascentium historia: ante biennium quidem Lusitanica lingua per dialogos conscripta*, trans. Carolus Clusius (Antwerp: Ex officina Christophori Plantini, 1567).

16 Christobal Acosta, *Tractado Delas drogas, y medicinas de las Indias Orientales, con sus Plantas debuxadas al biuo* (Burgos: Por Martin de Victoria impressor de su Magestad, 1578).

17 Richard Grove, "Indigenous Knowledge and the Significance of South-West India for Portuguese and Dutch Constructions of Tropical Nature", *Modern Asian Studies* 30, no. 1 (1996): 134.
18 Several works in the recent past have worked on the theme of Renaissance botany and have elucidated the efflorescence of botany in Europe spurred by the bioprospecting endeavours of officials of the European trading companies in the early modern period which not only led to a new interest in botany, but also a new pattern of understanding the plant-world. See for instance, Leah Knight, *Of Books and Botany in Early Modern England: Sixteenth-Century Plants and Print Culture* (Burlington: Ashgate, 2009). Also, Cristina Bellorini, *The World of Plants in Renaissance Tuscany; Medicine and Botany* (New York: Ashgate, 2016).
19 Van Rheede, *Hortus Malabaricus*, Vol.1. xx.
20 Ibid., xvi.
21 Ibid.
22 Ezhavas are mentioned as a 'lower'/oppressed caste group from the ninth century CE onwards in the history of South India. They are mentioned in the Tharisapalli Copper Plate of 849 CE issued by the local Venad (Quilon) ruler to the Christians in Malabar and they are traditionally represented as toddy tappers and brewers. In the medieval period, there are also references to them as physicians and middlemen in the spice trade. See M. R. Raghava Varier and Kesavan Veluthat, eds, *Tharisapalli Pattayam* (Trivandrum: NBS Publication, 2013) for further details on the antiquity of various caste groups in Kerala.
23 V. P. Chavan, *Vaishnavism of the Gowd Saraswat Brahmins: And a Few Konkani Folklore Tales* (New Delhi: Asian Educational Services, 1991), 10.
24 Van Rheede, *Hortus Malabaricus*, Vol.1, xv.
25 Ibid., xv.
26 Ibid., xxiii.
27 *Vyavahāramāla*, eds and annotated by S Paramesvara Aiyar (Trivandrum: Government Press, 1923). See the chapter on *Sāhasaprakaraṇam* for the severe regulations on professions based on caste. The text was used as a legal treatise until the adoption of Munroe Reform in the kingdom of Travancore.
28 Van Rheede, *Hortus Malabaricus*, Vol.3, xv.
29 Ibid., xvi.
30 Ibid.
31 Several scholars have worked on the impact of *Hortus Malabaricus* and *Colloqyies* on botany in Europe. These include, in the case of *Hortus*, J. Heniger, *Hendrik Adriaan Van Reede Tot Drakenstein (1636–1691) and Hortus Malabaricus; A Contribution to the History of Dutch Colonial Botany* (Rotterdam: A. A. Balkema, 1986) and K. S. Manilal, *Botany & History of Hortus Malabaricus* (Rotterdam: IBH, 1980). See also Grove, *Green Imperialism*; K. S. Manilal, *Hortus Malabaricus*

and Itty Achuden: A Study on the Role of Itty Achuden in the Compilation of Hortus Malabaricus (Kozhikode: Mentor Books, 1996); K. S. Manilal, Hortus Malabaricus and the Socio-Cultural Heritage of India (Kozhikode: Indian Association of Angiosperm Taxonomy, 2012) among many others. In the case of Colloquyies, some of the notable works are: Louis Pelner, "Garcia de Orta: Pioneer in Tropical Medicine and Botany", Journal of the American Medical Association 197, no. 12 (1966): 996–8; Palmira Fontes Da Costa and Teresa Nobre De Carvalho, 'Between East and West: Garcia de Orta's Colloquies and the Circulation of Medical Knowledge in the Sixteenth Century', Asclepio: Revista de Historia de la Medicina y de la Ciencia 65, no. 1 (2013): 35–53; Grove, 'Indigenous Knowledge'; Palmira Fontes Da Costa, ed., Medicine Trade and Empire: Garcia de Orta's Colloquies on the Simples and Drugs of India (1563) in Context (London: Routledge, 2016).

32 I am borrowing the term 'big science' from Londa Schiebinger who uses the term to refer to the focus given to the study of botany during this period and its close ties with business profits of the European trading companies. For a detailed analysis of botany as 'big science', see Londa Schiebinger and Claudia Swan, eds, Colonial Botany; Science, Commerce, and Politics in the Early Modern World (Pennsylvania: University of Pennsylvania Press, 2005).

33 Garcia Da Orta, Colloquyies, Thirty Sixth Colloquy, 310–13.

34 Da Orta, Colloquyies, Tenth Colloquy, 66–77.

35 Da Orta, Colloquyies, Fifty Sixth Colloquy, 452.

36 Da Orta, Colloquyies, Fourth Colloquy, 28–30.

37 Da Orta, Colloquyies, Fifty Second Colloquy, 420–1.

38 In several chapters in the Colloquyies, Garcia Da Orta mentions his observation of South-Indian medical practices and how he has learnt to use Indian and Arabic materia medica. See pp. 7, 29, 82, 306, 432, 452.

39 Van Rheede, Hortus Malabaricus.

40 Van Rheede, Hortus Malabaricus, Vol. 1, 1–29.

41 Quite a lot of works from the 1930s and well into the 1970s followed the pattern of glorifying the marvels of 'modern' science and Western medicine. For instance, see Herbert Butterfield, The Origins of Modern Science (London: G. Bell & Sons, 1949); Rupert A. Hall, The Scientific Revolution 1500–1800: The Formation of the Modern Scientific Attitude (London: Longmans & Co., 1954). Another appropriate example would be Joseph Needham, The Grand Titration: Science and Society in East and West (London: George Allen & Unwin, 1969).

42 Harold Cook, Matters of Exchange: Commerce, Medicine and Science in the Dutch Golden Age (New Haven and London: Yale University Press, 2007).

43 For detailed analyses on the theme of imperial knowledge networks, see Raj, Relocating Modern Science; Drayton, Nature's Government; McLeod, Nature and Empire; Arnold, Science, Technology and Medicine; Schiebinger, Plants and Empire; Chakrabarti, Materials and Medicine.

44 *Manipravalam* is a South-Indian language which is an admixture of Sanskrit and Tamil which was used mostly as a performative and courtly language from the early medieval period to about the sixteenth century CE.
45 *Caraka Samhitā, Vol.2, Sūtrasthāna*, Ch. 20, commentary and translation by Kashinath Sastri (Varanasi: Chaukambha Sanskrit Academy, 1991), 2.
46 Da Orta, *Colloquyies*, 6. Pages 51 and 100 have descriptions of Garcia Da Orta using the names and typology used by Malabari and Gujarati physicians.
47 Da Orta, *Colloquyies* 8, 53–7. Also, see *Colloquyies* 36, 308–10.
48 Extensive oral interviews, conducted by the present author, of twenty-four Ezhava Ayurveda practitioners in Kerala from the period between August 2018 and September 2019 have revealed a very rich tradition of medical practise extending to the seventeenth century CE among the Ezhavas.
49 Garcia Da Orta refers to all non-Semitic physicians as Gentoo or Gentio physicians. See, for instance, Da Orta, *Colloquyies* 2, 10–11.
50 Da Orta, *Colloquyies* 27, 231–3.
51 Ayurvedic compendia such as the *Bhavaprakasha Nigantu* and *Raja Marthanda* and *Sahasrayogam* have detailed chapters about the herbal uses and procedures involving the new products introduced as therapeutic commodities.
52 *Bāvaprakasha* of Bāva Misra composed in the sixteenth century has a detailed description of the *Śitalā* pox disease in its sixtieth chapter (vv. 70–82). *Bāvaprakasha* of Bāva Misra, chavanaprakah yantra, Indraprasth nagar, 1944, 331. *Yōgaratnākara* and *Yōgamṛutam* too have chapters dedicated to *phiraṅga roga* (syphilis) and *parangipuṁṅu*.
53 *Dhumṛapāna* (smoking) and bloodletting (*raktamokṣa/raktamokṣaṇa*) are mentioned in texts such as the seventeenth-century *Yōgaratnākara* and *Yōgamṛutam* and also in later eighteenth-century texts like *Bhaiṣjya Ratnavāli*.
54 *Phiraṅga roga* or syphilis is mentioned in the sixtieth chapter of *Bāvaprakasha* along with its medical treatment. It must be noted that in most South-Indian languages the term *phiraṅga* or *firangi* is used to refer to Europeans, particularly to the Portuguese. *Cōpacini* or China root finds mention as a therapeutic drug for it along with the use of *rasakarpura* or a chemical compound made of sulphur, camphor and mercury.
55 *Yōgaratnākara*, a seventeenth-century Sanskrit text, mentions the use of *tamākhu* or tobacco as a therapeutic commodity and describes its pungent and medical properties in its first chapter in about twelve verses.
56 *Raktamokṣa* or bloodletting is mentioned in *Yōgamrutam*, an Ayurvedic text, but only as a passing reference rather than as a recommended technique of healing some diseases like pox and tuberculosis.
57 Bhavamishra, *Bavaprakash Nighantu*, trans. G. S. Pandey and Mishra Prakarana (Varanasi: Chaukhambha Bharati Academy, 2004), 187.
58 *Yōgaratnākara, Vol.1*, eds and trans. Premavati Tiwari and Asa Kumari (Varanasi: Chaukhambha Visvabharati, 2010), 307–8.

59 Bhavamishra, *Bāvaprakaśa, Purvakhanda*, trans. and ed. Nirmal Saxena (Varanasi: Chaukhambha Bharati Academy, 2010), 17–18.
60 *Yōgaratnākara*, 117.
61 According to Zimmerman, Ayurveda's system of classification is based on a division of all land into *jungala* (dry land), *anūpa* (marshy land) and *sādharana* (an admixture of dry and marshy land). See Francis Zimmermann, *The Jungle and the Aroma of Meats: An Ecological Theme in Hindu Medicine* (Berkeley: University of California Press, 1987).
62 For a detailed analysis, see Zimmermann, *The Jungle and the Aroma of Meats*.

4

Rhubarb in the Indian Ocean world
The entangled itinerary of a material complex

Anne Gerritsen

Introduction

'An attractive hardy perennial with large leaves and pink, red or greenish leaf stalks that are used as a dessert, often in pies and crumbles.'[1] Few English gardeners would fail to recognize the plant in this Royal Horticultural Society description. Rhubarb makes an appearance in most English vegetable plots, with its dense semi-underground rhizome, forest of stalks and massive leaves. New rhubarb stalks appear in spring, long before other fruits ripen, and are appreciated for their fresh, sweet-sour taste when cooked properly. What these same gardeners might not be aware of, however, is how widely varied the names, meanings and uses associated with that same plant are. See, for example, this completely different way of seeing rhubarb, from a 2015 description in a journal of alternative medicine:

> Rhubarb (Da Huang), one of the most popular traditional Chinese medicines used to control various diseases for thousands of years, is made of roots and rhizomes of *Rheum palmatum* L., *Rheum tanguticum* Maxim. ex Balf., *Rheum undulatum*, or *Rheum officinale* Baill.[2]

Instead of focusing on the stem, and the desserts and pies they can be transformed into, the authors of this description focus on the roots of the plant, which form 'one of the most popular traditional Chinese medicines', used in this case for the treatment of sepsis. The authors of these two texts have very different answers to an ostensibly simple question: what is rhubarb? The divergent answers can be explained by the different uses of rhubarb: a horticulturalist looks at a plant differently from a specialist in alternative medicine.

The differences between answers to the same question are even greater when we add different historical periods. The Greek physician Dioscorides of the first century CE, for example, described a plant known to grow abundantly along the banks of the River Rha (the Scythian name for the Volga), with roots that were black, odourless, spongy and quite light, best when not 'worm-eaten':[3]

> It is good for flatulence in the stomach, for lack of energy, for all sorts of pains, spasms and ruptures, for patients with spleen, liver and kidney diseases, for the colicky, for disorders associated with the bladder and chest, for tension in the general area of the stomach, and for disorders in the area of the uterus, for hip ailments, blood-spitting, asthma, hiccups, dysentery, for bowel conditions, for fits of intermittent fever and for bites of wild animals.[4]

In an entirely unrelated time and place, the eighteenth-century Muslim physician Muhammad Sharîf Khân (1722–1807), based in Delhi, described rhubarb as follows:

> Rewind (راوند). *Rheum Palmatum*. Rhubarb. Laxative, stomachic, and astringent; and if taken after meals with rose water, it promotes digestion and strengthens the bowels. It removes mucus from the pylorus.[5]

Each of these sources has far more to say about rhubarb than I have quoted here, but even from these short extracts, we see some similarities but mainly differences: some focus on the root, others on the stems; some focus on its medicinal function, others on its edible aspects; some call it rhubarb, others various types of *rheum*, or rewind. The point here is that they encounter rhubarb and explain what it is from the perspective of very different contexts and intellectual frameworks.

Rather than approaching the history of rhubarb as the history of a physical commodity, I propose that we approach it as the history of an idea. Placing the emphasis on the idea of this commodity rather than on its physical identity means a shift towards cultural history, away from botany, economic history or the history of medicine. Rather than asking, 'Where was rhubarb from?', I ask, 'Where was rhubarb thought to come from?'; rather than asking, 'What was the medical efficacy of rhubarb?', I ask, 'What was rhubarb thought to be good for?'. This is a particularly suitable approach to the study of rhubarb, because in most parts of the world, the substance identified as rhubarb was not grown locally, but imported from elsewhere. Wherever and whenever medics, merchants or consumers encountered the imported commodity identified as 'rhubarb', they made sense of it by integrating it into their own frameworks of knowledge. Using this cultural history approach, we not only find traces of something referred to as rhubarb in many different parts of the world, but also almost as many different ways of naming it, categorizing it, valuing it and applying it. Rather than aiming to offer a complete overview of the use of the substance in all parts of the world and at all times, which has already been done by Clifford Foust and would go far beyond the confines of this essay, I focus mostly on understanding the idea of rhubarb in the wider context of the Indian Ocean world.[6]

To approach rhubarb less as a commodity and more as a concept draws on recent developments in material culture studies, as touched upon in the introduction to this volume. Historians have made extensive use of this interdisciplinary field of studies to demonstrate, for example, that an object, or a type of object, should be understood as a multi-layered complex rather than a single thing. Social and emotional relationships, skills and knowledge all form part of what an object 'is', as do the itineraries of objects through space and time.[7] Dorothy Ko has recently coined the term 'material-emotional complex' for the East Asian inkstones she has written about, which are entangled with 'the production of elite masculinity, texts, and the culture of *wen* 文 (culture, literature, civility)'.[8] To Ko, the idea of the inkstone as a 'material-emotional complex' makes sense because it is 'a conduit of such dynamic consternation of embodied skills and emotional investments'.[9] Rhubarb, too, as I will seek to demonstrate in this chapter, can be seen as a material-emotional complex.

The mobility of objects adds further depth to that complexity. Long-distance trade, travel, migration and gift-giving are just some of the multiple ways in which objects move, gaining new layers of meaning along the way. In the process of the object moving, technologies, designs and emotions also move, creating not only new materials and practices but also new knowledge systems. Pamela H. Smith refers to these processes as 'entangled itineraries'.[10] The mobility of objects forms an integral part of, and can help shed light on, the movement of people and ideas and the transformations such movement brings about. These movements or itineraries are nonlinear and uneven as much as the transformations are messy and entangled, transmitting old ideas as well as facilitating the creation of new knowledge. The term 'entangled itineraries' seeks to capture the ways in which the movements of object complexes through different material and spiritual worlds form and are part of ongoing entanglements. Again, for an imported commodity that reached the markets in India via a range of different routes, this is a particularly suitable approach.

The movement of objects also has an emotional dimension: the desire for goods from other places and the appeal of the exotic. There is an almost timeless element to this desire; archaeological excavations have revealed the presence of non-indigenous crops as well as high-value exotica among some of the earliest traces of human existence.[11] Christopher Bayly has referred to the intensification of such desires for luxury goods as archaic globalization, referring, for example, to the movement of goods along the Silk Roads.[12] While it is clear that the desire for exotic goods can be found from some of the earliest time periods and across the globe, it is also clear that at certain times in different parts of the world, the desire for exotic luxury goods and the long-distance trade to satisfy such desires intensified considerably.[13] The flourishing of the Silk Road trade and its flows of goods, people and ideas in the late thirteenth and early fourteenth centuries, or the emergence of the European trade companies in the seventeenth, and the intensification of maritime trade between Asia and Europe in the eighteenth centuries are just some well-known examples of this.[14] When we think of an object as an emotional-material complex, it captures this element of desire for the exotic that shapes the ways in which humans assign meanings to objects.

That consumer desire for exotic commodities also creates commercial opportunities. Goods are created in and shaped by the market; they become commodities in a process known as commodification. The producer's interest in the commodification of goods that can generate profit both feeds and is fed by that consumer desire. Value and meaning of goods are determined by the processes of exchange that are part of the social life of such goods, as scholars like Arjun Appadurai, Igor Kopytoff and others demonstrated many decades ago.[15] An object or substance might begin its social life in one context, in which its value and meaning are established, but may then be brought to a market in another, in which new values and meanings are established. This process of commodification across cultural boundaries created opportunities for profit and exploitation from which first the European trade companies and subsequently the colonial powers were especially well-positioned to benefit. Here, too, my focus lies in the cultural sphere rather than the economic one: I am interested in the extent to which these processes of commodification and attempts at the profitable cultivation of rhubarb by the British in India shaped the meanings of rhubarb.

In what follows, I will begin by introducing rhubarb by presenting some of the wide-ranging ideas held about rhubarb in China, India and Europe, to explore the ways in which rhubarb can be seen as an emotional-material complex. I will then map out some of the entangled itineraries along which rhubarb travelled. After a discussion of the ways in which the 'foreignness' of rhubarb formed part of its attraction for consumers, I will turn my attention to the ways in which producers sought to capitalize on that attraction to turn rhubarb into a marketable commodity in the context of the Indian Ocean world.[16]

The idea of rhubarb in Chinese, Indian and Western contexts

Some of the earliest references to rhubarb are found in Chinese sources. The medicinal qualities of rhubarb root (*dahuang* 大黃) are described in medical notes dating to the Han dynasty, allegedly from the herbal of the legendary Shennong emperor, the *Shennong bencao jing* 神農本草經. The medicinal properties of *dahuang* are given as follows:

> *Dahuang* is bitter, cold, and toxic. It mainly precipitates blood stasis, blood block, and cold and heat. It breaks concretions and conglomerations, accumulations and gatherings, and lodged rheum and abiding food. It flushes the stomach and intestines to weed out the stale and bring forth the new, disinhibits and frees the flow of water and grain, regulates the center to transform food, and quiets and harmonizes the five viscera. It grows in mountains and valleys.[17]

The main categorization of the efficacy of rhubarb root that emerges from this is that *dahuang* is a bitter-tasting drug, with a cooling function, meaning that it would be used in the context of the very broad category of 'cold damage disorders'. Moreover, Chinese medical knowledge established that *dahuang* has a purgative function, hence phrases like breaking up conglomerations, flushing the stomach and freeing the flow. In different ways, the many Chinese *materia medica* that emerged over the centuries all drew on this herbal of the Shennong emperor. So, for example, the eighth-century medical compendium *Waitai miyao fang*, a title usually translated as 'arcane essential formulas from the imperial library', relied heavily on the use of rhubarb root in prescriptions for a wide range of medical conditions, usually together with other ingredients, and always in connection either with cold damage disorders or for its purgative qualities.

As for Ayurvedic medicine, according to the nineteenth-century author, physician and Ayurvedic expert Udoy Chand Dutt (1834–84), rhubarb was 'not known to the ancient writers, and . . . not mentioned in their works'.[18] Dutt mentions this absence of rhubarb in the Ayurvedic tradition under his lemma for the haritaki tree in his 1877 compilation of translations from Sanskrit texts: *The Materia Medica of the Hindus: Compiled from Sanskrit Medical Works*.[19] The dried fruit of the haritaki tree is seen, not unlike rhubarb in the Dioscoridian tradition, almost as a panacea in Ayurvedic medicine, serving as: 'laxative, stomachic, tonic and alterative... and... used in fevers, cough, asthma, urinary diseases, piles, intestinal worms, chronic diarrhoea, costiveness, flatulence, vomiting, hiccup, heart disease, and so on.'[20] According to Dutt, it was only the 'Bengali practitioners' who use rhubarb.

Two specialists of Unani medicine, Misbahuddin Azhar and Nighat Anjum, published an article in 2019 on what they called 'Revand Chini' or 'Chinese rhubarb'.[21] They begin with an overview of the observations on rhubarb by some of the famous Islamic physicians of the past, such as Avicenna, Mesue the Younger and Haji Zayn Attar:

> Ibn-e-Sina (978-1023 AD)[22] notices both the plant 'Ribas' (Riwas, Persian) and the drug 'Rewand' (Rawand, Persian). The first an acid plant, and the second evidently Chinese Rhubarb. 'Mesue' (Masih),[23] early in the 11th century, distinguishes between Chinese and Khorasan Rhubarb.[24] 'Haji Zein-al-Attar' (1368 Hijri)[25] considered 'Rewand' to be the same as 'Ribas'. According to 'Ibn-e-Jazla',[26] there are two kinds of Rhubarb, China and Khorasan Rhubarb, and that the later is known as 'Rewand-aldawaab', and is used in veterinary practice, whilst the Chinese is reserved for human beings. The later is the best kind, and when powdered, is of a saffron colour. The fractured surface has the grain of a cow's hump and is friable; It is called 'Rewand-i-lahmi' (meaty Rhubarb), and should be in large pieces like a horse's hoof and not worm eaten.[27]

A lot of information is packed into these few lines: several different plants are mentioned (ribas and rewand), and by drawing on four of the foremost Islamic scholars of medicine, Misbahuddin Azhar and Nighat Anjum add legitimacy to their assessment of 'the best kind' of rhubarb and its appearance.

Within the Western context, the oldest reference to rhubarb probably stems from the first century CE, in the writings of the Greek physician Dioscorides, quoted earlier. Over the centuries that followed, physicians like Alexander of Tralles (Alexander Trallianus, *c.* 525–*c.* 605 CE), Paulus of Aegina (*c.* 625–690 CE) and Rufinus, author of a herbal dated after 1287, simply followed Dioscorides in their descriptions of rhubarb.[28] Pietro Mattioli (1501–77), botanist and commentator and translator of Dioscorides' *De Materia Medica*, too, followed Dioscorides' description of rhubarb closely. Until the late sixteenth century, rhubarb root was known in Europe mostly as a very valuable remedy, used both to purify the four Galenic humours so as to restore them to their natural state and to evacuate excessive or defective humours.[29] John Gerard (1545–1612), author of the famous 1597 *Herball* or *Generall historie of plantes*, described rhubarb root as having a 'mixt substance, temperature and facultie: some of the parts thereof are earthie, binding and drying, others thinne, aëreous hot, and purging'.[30] In what follows, he offers a medley of quotes on rhubarb drawn from Dioscorides and Galen, Paulus of Aegina and Mesue.[31] By the time the Linnaean system had become the established way of identifying plants in the eighteenth century, rhubarb acquired its now common Western botanical identity: a genus called 'rheum' of the Polygonaceae family. This genus has numerous different species, such as *R. australe* or *emodi*, *R. officinale*, *R. palmatum*, *R. tanguticum*, *R. rhaponticum* and *R. rhabarbarum*.

Far from complete, this brief overview has merely suggested that when we ask what rhubarb 'is', we find not one but many things. The descriptions quoted here stem from entirely different contexts, both chronologically and spatially. More importantly, they stem from different frameworks of knowledge. One might broadly group those here as Chinese, harking back to the *Shennong bencao jing*, Greek, with its origins in Dioscorides, laying the foundations for Western medicine, and Islamic (or Unani medicine), even though of course the idea of a clear separation between them is spurious, especially between 'Western' and 'Islamic' thought. None of these were closed thought systems; all of them benefited from the transmission and translation of ideas that had come from elsewhere, as we will see below. For now, the main point of presenting these different ways of identifying rhubarb is to show the extent to which the encounter with a plant like rhubarb was and is shaped by the cultural lens through which it is seen. When Linnaeus identifies one type of rhubarb as 'rheum palmatum', then that Linnaean framework determines how rhubarb appears: a species of a genus in the Polygonaceae family. The Linnaean framework provides the language of identification, and thereby situates the plant within the Linnaean knowledge system. When the authors of an alternative medicine journal write that rhubarb (*dahuang*) is 'one of the most popular traditional Chinese medicines used to control various diseases for thousands of years', they give the Chinese name and reference the Chinese way of seeing rhubarb: not a plant but a therapeutic substance that fulfils many functions in traditional Chinese medicine. When they add that this medicine 'is made of roots and rhizomes of *Rheum palmatum* L., *Rheum tanguticum* Maxim. ex Balf., *Rheum undulatum* or *Rheum officinale* Baill', they combine two frameworks of knowledge.[32] When John Gerard references both Dioscorides, Galen and Mesue in his description of rhubarb, he, too, combines different knowledge systems. The systems of knowledge within which botanists and physicians work are never hermetically sealed. But each description of rhubarb that begins with a claim about what rhubarb *is*, uses the legitimacy offered by one or more systems to determine rhubarb's identity. Rather than separating these, I follow authors like Pamela Smith, Dorothy Ko, Angela Ki Che Leung and Ming Chen to emphasize rhubarb as material complex rather than single thing.

Entangled itineraries

We find yet more complexity when we bring in the itineraries along which rhubarb travelled. Again, I am less interested here in identifying the actual place of origin of rhubarb or the routes along which the commodity was traded. Instead, I am interested in understanding where different people *thought* rhubarb came from and establishing the importance of rhubarb's putative place of origin and trade routes for the meanings they assigned to rhubarb.

Almost all writings about rhubarb make some mention of its place of origin and the routes along which it had travelled. When Dioscorides described rhubarb in the first century AD, he located its source as lying 'beyond the Bosphorus'. *Rha ponticum* (much like the common or garden rhubarb we know today) was the *rha* from Pontus, the region south of the Black Sea in northern Anatolia; the lesser known *rha*, from an unfamiliar origin even further to the east was identified as *rha barbarum*. The thirteenth-century Venetian Marco Polo, who mentioned rhubarb in the account of his travels through what is now the Chinese province of Gansu observed: 'In all the mountains of this region, rhubarb grows in great abundance; it is bought here by merchants, who export it far and wide.'[33] When Marco Polo travelled here, this area had not yet been brought under the control of the Chinese empire; he described it as inhabited by people 'subject to the Great Khan', and 'part of the major province of Tangut'.[34] For both Dioscorides and Polo, the place of origin mattered and was specific: the area south of the Black Sea and the province of Tangut were both part of the Silk Roads region, albeit at extreme ends of it. Criss-crossed by trade routes, this region would now more precisely be referred to as Central Asia, and features prominently, though not exclusively, in origin stories about rhubarb.

Duarte Barbosa (1480–1521), the Portuguese traveller and official who spent the early decades of the sixteenth century in India, wrote about 'rhubarb of Babilonia' in his *Book of Duarte Barbosa* around 1518, listing it along with silk and very fine musk among the goods found in the market in Hormuz, and brought there 'from the lands of the Xeque Ismael'.[35] According to the editor of Duarte Barbosa's book, Mansel Longworth Dames (1850–1922), 'rhubarb of

Babilonia' means it came from Baghdad, while the lands of Xeque Ismael refer to Persia. Dames further explained that when the Venetian Giovanni Battista Ramusio (1485–1557) included Duarte Barbosa's text in his collection of notable travellers entitled *Delle navigationi et viaggi* ('Some Voyages and Travels') between 1550 and 1559, he deleted the reference to 'the lands of Xeque Ismael' and replaced it with China.[36] In the mid-sixteenth century, Ramusio clearly felt it was unlikely that Barbosa could be right about the Persian origins of rhubarb. Barbosa also observed rhubarb for sale in markets elsewhere: in Malabar, in Malacca and in China.[37] Also noteworthy is the fact that Duarte Barbosa merely lists rhubarb as a marketable commodity; he does not say anything further about what he thinks 'rhubarb' is, or what it may be used for.

Garcia de Orta (1501?–68), another Portuguese based in India for some time, provided more information on what he thought rhubarb to be in his 1563 book entitled *Colóquios dos simples e drogas da India*, the earliest treatise on the medicinal and economic plants of India.[38] In the forty-eighth of the colloquies, he writes about rhubarb, although he confesses that he does 'not know much about it'.[39] Da Orta's interlocutor begins by asking 'about the tree yielding rhubarb, and what the leaves and fruit are like, and whether this root we see is true or false; for certainly I would give much to see the true one'.[40] Da Orta answers that he is certain that all rhubarb comes from China, apart from a certain variety that is associated with Samarkand, which he considers 'very bad and of little weight', and only good for the purging of horses.[41] Da Orta goes on to ascertain that what is available for sale in India has been brought there from Hormuz. Hormuz was already known as a place for buying rhubarb from a mid-century letter exchange between a Flemish Jesuit based in Hormuz named Jasper Bartzoen, better known as Gaspar Barzeus (1515–53), and St Ignatius of Loyola (1491–1556), the Spanish priest who had co-founded the Jesuit order in 1541. In 1551, Barzeus sent a letter to St Ignatius, in which he explained that he was sending a supply of rhubarb that had been delivered overland to Hormuz from the northwest of China.[42] Da Orta continued with this assumption, that all the rhubarb in Hormuz had all been brought overland to Hormuz from China, via what he called 'Uzbeg'. According to Da Orta, the rhubarb market in Hormuz, described earlier by Duarte Barbosa, also supplied rhubarb to consumers in Venice, Portugal, Castile and Seville.[43] Da Orta expanded further on how to preserve rhubarb from rotting in the humid environments where he encountered it, and on the months during which fresh rhubarb arrived in India. While he was interested in rhubarb as a commodity and concerned with where to source it and how to preserve it, he seemed to have little further interest in discussing any possible applications of rhubarb.

The Venetian editor of travel records, Ramusio, however, was very interested in rhubarb. When he included Marco Polo's writings in his anthology of travel writings, he prefaced Polo's text with an introductory text entitled 'Espositione' (Exposition), followed by an illustrated 'Dichiaratione' (Declaration) on the subject of rhubarb.[44] Ramusio considered such an explanation of rhubarb 'highly necessary' and 'well worthy of correct knowledge', especially 'seeing how universal the use of the article among sick people has become in our time', while he considered that there was not 'so much information regarding it in any book'.[45]

For this account of rhubarb, Ramusio based himself on another source: a lengthy account, provided to Ramusio by a man only identified as 'Chaggi Memet'.[46] Luckily for us, the account of 'Chaggi Memet' has been translated in full into English by Henry Yule, who entitled this text: 'Hajji Mahomed's Account of Cathay, as delivered to Messer Giov. Battista Ramusio' (c. 1550).[47] This man, variously referred to as Memet or Mahomed, was a hajji: a Muslim Persian from 'Chilan on the shores of the Caspian Sea' who had completed the pilgrimage to Mecca.[48] He had come to Venice to sell the large consignment of rhubarb he had bought himself in Suzhou (Ganzhou). Ramusio had met him over dinner in Murano, in the Venetian Lagoon, where a linguist called Michele Mambre served as translator for Memet as he told his story to Ramusio and the other dinner guests.

Ramusio's 'Declaration' on rhubarb probably represented the most detailed understanding of the plant and its growing environment available anywhere in Europe in the mid-sixteenth century. He describes the conditions in which the best rhubarb grows: in the 'lofty and rocky mountains' near Suzhou ('Succuir') in Ganzhou, where the trees grow to a great height and the very moist soil has a red colour. Memet also added a description of the use of rhubarb root in Cathay: pounded and burnt as a perfume in temples, or even used as fuel. In the paragraph that follows, Ramusio adds what has become well known as the first description of tea (leaves) in a European language, and concludes by saying that tea leaves are so highly valued in Cathay that 'people would gladly give (as he expressed it) a sack of rhubarb for an ounce of *Chiai Catai*'.[49] What rhubarb 'was', thus, for the Europeans who did not 'know' rhubarb, was closely connected to the place where it was found (it was a substance from such and such a place). The place where it was found was identified in European sources initially by Dioscorides, and later also by first-hand observers of rhubarb such as Marco Polo and Chaggi Memet. In the sixteenth century, the way rhubarb was used and how it 'worked' were of less interest to understanding what rhubarb was.

In the seventeenth century, when Sir John Chardin (1643-1713) travelled through Persia, he encountered a medicinal commodity, which he identified as rhubarb:

> The rhubarb grows in *Corasson*, which is the ancient Sogdiana. The best comes out of the Country of the Eastern Tartars, who are between the Caspian Sea and China. The one and the other is call'd *Rivend-Tchini*, the *Rhubarb* of *China*. They eat *rhubarb* in *Corasson*, as we do *Red-Beet*, and it grows there just in the same Manner.[50]

A few things are noteworthy in this late seventeenth-century description: the place of origin is located quite precisely, with the name of *Corasson*, and a political entity: Sogdiana. There is also a reference to classification on the basis of quality: 'the best' supply of rhubarb, which is associated with a different place: 'the Country of the Eastern Tartars', as opposed to the lesser quality, which came from China. And finally, Chardin observed rhubarb to be an edible substance, eaten 'as we do *Red-Beet*'.

When Da Orta was translated in the nineteenth century by Clements Markham (1830–1916), Markham added a footnote, offering first an identity based on the Linnaean system: 'Rhubarb, that is "Rha barbarum" . . . is the root of various species of *Rheum* – *R. palmatum*, Linn., *R. Rhaponticum*, Linn., and *R. officinale*, Bail., N.O. Polygonaceae'.[51] He followed this identification by an explanation of the trade routes by which rhubarb arrived in India: via 'natives of Tartary, Thibet and Western China'.[52] Hence, Markham explained, rhubarb was 'known in commerce as "Chinese," "East Indian," "Turkey," and "Russian" Rhubarb, according to the route by which the drug is imported into Europe'.[53]

In the late nineteenth century, the journeys associated with rhubarb became even more entangled. In the *Pharmacographia Indica*, compiled in 1892 by Dymock, Warden and Hooper, the following description of rhubarb was included:

> The rhubarb found in the Indian bazars is of a very inferior kind, in long stick-like pieces, shipped to Calcutta and Bombay from the Eastern ports. It comes from China, and has hardly any aroma, a bitterish taste, and but slight purgative action. When fresh, it is covered with a yellow dust, like ordinary rhubarb. The natives use it as a tonic and stomachic. None of the commercial rhubarb known as East Indian is imported into Bombay unless specially ordered from China, but it often passes through the port on board the P. and O. Company's steamers. Bombay druggists, Native and European, usually obtain their rhubarb from London. On account of its low price, the former always import English rhubarb.[54]

This description points to the presence of rhubarb in several different qualities: an 'inferior kind' found in 'Indian bazars', but also a 'fresh' kind, an 'ordinary' kind, and a 'commercial' kind. Rhubarb arrives in the Indian marketplace via different commercial routes, sometimes directly from China, but also 'from London'. This shows the complex entanglements of the itinerary: the place of origin may well be China, or indeed a Central Asian location beyond the boundaries of the Chinese empire. Having reached the southern coast of China, from either Central Asia or the far Western reaches of the Chinese empire, it was shipped to London, and from there, placed onto British ships sailing to India on behalf of the Bombay druggists, their desire for rhubarb from London ostensibly 'on account of its low price'. Might part of its appeal not also have been the 'Britishness' that was added to its multiple layers of identity and meaning, on its journey via London on the steamers of the P. and O. Company?

These accounts, taken from many different times and places, offer no great insights into the actual 'origins' of rhubarb. For Dioscorides, it was the unknown world beyond the Rha, for Polo the province of Tangut, for Duarte Barbose the 'lands of Xeque Ismael', for Da Orta China, for Barzeus Uzbeg, for Hajji Mahomed Suzhou and for Chardin Corasson. Markham added the clarification that it was not the origins of the plant, but the routes via which it had travelled that explained the differences between 'Chinese', 'East Indian', 'Turkey', and 'Russian' Rhubarb. Clearly, all those who encountered rhubarb along their travels tried to make some sense of what rhubarb was, and thereby placed rhubarb within their own system of knowledge. If we want to understand what rhubarb meant in different times and places, we need to consider not a single, simple origin story, but the multiple, complex ways in which rhubarb was understood. The entangled itineraries along which rhubarb travelled form an inextricable part of rhubarb's complex of meanings.

Making the exotic known

We have established that the idea of rhubarb existed in many different cultural contexts. In each of those, rhubarb gained a different story, about where it came from, along which routes it had travelled, what it was for and how different types and qualities of rhubarb could be distinguished. There are overlaps and shared elements within these stories, but there are also significant differences. Rather than searching for some kind of fundamental truth about rhubarb among these, I have focused on the ways in which stories were told, and how they made rhubarb knowable. For consumers, the distant origins, the entangled itineraries and the multiple therapeutic uses of rhubarb were all part of the attraction. For those interested in profiting from this interest in rhubarb, such as producers and traders, making rhubarb knowable was the first step towards asserting some kind of control over it. In the British–Indian context, colonial officers often began their attempts to turn locally grown rhubarb into a profitable therapeutic commodity so as to satisfy the desire for rhubarb in Britain by establishing the many linguistic variations in the nomenclature.

The colonial botanist John Forbes Royle (1798–1859), for example, began his explanation of what rhubarb 'was' by detailing the many languages in which it was known. Born in India, Royle served as a military surgeon, but became a naturalist, ultimately taking up a professorship in materia medica and therapeutics at King's College London. In 1839, Royle's *Illustrations of the botany and other branches of the natural history of the Himalayan mountains, and of the flora of Cashmere* was published, which included a description of the various 'denominations' of rhubarb:

> Rhubarb is, in India, commonly denominated *rewund-cheenee* (*rivend-tchini* in Persia, *Chardin*), with *rawund* assigned as its Arabic, and *reon* (ρέον) as its Greek name. The above are evidently the *rewund* of Avicenna, and the *ravedseni* of the translators of Mesue. Three kinds are described in Persian works on Material Medica. 1. *Cheenee*; 2. *Khorassanee*; 3. *Hindee*.[55]

By presenting the terms used for rhubarb 'in India', and reducing these to their shared linguistic roots (*rawund* in Arabic, and *reon* in Greek), Royle emphasized the non-Hindu roots of rhubarb. Linking these, as he says, 'evidently', to the knowledge systems provided by Avicenna and Mesue, serves to strengthen that impression. Rhubarb, this passage suggests, is known in India, but far better known in other medical traditions than the Hindu one. Drawing on Persian works, then, he identifies three separate varieties, depending on their location: *Cheenee*, i.e. from China, *Khorassanee*, i.e. from Sogdiania (as Chardin had established much earlier, and Misbahuddin Azhar and Nighat Anjum did recently in the context of Unani medicine), and finally, a *Hindee* (Hindu) variety. Royle may well have thought he identified 'three kinds' of rhubarb, but arguably, Royle was pointing to three different medical knowledge systems in which rhubarb featured: Chinese, Islamic and Hindu.

Over the course of the nineteenth century, rhubarb frequently appeared on British–Indian lists of what came to be referred to as 'economic products'. It was included, for example, among the drugs listed in the 1862 *Catalogue of Economic products of the Presidency of Bombay* by the British–Indian official and naturalist George Birdwood (1832–1917). As had become common practice, Birdwood added what he assumed to be the linguistic equivalents: 'Rewund-chenee, Hind. Rawund, Reebass, Arab. Rivend-tchini, Pers'.[56] The Arabic root of the name (*rewund, rawund, rivend*) refers to the plant itself, accompanied by an indication of its origins in China (*chenee* or *tchini*). The *Reebass* or *ribas* that he inserts in that list refers in fact to a different plant, but as discussed earlier, the fourteenth-century Persian physician Haji Zayn Attar already assumed these were the same plant, and it seems Birdwood simply follows in that tradition.

Over time, the linguistic equivalents were expanded. In a description included in *Indian Medicinal Plants* (1918), the entry for one variety of the rhubarb plant, *Rheum emodi*, is given:

> Revand-chini (H. and B.); Révande-hindi (Pers.); Variyâttu (Tam.); Natturéval-chinni (Tel.); Gamni-revan-chini (Guz.); Padam-chal (Nepal); Archu (Garhwal); Mulka-cha-reval-chini (Mar.); Nat-reva-chinni (Kan.).[57]

In other words, the plant in question is identified with a distinct language marker in Hindi and Bengali, Persian, Tamil, Telugu, Gujarati, Nepali, Garhwal, Marathi and Kannada, the language spoken in the south-western region of India. The Persian linguistic root, *revand*, is present in seven of the ten linguistic forms mentioned here. Only in Tamil, Nepali and the Garhwal language do we find a term that has no reference to the Persian root. Moreover, in five of the ten terms, the connection with China is made by way of the suffix 'chini' or 'chinni'. The four that do not indicate the reference to China are Nepal (Padam-chal), Garhwal (Archu) and Tamil (Variyâttu). In the Linnaean system, the Nepali Padam-chal has been identified as 'rheum australe D. don', commonly known in English as 'Himalayan rhubarb', harvested in the wild in Nepal.[58] According to the compilers of this source, the Persians located this plant within the Hindu context ('Révande-hindi'). The addition of further linguistic varieties in the lemma on rhubarb confirms several things at once: the presence of knowledge about rhubarb across linguistically diverse spaces of India, the dominance of the Persian roots of that knowledge, and the association of rhubarb with spaces other than one's own, including China in the Indian-language context and Indian for the Persian language context.

When Clements Markham commented on Da Orta's passage on rhubarb in a note, he also pointed to that quality of the 'foreign':

> In India the natives use also the root of *R. Emodi*, Wallich, *R. moorcroftianum*, Royle, and *R. webbianum*, Royle, of the Himalayas. *Ravaud-chini* is the Indian

name of the foreign, *i.e.* 'Chinese' rhubarb, and *ravaud-chini-hindi* of native Indian rhubarb.[59]

Markham's footnote validates the knowledge of the local users, which imposes a distinction between 'native Indian rhubarb' sourced in the Himalayas and Chinese rhubarb, which is identified as 'foreign'. At the same time, Markham distances himself from that local knowledge, by imposing the Linnaean classification system upon the varieties that are distinguished locally.

This points to a tension that is pervasive in much of the colonial writing about rhubarb. On the one hand, the inclusion of numerous linguistic forms of the name of the plant serves as an acknowledgement of locally held knowledge, which regularly emphasizes the non-local origins of rhubarb, and reveals the attraction of rhubarb's 'foreign' or exotic identity. On the other hand, the translation of the terms and the inclusion of what these authors consider to be their Linnaean equivalents suggests a hierarchical ordering of knowledge systems, in which Western knowledge of what rhubarb is appears as the more authoritative. The German anthropologist Berthold Laufer, based at the Field Museum in Chicago, added to these distinctions between different knowledge systems the differentiation of quality. In 1919, he published details of the cultivated plants and products that formed part of the 'Chinese contributions to the history of civilization in ancient Iran'.[60] He included rhubarb,[61] which he describes as follows:

> WATT gives a Persian term *revande-hindi* ('Indian rhubarb') for *Rheum emodi*. Curiously, in Hindustani this is called *Hindi-revand cini* ('Chinese rhubarb of India'), and in Bengali *Bangla-revan cini* ('Chinese rhubarb of Bengal'), indicating that the Chinese product was prominently in the minds of the people, and that the Himalayan rhubarbs were only secondary substitutes.[62]

Quoting the botanist George Watt, Laufer explains these entangled origins in his own way, seeing them as evidence of the pre-eminence of 'the Chinese product'. In nineteenth-century Europe and America, 'Chinese rhubarb' was understood as the foremost in quality, an identification that went back to the likes of the sixteenth-century naturalists like John Gerard, as we saw earlier. Writing in the early twentieth century, Laufer assumed this was a value judgement shared by Hindustani and Bengali alike. It seems equally possible, however, to understand all three terms, *revande-hindi* ('Indian rhubarb'), *Hindi-revand cini* ('Chinese rhubarb of India'), and *Bangla-revan cini* ('Chinese rhubarb of Bengal') as emphasizing the non-local quality of the plant. In all three languages mentioned by Laufer, it concerns a plant that was thought of as coming from elsewhere: from

India for the Persians, and from China for its Hindu and Bengali consumers. It was this otherness, this origin that lies elsewhere, that those who encountered rhubarb often saw as key to defining it. As we will see, it was this idea of 'coming from elsewhere' that contributed to making the local cultivation of rhubarb a challenging proposition.

The creation of a profitable commodity

The British colonial approach to rhubarb in India consisted of a search for a reliable supply of the product from land within or near British-controlled territory, so that the plant could be cultivated for commercial purposes. The mountainous regions in the north seemed to offer such an opportunity. So, when the British explorer in the service of the East India Company William Moorcroft (1767–1825) travelled to Tibet in 1812, his purpose was the development of trade relations between India and Central Asia. He encountered rhubarb on his travels in the mountains and described it as follows:

> In respect to game, my search was unsuccessful, but I met with many plants, amongst others were two kinds of rhubarb. – One I took for the Rheum palmatum, the other was much smaller. I cut up the roots of many large plants. . . . I presume, that the best time for taking up the roots is in September. If the quality of this root should be found to equal that of the Levant, the quantity procurable here at an easy rate would be very great.[63]

Rhubarb was not what Moorcroft had set out to find, game was, but he was clearly hopeful that the mountainous region on the northern borders of the British empire could yield a good quantity of a commodity for which he knew there was demand. A few years later, in 1815, the border was extended towards Tibet, which brought more opportunities. In 1828, rhubarb was included in a list of 'exports from the hills to the plains' in the 'Statistical Report of Kamaon'.[64] This report, by G. W. Traill, who served as the second commissioner of this region (Kamaon, or Kumaon), was one of the first detailed colonial studies of the Himalayas.

Despite their optimism, it turned out to be rather difficult to grow rhubarb with the right kind of properties, that is the purgative function for which the root was so popular in Britain, in British-controlled territory. The botanist John Forbes Royle, too, sought to identify a location in the region of the Himalayas where this crop, 'so important in a commercial point of view' could be grown.[65]

His 1839 *Illustrations of the botany and other branches of the natural history of the Himalayan mountains* was the first of a series of publications focused on commercial crops in British India, and his discussion on rhubarb provides an insight into the colonial mindset of the time. Royle provides geographical references for some of the places where rhubarb is grown: in Gansu ('Russian Rhubarb') and in Sichuan ('China Rhubarb').[66] He then asks 'how near it approaches the British territories in India, in order to share in the trade, or attempt the cultivation'.[67] Happily for him, he claims that '[t]here can . . . be no rational doubt about the successful cultivation of the true Rhubarb in territories within British influence'.[68] The process he envisages would involve several separate steps: 'obtaining specimens or seeds of the true Rhubarb', which he thinks could be done in 'Kemaon and Nepal', and 'establishing a trade in Rhubarb with Tibet . . . by means of the Tatars', who sell most but not all of their rhubarb to the Russians. The trade with Tibet, in turn, could be encouraged by 'the government purchasing all the Rhubarb it requires . . . for hospital use'.[69] Unfortunately, Royle's account does not confirm whether any of these steps were ever completed successfully.

In other places, attempts were made at the commercial cultivation of rhubarb. In 1839, Rheum rhaponticum was described as follows: 'Common *Rhubarb*; – in Dr Elliot's garden at Dhoolea'.[70] Dhoolea, also known as Dhulia or Dhule in Khandesh, had come under British control in 1818. In 1827, the collector of Khandesh, an Indian Civil Servant named George Giberne (*c*. 1797–1876), had established a mulberry garden here, to try and get the silk production off the ground. In the end, no silk industry was established in Dhule, and although over the decades that followed, the gardens in and around Dhule were productive, especially thanks to the extensive use of convict labour, no mention is made of a successful rhubarb production.

In the early twentieth century, the botanist George Watt (1851–1930) published *The Commercial Products of India*.[71] One of the examples of economic botany he discussed in this volume was the Himalayan rhubarb:

> Himalayan rhubarb is usually stated to be of little commercial importance, and the rhubarb sold in the bazars of the plains is ordinarily affirmed to be of an inferior grade to the Chinese drug, and still more to that imported from London. Considerable quantities are, however, annually conveyed to the plains from the Kangra district of the Panjáb. . . . It is remarked in the *Pharmacopoeia of India* that were the Himalayan rhubarb cultivated with due care, there is reason to believe a drug equal to the Chinese or Turkey rhubarb might be obtained.[72]

This short extract confirms the ongoing lack of commercial success with the local cultivation of rhubarb, and the ongoing success of the Chinese import. The enduring appeal of rhubarb that arrived in India via the London market is revealed here, too. But the extract also shows the ongoing faith that colonial botanists had in their own endeavours to cultivate a local crop that could be equal, or even better surpass, any imported variety. The authority Watt uses to legitimize his view on rhubarb is the *Pharmacopoeia of India*, compiled forty years earlier by E. J. Waring in 1868.[73] As a reporter on economic products, it was probably in Watt's job description to be optimistic about the commercial potential of Himalayan rhubarb. But perhaps he should have paid more attention to what consumers in India and Britain actually wanted, a therapeutic commodity that had reached them from a remote location along a complex itinerary, rather than overestimating British abilities to create commercially successful commodities.

Concluding thoughts

Rhubarb has attracted a great deal of research to date. Much of the more recent scholarship in Western languages on rhubarb has been focused on rhubarb in a single country. Matt Romaniello, for example, focused on Russian rhubarb in his discussion on 'true rhubarb'.[74] Lin Rizhang considered rhubarb by means of Jesuit writings within the Chinese context.[75] Chang Che-chia discussed rhubarb in the political space between Britain and China.[76] Erika Monahan considered the early modern European history rhubarb.[77] India has been largely absent in this literature. Clifford Foust's study of rhubarb, for example, which aims at offering a comprehensive 'biography of a plant', 'from earliest times down to the present day', does not include India as a separate space.[78] In one-way or another, all of these studies are concerned with discussing the actual social and economic histories associated with rhubarb.

Instead, I have focused on the idea of rhubarb and on the stories told about rhubarb in different cultural contexts. In this sense, this draws on recent developments in the field of history, where material culture studies have become more prominent. This has not brought us any closer to understanding the history of the actual plant in its native context, nor its transition to a commercial product, cultivated in British India. But it has shown that the stories told about rhubarb, including those that told of its remote origins and its complex itineraries, were key to its appeal. Despite extensive efforts to bring rhubarb under control, by naming it, classifying it and by trying to commercialize its cultivation, the appeal of these stories and their remote origins remained the more enduring.

Notes

1. 'How to Grow Rhubarb/RHS Gardening', https://www.rhs.org.uk/advice/grow-your-own/vegetables/rhubarb (accessed 16 September 2020).
2. Fang Lai et al., 'A Systematic Review of Rhubarb (a Traditional Chinese Medicine) Used for the Treatment of Experimental Sepsis', *Evidence-Based Complementary and Alternative Medicine* 2015 (2015): 1.
3. John M. Riddle, *Dioscorides on Pharmacy and Medicine* (Austin: University of Texas Press, 1985), 37.
4. Dioscorides, *De materia medica*, trans. Lili Beck, 3rd rev. ed. (Hildesheim: Olms-Weidmann, 2017), 175.
5. Muḥammad Sharîf Khân, *The Taleef Shereef, or Indian Materia Medica*, trans. George Playfair (Calcutta: Baptist Mission Press, 1833), 89.
6. Clifford M. Foust, *Rhubarb: The Wondrous Drug* (Princeton: Princeton University Press, 1992). India and the Indian Ocean World do not feature prominently in this study.
7. For a brief overview, see the introduction in Anne Gerritsen and Giorgio Riello, eds, *Writing Material Culture History*, 2nd ed. (London: Bloomsbury Academic, 2021), 1–19.
8. Dorothy Ko, 'Itineraries of Inkstones in Early Modern China', in *Entangled Itineraries: Materials, Practices, and Knowledges across Eurasia*, ed. Pamela H. Smith (Pittsburgh: University of Pittsburgh Press, 2019), 202.
9. Ibid., 202.
10. Pamela H. Smith, 'Nodes of Convergence, Material Complexes, and Entangled Itineraries', in *Entangled Itineraries: Materials, Practices, and Knowledges across Eurasia*, ed. Pamela H. Smith (Pittsburgh: University of Pittsburgh Press, 2019), 5–24.
11. Andrea Vianello, *Exotica in the Prehistoric Mediterranean* (Oxford: Oxbow Books, 2011); Nicole Boivin, Dorian Fuller, and Alison Crowther, 'Old World Globalization and the Columbian Exchange: Comparison and Contrast', *World Archaeology* 44, no. 3 (2012): 452–69.
12. Christopher Bayly, '"Archaic" and "Modern" Globalization in the Eurasian and African Arena, ca. 1750-1850', in *Globalization in World History*, ed. Anthony Hopkins (New York: W.W. Norton, 2002), 47–73.
13. Peter McNeil and Giorgio Riello, *Luxury: A Rich History* (Oxford: Oxford University Press, 2016); Karin Hofmeester and Bernd-Stefan Grewe, eds, *Luxury*

in Global Perspective: Objects and Practices, 1600–2000 (Cambridge: Cambridge University Press, 2017).
14 Janet Lippman Abu-Lughod, *Before European Hegemony: The World System A.D. 1250-1350* (New York: Oxford University Press, 1989); Maxine Berg, 'In Pursuit of Luxury: Global History and British Consumer Goods in the Eighteenth Century', *Past & Present* 182, no. 1 (2004): 85–142; Maxine Berg, ed., *Goods from the East, 1600–1800: Trading Eurasia* (Basingstoke: Palgrave Macmillan, 2015).
15 Arjun Appadurai, 'Introduction: Commodities and the Politics of Value', in *The Social Life of Things: Commodities in Cultural Perspective*, ed. Arjun Appadurai (Cambridge: Cambridge University Press, 1986), 3–63; Igor Kopytoff, 'The Cultural Biography of Things: Commoditization as Process', in *The Social Life of Things: Commodities in Cultural Perspective*, ed. Arjun Appadurai (Cambridge: Cambridge University Press, 1986), 64–92; Wim M. J. van Binsbergen, 'Commodification: Things, Agency, and Identities: Introduction', in *Commodification: Things, Agency, and Identities (The Social Life of Things Revisited)*, ed W. M. J. van Binsbergen and P. L. Geschiere (Münster: Lit Verlag, 2005), 9–51.
16 This will regrettably be an extremely limited approach to the topic due to my lack of access to the multiple linguistic contexts in which rhubarb was discussed in the Indian Ocean world.
17 Translation from Shouzhong Yang, *The Divine Farmer's Materia Medica: A Translation of the Shennong Bencaojing* (Boulder: Blue Poppy Press, 1998), 69; A slightly different translation appears in He Bian, 'Assembling the Cure: Materia Medica and the Culture of Healing in Late Imperial China' (PhD diss., Harvard University, 2014), 110; see also: He Bian, *Know Your Remedies: Pharmacy and Culture in Early Modern China* (Princeton: Princeton University Press, 2020).
18 Udoy Chand Dutt, *The Materia Medica of the Hindus, Compiled from Sanskrit Medical Works* (Calcutta: Thacker, Spink & Co, 1877), 161.
19 The haritaki tree is also known (in Western scientific terms) as *Terminalia chebula*. Bhagwan Dash and Acharya Manfred M. Jounious, *Handbook of Ayurveda* (New Delhi: Concept Publishing, 1983), 84–8. The fruit is known as chebulic myrobalan.
20 Dutt, *The Materia Medica of the Hindus*, 161.
21 Misbahuddin Azhar and Nighat Anjum, 'Revand Chini (Chinese Rhubarb): A Review on Historical and Unani Classical Prospect', *International Journal of Unani and Integrative Medicine* 3, no. 1 (2019): 11–18.
22 Ibn-e-Sina is also known as Avicenna.
23 Mesue (or Mesue the Younger) is also known as Masawaih al-Mardini, or Yaḥyā ibn Masawaih al-Mardini. He was a Syrian physician who worked in Baghdad.
24 Khorasan refers to the historical region encompassed by north-eastern Iran, southern Turkmenistan and northern Afghanistan.
25 Haji Zayn Attar (died *c.*1403) was a fourteenth-century Persian physician. His name is also rendered as Ali ibn Husayn Ansari Shirazi. Farid Ramezany and Mohammad

Reza Shams Ardakani, 'Ali Ibn Hosein Ansari (1330–1404): A Persian Pharmacist and His Pharmacopoeia, Ekhtiyarat i Badi i', *Journal of Medical Biography* 19, no. 2 (2011): 80–3.
26 Ibn Jazla was an eleventh-century Arab physician of Baghdad.
27 Azhar and Anjum, 'Revand Chini (Chinese Rhubarb)', 11.
28 Foust, *Rhubarb*, 6.
29 Ibid., 15–16.
30 John Gerard, *The Herball or Generall Historie of Plantes* (London: Iohn Norton, 1597), 317.
31 Gerard, *The Herball*, 317–18.
32 Lai et al., 'A Systematic Review'.
33 Marco Polo, *The Travels of Marco Polo*, trans. R. E. Latham (Harmondsworth, Middlesex: Penguin Books, 1958), 90.
34 Polo, *The Travels*, 90; Frances Wood, *The Silk Road: Two Thousand Years in the Heart of Asia* (Berkeley: University of California Press, 2002), 111.
35 Duarte Barbosa, *The Book of Duarte Barbosa: An Account of the Countries Bordering on the Indian Ocean and Their Inhabitants, Written by Duarte Barbosa, and Completed about the Year 1518 A.D.*, ed. Mansel Longworth Dames, vol. 1 (London: Hakluyt Society, 1918), 93.
36 Ibid., 1:93–94, footnote 3.
37 Duarte Barbosa, *The Book of Duarte Barbosa: An Account of the Countries Bordering on the Indian Ocean and Their Inhabitants, Written by Duarte Barbosa, and Completed about the Year 1518 A.D.*, ed. Mansel Longworth Dames, vol. 2 (London: Hakluyt Society, 1921), 77 (Malabar), 173 (Malaca) and 214 (China).
38 The text has been translated into English. See Garcia de Orta, *Colloquies on the Simples and Drugs of India*, trans. Clements Markham (London: H. Sotheran, 1913).
39 Orta, *Colloquies*, 392.
40 Ibid., 390.
41 Ibid.
42 António da Silva Rêgo, *Documentação para a história das missões do padroado português do Oriente*, vol. 7 (Lisboa: Agência geral do ultramar, Divisão de publicacões e biblioteca, 1947), 83. The letter, written on 16 December 1551, was originally included in *Documenta India II*, 245–67.
43 Orta, *Colloquies*, 291.
44 Giovanni Battista Ramusio, *Delle Navigationi et Viaggi*, vol. 2 (Venetia: Giunti, 1559), 9v–13v.
45 Henry Yule, *Cathay and the Way Thither; Being a Collection of Medieval Notices of China: Translated and Ed. with a Preliminary Essay on the Intercourse between China and the Western Nations Previous to the Discovery of the Cape Route*, vol. 1 (London: Hakluyt Society, 1866), ccxiv.

46 Ramusio, *Delle Navigationi et Viaggi*, 2:folii 13v–17v. The section on rhubarb is entitled 'Dichiaratione d'alcuni luoghi ne libri di M. Marco Polo con l'Historia del Rheubarbaro'. The account provided by Chaggi Memet to Ramusio starts on folio 14v and ends on folio 16v.
47 Yule, *Cathay and the Way Thither*, 1:ccxiv–ccxx.
48 Ibid., 1:ccxiv.
49 Ibid., 1:ccxvi.
50 Sir John Chardin, *Travels in Persia, 1673–1677* (Newburyport: Dover Publications, 2012).
51 Orta, *Colloquies*, 392.
52 Ibid.
53 Ibid.
54 William Dymock, C. J. H. Warden, and David Hooper, *Pharmacographia Indica: A History of the Principal Drugs of Vegetable Origin, Met with in British India*, vol. 3 (London: K. Paul, Trench, Trübner & co., 1892), 155.
55 John Forbes Royle, *Illustrations of the Botany and Other Branches of the Natural History of the Himalayan Mountains, and of the Flora of Cashmere*, vol. 1 (London: Allen, 1839), 317.
56 George C. M. Birdwood, *Catalogue of the Economic Products of the Presidency of Bombay* (Bombay: Education Society's Press, 1862), 70.
57 Kanhoba Ranchoddas Kirtikar and Baman Das Basu, *Indian Medicinal Plants*, vol. 2 (Bahadurganj, India: Sudhindra Nath Basu, Pâninî office, 1918), 1079–80.
58 Carsten Smith Olsen and Finn Helles, 'Medicinal Plants, Markets, and Margins in the Nepal Himalaya: Trouble in Paradise', *Mountain Research and Development* 17, no. 4 (1997): 363–74.
59 Orta, *Colloquies*, 392.
60 Berthold Laufer, *Sino-Iranica: Chinese Contributions to the History of Civilization in Ancient Iran, with Special Reference to the History of Cultivated Plants and Products* (Chicago: Field Museum of Natural History, 1919).
61 Ibid., 547–51.
62 Ibid., 551.
63 William Moorcroft, 'A Journey to Lake Mánasaróvara in Úndés, a Province of Little Tibet', *Asiatic Researches* 12 (1816): 407–8.
64 George William Traill, 'Statistical Sketch of Kamaon', *Asiatic Researches* 16 (1828): 226.
65 Royle, *Botany of the Himalayan Mountains*, 1:314.
66 Ibid.
67 Ibid., 1:315.
68 Ibid., 1:316.
69 Ibid., 1:317.

70 John Graham, *A Catalogue of the Plants Growing in Bombay and Its Vicinity: Spontaneous, Cultivated or Introduced, as Far as They Have Been Ascertained* (Bombay: Government Press, 1839), 172.

71 George Watt, *The Commercial Products of India: Being an Abridgement of 'The Dictionary of the Economic Products of India'*, 1908; this was a shortened version of his six-volume *A Dictionary of the Economic Products of India* (Calcutta: The Superintendent of Government Printing, 1883); see also David Arnold, *Science, Technology and Medicine in Colonial India* (Cambridge: Cambridge University Press, 2000), 132.

72 Watt, *The Commercial Products of India*, 913.

73 Edward John Waring, *Pharmacopoeia of India* (London: W.H. Allen & Co, 1868).

74 Matthew P. Romaniello, 'True Rhubarb? Trading Eurasian Botanical and Medical Knowledge in the Eighteenth Century', *Journal of Global History* 11, no. 1 (2016): 3–23.

75 Lin Rizhang 林日杖, 'Ming Qing Shiqi Lai Hua Yesu Huishi Dui Zhongguo Dahuang de Jishu Ji Qi Yuanlai 明清时期来华耶稣会士对中国大黄的记述及其原因 [On the Narratives of the Jesuits in China on Chinese Rhubarb and Its Reasons]', *Journal of Fujian Normal University* 2 (2011): 128–34.

76 Chang Che-Chia, 'Origins of a Misunderstanding: The Qianlong Emperor's Embargo on Rhubarb Exports to Russia, the Scenario and Its Consequences', *Asian Medicine* 1, no. 2 (2005): 335–54.

77 Erika Monahan, 'Locating Rhubarb: Early Modernity's Relevant Obscurity', in *Early Modern Things: Objects and Their Histories, 1500–1800*, ed. Paula Findlen (London: Routledge, 2013), 227–51.

78 Foust, *Rhubarb*, xv.

5

Perfumes in early modern India
Ephemeral materiality and aromatic mobility
Amrita Chattopadhyay[1]

Introduction

The 'material turn' in historical studies has paved the way for the study of material artefacts, even those with short lives and a transient presence in human lives such as perfumes.[2] Perfume as a material, despite its volatility and intangibility, has been the focus of scholarly engagement in the last few decades both in the global[3] and Indian[4] contexts. This article attempts to engage with the ephemeral materiality of perfumes in early modern[5] India and study its role in the making of a 'history of a fleeting moment'[6] from this period.[7] It brings to fore how the transformative and therapeutic properties of perfumes endowed with unique 'material-life'[8] played an important participatory role in shaping Mughal court culture.[9] Intrinsic to this was the Persianate medical philosophy and the imperial ideology linking the health of the Mughal body-politic to the well-being of an individual.[10] The presence and employment of external material-stimulants like perfumes aided the maintenance of health. As enhancers of beauty and restorers of balance, perfumes also came to determine bodily practices and consumption patterns in the imperial and noble households during this period. Laced with sensory experience and cultural significance, aromatics came to be integrated into the global economy through networks of procurement and circulation along the littoral spaces of the Indian Ocean. With these aspects in focus, the article primarily looks beyond the matter or form of perfume and assigns it with an agency of its own.[11] It foregrounds the materiality of perfumes and positions them as important determinants of socio-cultural praxis and economic activities of the period under study.

Perfumes: Materiality and body

The role of aromatics in both Ayurvedic and Unani medical traditions was well-recognized and was put into practice for therapeutic purposes. Olfactants were considered aromatic ingredients with medical properties in the various Sanskrit treatises, texts composed in other Indic languages, as well as in the Persian–Arabic texts composed in India.[12] Consequently, every aromatic ingredient had significance in Indian medical history and played as important a role in medical cures as it did in aesthetic regimes.[13] The different constituent aromatic ingredients with their respective distinctive properties could have a significant transformative effect on humans, their physical health, bodily humours and emotions.[14] The significance of fragrance was derived from the role of 'exhilarating' scent in maintaining the balance and harmony of bodily humours or bodily fluids (namely: blood, phlegm, black and yellow bile) which lead to the refinement of *mizaj*, or temperament.[15] As Indo-Islamicate medical thought was based on the humoral system, the body and everything consumed by the body, including food, drink, perfumes and medicines, were all classified in terms of their humoral properties: whether they were cold, hot, dry or wet.[16] The disease was caused by an imbalance, which could only be rectified by the consumption of something with the opposite properties. Emotions too were understood to be caused by the changes in bodily humours and could thus be manipulated by the application of particular substances with the right humoral characteristics. Perfume was particularly well placed to do this.[17]

Materially, perfumes are said to be 'internal-external bodily ornaments'[18] and this is presumably because they are applied to the actual surface of the body, while they affect it internally and physiologically in a variety of ways. According to Ibn Sīnā (980–1037), one of the most influential physician-philosophers of classical Islam, certain fragrances, which he referred to as exhilarants (*mufarriḥ*), would act physiologically upon the heart (*dil*) causing it to expand, with direct ameliorating consequences for both the emotional state of a person and for their physical health. Apparently, exhilaration describes a state of well-being that arises in the 'refreshment' of the spirit and the restoration of the body's equilibrium.[19] Essentially, underlying these pervasive theories of the transformative powers of smell was a conception of the body as a porous entity, one which could be moulded by outside forces, including forces invisible to the human eye like olfactants; both those rubbed onto the body, and those inhaled through the nose or mouth.[20] Here, we find one such instance as the introduction to the fifteenth/sixteenth-century Persian text produced in the Malwa Sultanate of central India, *Ni'matnama* (The Book of Delicacies by Nasir Shah) states:

> However, if the *pān*[21] is perfumed and if flowers and scent are rubbed into it, the benefits are as follows: seminal fluid increases, well-being is established, the body becomes comfortable, bad sight is prevented and feverishness, restlessness and stiffness are reduced.[22]

Thus, material properties of perfumes – their exhilarating nature, pervasiveness, sensory-aesthetics, pleasure-awakening and healing effects on body and mind – have guided the patterns of consumption during the period under consideration. The same source *Ni'matnama* further describes:

> Rub perfume separately into each joint. *(Use)* pellets of perfumed paste. Wash the hands in rosewater. Take the sap from the bark of the mango tree and from the bark of the wild fig tree and from the *pīpal* tree and wash the body *(with it)*. Rub aromatic paste, perfume and musk into the armpits. Rub *chūva,* rosewater and musk onto the private parts and rub sandal on the throat. Essence of musk is good for the mouth, *(also)* put aloes perfume into the mouth. Rub ointment made from bodily oils on the face, rub rosewater on the forehead, sniff flowers, scatter spikenard on the head, rub saffron on the face, use scented flower oils of every kind, make *'abīr (scented powder)* with the sweet scent of jasmine flowers, polish the two front teeth, rub perfume into the handkerchief, wash the whole body with rosewater. Put on a white *chādor* and apply scent to it. Rub the body with twigs and wash in cold water.[23]

Ni'matnama foregrounds that perfumes played an important role in sensory stimulation and enhancing physical as well as emotional intimacy between individuals and collectively. These material properties would continue to influence and inform the patterns of perfume consumption in private chambers, public settings of courtly ceremonies, religious festivals and special occasions throughout the Mughal empire. Creating the right ambience of fragrant air and bodily anointment of the right perfumes became part of the Mughal courtly culture and the consumption practices of the royals and the elites during this time.

The physical consumption of perfumes for their therapeutic and transformative purposes was encouraged by the Mughal emperor Akbar (reign: 1556–1605). Akbar preferred perfumes both for personal use, religious motives as well as for burning in the household and in the court-hall which were continually scented with *ambar* (ambergris), *agar* (aloeswood) and other incenses. *Araqs,*[24] *itrs*[25] and oils were extracted from flowers and used for skin and hair.[26]

The autobiography of the Mughal emperor Jahangir(reign: 1605–27), *Tuzuk-i-Jahangiri*, mentions the strength and quality of the special Mughal rose-perfume invented and named as *itr-i-Jahangiri*[27] as follows:

> Fragrance and perfume is of such a degree that if one drop is rubbed on the palm of the hand (که اگر یک قطره از آن بر کف مالیده شود /*ke agar yek qatrah az an bar kaf malideh shud*), it will perfume an entire assembly (مخلسی را معطر می سازد/ *majlisi ra muattar mi sazad*) and manifest in a way as if many red rose-buds had bloomed at once. (و چنان ظاهر می شود که چندین غنچه گل سرخ یکی بار در شگفتن آمده/ *wa chanan zahar mi shud ke chandin ghunche gul-e-surkh yeki bar dar shaguftan amade*).[28]

In the seventeenth century, yet another treatise on perfumery, *Bayaz i Khushbui*, in the form of a diary or a guidebook on art and administration lays out the method of preparation for perfume in the first chapter. It emphasizes the nuances of the craft of perfume-making, the various forms of perfumes that can be prepared, and the multiple ways of consuming them. According to the text, perfumes could either be made into globules and consumed orally for scented breath or prepared for external application in the form of a powder or a paste or a liquid to be applied directly on the individual's body.[29]

Examples of distinct Mughal perfumes show that they were consumed as an object of pleasure and a tool for enhancing the intimacy between lovers. Perfumes contributed to the enhancement of sensual pleasures in the spaces of early medieval court, as shown in the work of Daud Ali.[30] In the context of the Mughal setting, seventeenth-century Dutch traveller Francisco Pelsaert (1595–1630) observes that notable perfumes like *mossari* or *falanj* were used by the nobles and the elites for their private bodily consumption.[31] The wives of the nobles spent night and day studying the method of preparing 'such exciting perfumes, which were composed of amber, gold, opium, pearls and other stimulants'. According to Pelsaert, these were mostly for their own use, occasionally eaten in the daytime because they produce a pleasant elevation of the spirit. These perfumes, mostly in the form of oil, were applied on the bodies of men by slave girls to enhance pleasure and love-making.[32] Detailed descriptions are available of the lives of the noble women[33] and eunuchs in the harems and in the possession of Mughal nobles like Nawab Said Khan,[34] which suggests that among many other arts, the use of perfumes was an essential part of their opulent and elite presence. Their bodies, hairs and dresses were always perfumed with sweetly scented oils, mainly essence of rose, amber and musk.[35] *Chua* was also another very rich perfume, made of liquid, distilled from aloe-wood, black in colour and was commonly put under the armpits and many times over the bosoms and back, mainly by the dancing women and women of the noble households.[36]

While the application of perfumes on the body enhanced the health of the individual and delighted the sensory experiences, the consumption of oiled perfumes often caused ailments. The seventeenth-century English traveller Peter Mundy (1597–1667)[37] as well as the Italian traveller Niccolao Manucci (1638–1717)[38] mention accidents caused by fire at the Mughal court or in private chambers, as the women's linens doused in sweet oily perfume like *Chua* enhanced the spread of the fire and intensified the degree of the burn. Mughal chronicler Inayat Khan (1628–71) in *Shahjahannama* mentions how the Mughal princess Jahanara Begum was a victim of a similar fire accident and her treatment required specialized *hakims*, or physicians, the administration of powerful remedies and unique dressings for quick healing.[39]

Perfumes and the use of fragrance became part of the intrigues at the Mughal court in Aurangzeb's (1658–1707) bid for succession to the throne. He invited his brother and a rival claimant to the throne, Murad, to the tent before his coronation and welcomed him with an embrace displaying love and brotherhood. This was followed by cajoling and enticing him with all kinds of entertainments, comforts and bodily pleasures. Aurangzeb applied perfumes to his body, relaxing his senses. Murad was charmed and besotted by the sensuality of the atmosphere, whereafter he was disarmed and imprisoned and this was followed by Aurangzeb's coronation ceremony.[40]

Mughal fragrance also played an important role in the consolidation and embodiment of an elite class of urbane gentry of seventeenth-century *Mirzas*[41] through the 'conspicuous consumption'[42] of choicest, high-class perfume like *Jahangiri argaja* and finest smells of aloe-wood, *argaja* and *fitna*.[43] All these perfumes had properties of sensorial gratification and regulating humoral balance of the bodies of *Mirzas* when consumed. *Mirza*'s material choice and collective appropriation of specific exquisite perfumes into their consumption practices resonated with the Mughal imperial ideology as envisioned since Akbar's rule (1556–1605). As the norms of equilibrium and harmony were implicit in the idea of the 'empire',[44] perfumes played a decisive role in the material appropriation of these values into the political culture of the Mughals. The imperial vision of social-cohesion and the well-being of the empire came to be demonstrated at a microcosm-level in the life and character of *Mirza*. Group solidarity was being forged through the act of consorted and collective consumption of an object of the highest sensory capabilities to make a public statement of exclusivity as a culturally refined 'collective body' of perfume connoisseurs.

Perfume was believed to have the power to please and attract those to whom the scent is directed – the deities, the guests at a festival, a lover and so on. An integrative power is also usually attributed to smell, making scent an excellent means of uniting the participants in a ritual, who all breathe in and are enveloped by the same aroma.[45] Thus, perfumes in the Mughal empire were not just an object of personal consumption of the royal figures for the aspect of bodily anointment, beautification, love-making and sensuality but they also came to be consumed in various forms: as materials of exchange, as royal gifts with transactional symbolic value, and as items of distribution to the guests in special occasions and royal ceremonies. In this more transactional form, perfumes ensured the incorporation of a larger and more cosmopolitan nobility to ensure harmony and balanced health of the empire.

Rare and high-value perfumes from the Mughal empire such as *itr-i-jahangiri*, *atr of fitna*,[46] *bid-i-mishk*,[47] *argacha/argaja*[48] and other aromatic substances such as sandalwood, camphor and musk were endowed with transformative effects, royal value and aesthetic significance. For example, fragrant *argaja* placed within a gold cup with a cover and a saucer, whose worth varied between 20,000 and 40,000 rupees, was bestowed as a gift upon important political messengers such as Budaq Beg, the envoy of Persia, 'Abdussamad Amudi, the Sharif of Mecca's messenger and Muhammad 'Ali Beg, the ambassador from Iran.[49] Perfumed *itr-i-Jahangiri* poured into a large crystal hookah was also a lavish gift dispatched for the Qaisar of Rum by the Emperor Shahjahan.[50]

While perfume was integrated in the domestic economy through massive spending on 'luxuries' by the elites and other urban consumers, on the other hand, the integration of perfumes in the domestic economy would not have been possible without the circulation of luxury ingredients throughout the Indian Ocean world. Both of these contributed in determining perfumes and their ingredients as a commodity in the early modern world.

Perfumes and the Indian Ocean: Material mobility

The Indian Ocean world was a littoral space of production, trade, movement and exchange of goods, ideas, people, values[51] as well as social and political processes.[52] Perfumes came to chart their own journeys through the maritime networks, port cities and inland spaces of the Indian Ocean world.[53] Indian spices,⁵⁴ indigo⁵⁵ and textiles⁵⁶ have received considerable scholarly attention in the writings on the Indian Ocean trade. Although perfumes played a significant role in the history of Indian Ocean trade, they have been relatively overlooked.⁵⁷ Of late, scholars like K. N. Chaudhuri (1985) have located perfumes and aromatics in the 'geographical map of commodity exchange' between India and China and suggested certain regional imbalances that this exchange revealed in the Indian Ocean region.⁵⁸ Genevieve Bouchon and Denys Lombard (1987) further revealed that 'the demand of perfumes during fifteenth century was considerable'.⁵⁹ They also hinted at the circulation patterns of aromatics that made their way into the subcontinent from various parts of the Middle East, China and South-east Asia during this period.⁶⁰ Despite these notable mentions, the circulation patterns of aromatics in the subsequent periods as materials of exchange in the 'circuits of the Indian Ocean' still remain an almost uncharted territory.⁶¹ The following sections intervene in this gap and attempt to chart the networks of aromatic mobility during the period under consideration.

Perfumes of various aromatic ingredients, obtained from both plant and animal sources and procured from various geographical regions, were processed at perfume factories known as *karkhana*.⁶² Various aromatic ingredients like civet, musk, saffron, lignum aloes, sandalwood, camphor, each with their distinct fragrant properties and cultural significance, were spatially distributed depending on the nature of the soil and the climatic conditions favouring the properties of each ingredient. This procurement entailed a complex network of circulation and mobility over great distances, thereby integrating the various ecological regions with each other and with the global economy.⁶³ For example, saffron or *zafran* was mostly procured inland from the saffron-growing valley of Kashmir.⁶⁴ Saffron was also grown in and around Kishtawar, 'a Himalayan Rajput state lying in very beautiful country to the south-east of Kashmir Valley'⁶⁵, according to Sir Richard Carnac Temple, the twentieth-century editor of Peter Mundy's travel account. It was called 'Saffron Kestwally or *Kishtwari*' whose price was '16 rupees per *ser*'⁶⁶, as noted by Peter Mundy.⁶⁷ Pelsaert noted that Kashmir yields nothing for export to Agra except saffron, of which there are two kinds. That which grows near the city 'sells in Agra at 20 to 24 rupees the *ser*; the other kind, which grows at Casstuwary, 10 *kos*⁶⁸ distant, is the best, and usually fetches 28 to 32 rupees the *ser*'.⁶⁹ John Marshall, the English traveller in India from 1668 to 1672 also pointed out saffron 'was brought from Kashmir (where it grew in abundance) and Nepal to Pattana [Patna] where it is sold for 25 or 30 rupees per *ser*'.⁷⁰

The best of camphor was brought into the Indian subcontinent from Borneo,[71] China (*cina* camphor)[72] and Ceylon (*Ribahi* or *Qaichuri*).[73] It can be argued that the camphor trade was conducted in two routes during this period. One, the route through which camphor travelled from the Borneo and Sumatra islands, the other, the route through which it travelled from China into the manufacturing centres run by the Mughals in India. And distinctly Borneo camphor travelled by sea, from Borneo through Bengal and Masulipatan to Pegu.[74]

Zabad, or civet, came from the territory of Achin of Sumatra, and also made its way into the Mughal court from Africa.[75] The finest quality of musk was obtained from the land of Great Tibet,[76] Bhutan[77] or Kashghar,[78] from where it reached Patna, the principal town of Bengal following the Patna-China route.[79] Ambergris, lignum aloes and frankincense came from the Arabian Peninsula and were traded between 'Islamicate Eurasia'[80] and the Meghna–Brahmaputra Region in the East by the European companies through the port-town of Surat[81] in a 'braided network'.[82] The bulk of sandalwood came from China[83] and the surrounding Timor islands.[84] The European merchants, that is the Portuguese, Dutch and English, were involved in the overseas sandalwood trade in India. Sandalwood was also brought to Agra by the Dutch merchants in moderate quantity from the Portuguese, who obtained it in Timor, and transported it to Malacca, from where it was shipped to Goa and Cambay.[85] The English Factory records suggest that during the middle of the seventeenth century at Surat, the English merchants were actively engaged in the sandalwood trade as part of their 'bulk goods' between Surat and Bantam.[86] There was also a high demand for sandalwood in Basra and it fetched a high price. The Dutch merchants based at Surat in the year 1647 made an attempt to tap the sandalwood market by sending some in a hired vessel.[87] The trade pattern of these aromatics radiated in all directions and depended on the geographical conditions and natural environments in which these raw materials were available. Perfume remained highly dependent on these channels of circulation and modes of procurement.

Tomé Pires, the sixteenth-century Portuguese traveller in India from 1512 to 1515, also noted that great quantities of aromatic ingredients like Borneo camphor, sandalwood and nutmeg were shipped from Malacca to Bengal in four or five ships each year. Merchants from Malacca who went to Bengal had to pay a substantial amount of tax. This was because these goods were of so much value in Bengal and the things they took back were of such high value and so small in bulk that these merchants affirmed that when the goods were brought safely to the harbour and sold, 'the profit on one is from two and half to three'.[88] This trade between Bengal and Malacca was conducted continuously between the months of August and February during the early decades of the sixteenth century.[89]

The early modern port cities[90] of the Indian Ocean region like Surat, Cambay, Goa, Patna and Pegu came to play crucial roles as 'gateways' or 'catalysts' in the movement of the aromatic ingredients across the water as well as further inland to the factories and the workshops. Pegu served as a major entrepot for this trade. To the port of Martaban in the kingdom of Pegu came many ships from Malacca laden with sandalwood, porcelains, frankincense, camphor of Borneo[91] and musk of Arakan.[92] From the mountainous tracts,[93] musk of Arakan was brought to the city of Ava, chief city in the Kingdom of Arakan; from there it was transported to Pegu and from there distributed to Bengal and even to Malacca through inland water routes. Goods passing to and fro in this trade were transported under escorts in boats or carts carrying usually about half a tonne. These aromatic ingredients were then transported from Bengal to Agra by land transport which took around twenty-five to thirty days, often incurring losses due to robbery or damage by rains.[94] The city of Patna had two factories, one English and one Dutch. It was a large city with *bazars* inhabited by merchants. Apart from silk and cotton cloth, the city was known for two other commodities, both of them related to perfumes. One of these was saltpetre, which was produced locally and sent to be stored in Bengal, where it was loaded onto ships destined for various parts of Europe. The other item was one of the rare curiosities that were carried all over the world: perfume bottles and cups of clay. These were made finer than glass and lighter than paper, and usually highly scented.[95] Surat in western India was also another city of commercial significance during this period. Aromatic commodities like musk, amber, myrrh and incense that came to India from the Levant and elsewhere were assembled in Surat, bought by foreign merchants and transported to all parts of the world.[96] The town of Cambay in Gujarat which was as big as Surat but less populous had shops 'full of aromatic perfumes, spices, silk and other stuffs'.[97] Integrating the aromatics into the mercantile environment through the urban and commercial conduits, these port cities formed 'gateways' to a connected and navigable world of material circulation.

Amar Zohar and Efraim Lev have argued that there was a rise of 'New Perfumes' from India with 'the Islamic conquests that opened new trading centres that flooded the markets with goods and prestigious products from all over the world, mainly from South and East Asia'.[98] They suggest that new perfumes in the form of compounds and liquid perfumes were becoming popular in this period, especially with the circulation of aromatics such as camphor, sandalwood, ambergris, saffron and musk within the shared world of commerce and cultural interactions between the Arab world and Asia, particularly India. It was through the tradition of gift-giving and increasing mercantile activities that the 'New Perfume' culture became widespread, replacing and pushing aside two of the most prestigious perfumes of the classical Arabic period and culture: balsam and myrrh.[99] The introduction of rose from Persia in India and the proliferation of rose cultivation was also new to this time and led to the dissemination of the *itr-i-jahangiri*, unique to the Mughal empire.

As a consequence of these developments, aromatic materials in this period were not just objects of sensory pleasure and beauty but players in the South Asian trade networks of the Indian Ocean region. The constant processes of circulation and exchange contributed to the most important step in crediting perfume with the economic status of a recognizable commodity, suggesting early modern India's economic vibrancy and plurality.[100] Moreover, the interconnectedness of the littoral spaces with further inland areas was greased through the constant circulation of aromatics and the people[101] and ideas associated with it. This led to the creation of a space of great aromatic mobility, shared and additionally perfumed by the Indian spices.

Perfumes as a luxury commodity entered the factory system or the *karkhanas* under the patronage of Mughal emperor Akbar, constituting a state-run production economy. The demand for perfumes and the royal pattern of consumption is reflected in the *Ain-i Akbari*'s attestation of the importance of the perfume department of Akbar, the *khushbukhana*, and its inclusion of scents as a luxury commodity for royal use and religious consumption.[102] The *khushbukhana karkhana* was connected to the market by the very processes of acquiring and employing raw materials and craftsmen. Raw materials were purchased from the market and so were craftsmen, hired and paid by the *karkhana*.[103] Due to state-run production or *karkhana* catering to the demands of the court, it was not just a marketed commodity of the period but also an important constituent of the Mughal economy.

The aromatics were progressively integrating with the overall economy both in the form of raw materials as well as finished products of consumption and exchange. By the eighteenth century, perfume was identified as a popular commodity in the *bazaars* of Shahjahanabad.[104] Besides a diverse range of commodities like expensive clothes, carpets, medicinal powders, laxatives, designed cages, exotic birds and animals, large varieties of aromatic compounds were displayed in the *Chowk Sa'adullah Khan* and made available to all buyers.[105] The eighteenth-century Persian text *Muraqqa e Dehli*[106] describes the sale of perfumes (*itryat*) and the activities of the perfume sellers in Delhi with the help of agents (*dalalan*), unnecessary conversations (*fazuli guftuguyei*) and by extending the perfumes to the nostrils of those who wished to visit (*wasayat pishgan be masham arbab khawahsh payam rasan*).[107] This section has been translated by Chander Shekhar and Shama Mitra Chenoy and it states:

> The *Attarwalas*[108] sold varieties of perfumes and essence, and carried out a brisk trade with the help of their agents and smooth talk. Their perfumes send vapours to the minds of its lovers who come to buy them without any beckoning on the part of its shopkeepers.[109]

Sites of perfume-transactions in these urban spaces attracted people for their material properties, sensory qualities, desirability and other use-value. As Farhat Hasan has convincingly demonstrated, *qahwakhanas*, or coffee-houses in Shahjahanabad, Faizabad and other urban centres in the Mughal period were 'sites of sociability' and 'performative public spaces'[110] where people engaged in public opinions, and something similar can be assumed for the spaces selling perfumes at the corner of the streets. These fragrant *itrs*, or perfumes, with their striking properties further helped in attracting greater numbers of people and diverse populations to these vibrant, well-demarcated 'public spaces'. This encouraged more debates, discussions and deliberations, thereby making these spaces even more inclusive, diverse and plural in nature.[111] Coffee carries and dissipates a distinct aroma that can attract people to these sites of friendship. The smell of coffee defined a public culture that grew around the *qahwakhanas*[112] and contributed to the smellscapes of these cities. While fragrance and perfumes created an environment of exchange and camaraderie, there was also the presence of foul[113] smells in the city like that of the stench of the decomposing bodies of those killed during Nadir Shah's invasion of Delhi in 1739, highlighting the urban anxieties. Abhishek Kaicker[114] has described the 'dreadful spectacle' of the city in the aftermath of the invasion and associated the massacre with 'stench of death',[115] where 'putrefying corpses littered the streets for more than a month', 'bodies gnawed on by dogs and cats, choked the streets', some corpses were thrown in the river of Jamuna and it was impossible to conduct proper funeral rites of the rest of the burnt and rotting corpses. The remains of many who had been trapped inside their burning houses could not be excavated from the rubble, and the stench of death 'was a source of discomfort to the people' in some neighbourhoods for six months or a year'.[116] Najaf Haider also pointed out how during the 1729 shoe sellers' riot in Shahjahanabad (Mughal India), the dead body of the murdered shoe-seller Haji Hafiz was decided not to be buried and left at the door of the murderer till justice was met.[117] Even though the smell is not explicitly discussed in the account but it can be assumed from these recurrent narratives of conflict and massacre that the stench of decomposing bodies was integral to the smellscape of the city. Adding to it, the diverse range of commodities housed and sold in the market like food items, cooked food, aphrodisiacs, laxatives, glass objects, clothes,[118] fruits, shoe and other leather objects[119] had their own distinct smells further accentuating the olfactory identity of these public spaces.

As integral to public spaces and as urban hubs of mercantile activities, these great central *bazaars* of *Chandni Chawk*, *Faiz Bazar* and *Chawk Sa'adullah Khan* catered to the entire city of Shahjahanabad, the 'sovereign city of the Mughal empire', as described by Stephen Blake. At the apex of the urban hierarchy, they catered to the imperial household, the *amirs* and the nobles.[120] At the same time, they performed the role of markets and the economic functions unique to the city which drew customers from the entire empire as well as from the city at large.[121] With regards to the merchants, the foreign and domestic merchants who supplied these *bazaars* were not members of elite households. Unlike client merchants who worked only with household officials to obtain grains, vegetables, fruits and likes, these men arranged their own schedules, controlled their own goods and sold to many customers. And in a pursuit to find personal niches in the marketplace, the merchants particularly trading in materials like jewels, precious clothes and perfumes developed manners and ways to attach themselves to the great households and great men. Within this economic milieu, perfumes featured as an affordable and desirable commodity to these men and alliances with at least three to four such households rendered profit to these merchants.[122] These markets in which perfume had been commercialized increasingly became spaces for the confluence of people and a diverse range of goods.[123]

While perfume was a recognizable commodity during the Mughal period, there was the possibility of an identifiable professional group of perfumers or perfume-trader during this period. Banarasidas, a local Jain Merchant primarily trading in precious stones, based in Jaunpur during the heyday of Mughal rule in 1641, can be seen in the seventeenth-century autobiographical account *The Ardhakathanaka* (Half A Tale), carrying and exchanging seven kilos of costly perfume-*phulel*. It was perfumed oil with the essence of flower and exchanged for appeasement to the *hakim*, the *diwan* and the *kotwal*, 'giving to each a share keeping with his rank' to settle trade disputes.[124] Although often denigrated for their liminality and having their own forms of social honours which were embedded not in economic activities or profit-making ventures but in the religious traditions of pleasing and displeasing goddesses, the mere presence of

Hindu or Jain merchants in the commercial milieu is noteworthy here.[125] Even as late as the eighteenth century, perfume sellers and distillers continued to thrive in the big towns of Bengal such as Dhaka, as a significant professional group among a wide array of specialized groups dealing in a wide range of commodities and services, making up a sizeable proportion of the population.[126] Manucci mentions a story where one of Ja'far Khan's[127] grooms made a profit by selling twenty-five ounces of rosewater perfume that he had accumulated during the years of its abundance. During the early years of the eighteenth century, he sold that quantity at fifty rupees per ounce during a period of scarcity 'which placed him in easy circumstances, to the astonishment of those who heard the story'.[128] The relevance of this episode lies in the economic quantification and transaction of perfumes that assigns an exchange-value to the commodity in the urban milieu of trade and mercantilism of the period.

Besides the growing trade in perfumes and proliferation of markets[129] selling perfumes, there were also instances of periodical consumption of perfumes[130] reflected in ballads, court literature, travel accounts and other archival records, even at the regional level, like in eighteenth-century Bengal.[131] Mercantile activities catering to the demand and consumption of perfumes suggest the emergence of a vibrant market economy for perfumes during this period. A 'deodorized'[132] mercantilism contributed to the overall mercantile early modern environment, marked by urbanization and commercial growth.

Conclusion

Perfume represented in the various historical sources produced in this period has a distinct material identity and function of its own. Despite their ephemerality, perfumes assumed a sociocultural material presence, their healing effect and bodily affect valued by the Mughal authority and the imperial nobility during this period. The Mughals held the sensory-stimulus of perfume essential for their curative and remedial measures to maintain the good health of individual and collective bodies. Usage of various aromatics and their associated bodily practices, thereby, remained integral to the Persianate aesthetics and cultural regimes of the Mughals. 'Aristocratic culture and political power'[133] further facilitated the consumption practices and commercial activities of the perfumes. This not only boosted the social position of the ruling authorities but also strengthened the economic resilience of agriculture-based artisanal products and the craftsmanship associated with them.[134] Perfume actively participated in the early modern trade and commerce that integrated the merchants, markets and trade routes into a shared aromatic network along the Indian Ocean littoral arc. Famed perfumes like *argaja, itr-i-jahangiri* and *bid-i-mushk* became a part of the material-cultural identity of the early modern commercial milieu and urban public spaces catering to larger consumer demands. Urban public spaces in early modern India came to be gradually defined, culturally and commercially, by smell.

With this 'olfactory flashback', the article has foregrounded the materiality and mobility of Mughal perfumes as therapeutic commodities. By focusing on the various instances of sensory experiences, perfumery practices and aromatic circulations enacted in the Mughal polity and maritime spaces of exchange, the study has revealed the importance of ephemeral objects in the material culture of the early modern world.

Notes

1 This article is part of my MPhil dissertation on the Perfumery Culture in Mughal India done under the supervision of Professor Syed Najaf Haider. I am indebted to him for his continuous guidance and support in the course of the work. Grateful thanks to Professors Chander Shekhar, Rajat Datta, Pius Malekandathil, Yogesh Sharma and Tilottama Mukherjee for their constant encouragement and comments over the years. A section of this article was presented at the international workshop on 'Health and Materiality: Histories of Health, Medicine and Trade across Cultures, 1600–2000' organized in collaboration with the University of Warwick and the Centre for Historical Studies, Jawaharlal Nehru University (JNU), and held at JNU, 2018. I am thankful to Professor David Arnold for his valuable suggestions. Professors Burton Cleetus and Anne Gerritsen have guided me to develop the final paper with their minute readings, insights and detailed comments. I am deeply grateful to them.

2 Anne Gerritsen and Giorgio Riello, 'Introduction', in *Writing Material Culture History*, ed. Anne Gerritsen and Giorgio Riello (London and New York: Bloomsbury, 2015), 3.

3 Alain Corbin, *The Foul and The Fragrant: Odor and the French Social Imagination* (Cambridge, MA: Harvard University Press, 1986); Constance Classen, David Howes and Anthony Synnott, *Aroma: The Cultural History of Smell* (London: Routledge, 1994); Holly Dugan, *Ephemeral History of Perfume: Scent and Sense in Early Modern England* (Baltimore: John Hopkins University Press, 2011).

4 Parashuram Krishna Gode, *Studies in Indian Cultural History Vol. 1* (Hoshiarpur: Vishveshvaranand Vedic Research Institute, 1961); David Shulman, 'The Scent of

Memory in Hindu South India', *RES: Anthropology and Aesthetics* 13 (1987): 122–33; Ali Akbar Husain, *Scent in the Islamic Garden: A Study of Deccani Urdu Literary Sources* (Karachi: Oxford University Press, 2000); James McHugh, *Sandalwood and Carrion: Smell in Indian Religion and Culture* (New York: Oxford University Press, 2012); Emma J. Flatt, 'Spices, Smell and Spells: The Use of Olfactory Substances in the Conjuring of Spirits' *South Asian Studies* 32, no. 1 (2016): 3–21.

5 Despite the limitation of the term and problems of the periodization of 'early modern', in India it is used to bracket 'the years from the onset of Mughal rule in 1526 to the final victory of the British Raj in the Mutiny of 1857–58'. Jack A. Goldstone, 'The Problem of the "Early Modern" World', *Journal of the Economic and Social History of the Orient* 41, no. 3 (1998): 255.

6 Claude Levi-Strauss, 'History and Anthropology', in Claude Levi-Strauss, *Structural Anthropology, Volume I*, trans. Clair Jacobson and Brooke Grundfest Shoepf (New York: Basic Books, 1963), 9.

7 Here, the chapter focuses on the period between sixteenth to eighteenth century in India, when the Mughal empire was at the helm of political affairs.

8 At the heart of this term resides Appudurai and Kopytoff's concept of 'object-biography'. The basic tenet of this biographical approach is that all artefacts had, and indeed have social lives, a study of that links people and things and how objects are understood to accumulate lives as they repeatedly move between people; see Arjun Appadurai, 'Introduction: Commodities and the Politics of Value', in *The Social Life of Things: Commodities in Cultural Perspectives*, ed. Arjun Appadurai (Cambridge: Cambridge University Press, 1986), 3–63; Igor Kopytoff, 'The Cultural Biography of Things: Commoditization as Process', in *The Social Life of Things: Commodities in Cultural Perspective*, ed. Arjun Appadurai (Cambridge: Cambridge University Press, 1986), 64; Chris Gosden and Yvonne Marshall, 'The Cultural Biography of Objects', *World Archaeology* 31, no. 2 (1991): 169–78; Harold Mytum, 'Artefact Biography as an Approach to Material Culture: Irish Gravestones as a Material Form of Genealogy', *The Journal of Irish Archaeology* 12/13 (2003–2004): 111–27.

9 Flatt, 'Spices, Smell and Spells', 9.

10 See Muzaffar Alam, 'Sharia, Akhlaaq & Governance', in *The Language of Political Islam in Indian 1200–1800*, ed. Muzaffar Alam (New Delhi: Permanent Black, 2004), 26–80; Seema Alavi, 'Medical Culture in Transition: Mughal Gentleman Physician and the Native Doctor in Early Colonial India', *Modern Asian Studies* 42, no. 5 (September 2008): 853–97.

11 Bruno Latour, 'The Berlin Key or How to Do Words with Things', in *Matter, Materiality and Modern Culture*, ed. P. Graves-Brown (London: Routledge, 2000), 10–21.

12 P. K. Gode in his work draws upon a wide range of texts to show the cultural and medical presence of aromatics in Indian history; Gode, *Studies in Indian Cultural History*, 3–100.

13 Ibid., 5.
14 Husain, *Scent in the Islamic Garden*, 73–5.
15 Ibid., 71.
16 David Gilmartin and Bruce B. Lawrence, eds, *Beyond Turk and Hindu: Rethinking Religious Identities in Islamicate South Asia* (Gainesville, FL: University Press of Florida, 2000), 2.
17 Flatt, 'Spices, Smell and Spells'.
18 See McHugh, *Sandalwood and Carrion*, 3.
19 Ibid., 73–5.
20 Husain, *Scent in the Islamic Garden,* 131; Also in Flatt, 'Spices, Smell and Spells'.
21 It is an Indic word for betel leaves and betel leaf preparations that act as a stimulant consumed orally.
22 Anonymous, 'Introduction', in *The Ni'matnama Manuscript of the Sultans of Mandu: The Sultan's Book of Delight*, trans. Norah Titley (London and New York: Routledge Curzon, 2005), 50.
23 Ibid., 53.
24 It refers to any form of distilled liquid.
25 *Itr* or *attar* is the Persian word for perfume, scents, essences or essential oils.
26 Abul Fazl, *The Ain-i-Akbari,* Vol. 1, trans. H. Blochmann and H. S. Jarrett (Calcutta: Baptist Mission Press, 1873), 73–74; also in R. Nath, *Private Life of The Mughals of India (1526–1803 A.D.)* (New Delhi: Rupa Publications, 2013), 108.
27 Rose-perfume was discovered by the Mughal Empress Noor Jahan and named after Emperor Jahangir, signifying and immortalizing his rule.
28 Nur-al-din Muhammad Jahangir Gur Kani, *Tuzuk-i-Jahangiri/Jahangirnama (1628)* (Tehran: Iran Cultural Foundation/*Bunyad-i-Farhang-i-Iran*, 2000), 154. My translation of this section has drawn on the following translations: Jahangir, *The Tuzuk-i-Jahangiri*; 2 Vols, ed. Syed Ahmed Aligarh, 1863–1864; trans. Alexander Rogers and Henry Beveridge (London: Royal Asiatic Society, 1909–1914, reprint, Delhi, 1989), 271–2; Jahangir, *The Jahangirnama: Memoirs of Jahangir, Emperor of India*, trans. and ed. Wheeler M. Thackston (Oxford and New York: Oxford University Press, 1999), 163.
29 Anonymous, *Bayaz i Khushbui,* British Library, MS Or. 828, ff. 5a-12a. Here, I extend my heartfelt gratitude to Professor Chandershekhar for his generousness and constant encouragement in helping me translate this section of the manuscript and carefully pointing out the delicacy of it.
30 See Daud Ali, 'Padmasri's Nagarasarvasva and the World of Medieval Kamasastra', *Journal of Indian Philosophy* 39, no. 1 (2011): 45; Padmasri, *Nagarasarvasva*, ed. Bhagirathwami and Rajdhar Jha (Kalkutta: Srivenkateswar Pustak Agency, 1929), 23–4.
31 *Falanj* or فلنجه (A red seed used as a perfume), Francis Joseph Steingass, *A Comprehensive Persian-English Dictionary* (New Delhi: Manohar, 2008), 938.

32 Francisco Palsaert, *Jahangir's India: The Remonstratie of F. Palsaert*, ed. W. H. Moreland and P. Geyl (Cambridge: W. Heffer & Sons, Ltd., 1925), 64.

33 Niccolao Manucci, *Storio do Mogor*, Vol. II, trans. William Irwine (London: Royal Asiatic Society, 1907), 340–1.

34 Shaikh Farid Bhakkari, *The Dhakhirat Ul-Khawanin of Shaikh Farid Bhakkari: A Biographical Dictionary of Mughal Noblemen Part One*, trans. Ziyaud-Din A. Desai (Delhi: Idarah-I Adabiyat-I Delli, 2009), 139–40.

35 Francois Bernier, *Travels in the Mogul Empire 1656–1668*, trans. Irving Broke, annotated Archibald Constable, 2nd rev. ed. Vincent A. Smith (London: Oxford University Press, 1916), 222.

36 Peter Mundy, *The Travels of Peter Mundy in Europe and Asia 1608–1667* Vol. II, ed. R. C. Temple (London: Hakluyt Society, 1914), 161–2.

37 Ibid.

38 Manucci, *Storio do Mogor*, Vol. I, 219.

39 Inayat Khan, *The Shahjahannama: An Abridged History of the Mughal Emperor Shah Jahan*, trans. A. R. Fuller, ed. and completed W. E. Begley and Z. A. Desai (Delhi: Oxford University Press, 1990), 309–10.

40 Manucci, *Storio do Mogor*, Vol. I, 301–4.

41 Rosalind O'Hanlon and Aziz Ahmed in their respective works draw upon a range of sources, biographical accounts of noblemen, and lexicons to define *mirza* as 'an abbreviation of the word *amir*, the term from the fifteenth century onwards in the Islamicate world has been used as a suffixed title for kings, princes and later by noblemen. In India, it was particularly added to close kinsmen of the Mughals and to others with Timurid and Safavid ancestry. The title was sometimes simply assumed by men who were high born, pretended to the right lineage; it could also be granted by the emperor. In India, however, *mirza* and the qualities of *mirzai* associated with it came increasingly to have a rather different secondary sense, which brought it close to the sense of personal and moral cultivation in *adab* and refinement in civility, manners, taste and connoisseurship'. Rosalind O'Hanlon, 'Manliness and Imperial Service In Mughal North India', *Journal Of The Economic And Social History of the Orient* 42, no. 1 (1999): 70–1; Aziz Ahmed, 'The British Museum Mirzanama and the Seventeenth Century Mirza In India', *Iran* 13 (1975): 108.

42 Thorstein Veblen, *The Theory of Leisure Class* (London: Transaction Publishers, 1929), 41–75.

43 O'Hanlon, 'Manliness and Imperial Service', 82.

44 See Muzaffar Alam, *The Languages of Political Islam, India 1200–1800* (London: Hurst and Company, 2004) and Rosalind O'Hanlon, 'Kingdom, Household and Body History, Gender and Imperial Service under Akbar', *Modern Asian Studies* 41, no. 5 (2007): 889–923.

45 Classen, Howes, and Synnott, *Aroma*, 123.
46 Scent or essence of the flower *fitna*. A species of mimosa or acacia, bearing flowers and having a powerful scent.
47 Musk-willow, celebrated for its fragrance. Duncan Forbes, *A Dictionary, Hindustani and English*, 2nd ed. (London: W. H. Allen & Co., 1866), 155.
48 A perfume of a yellowish colour compounded of several scented ingredients (one receipt specifies *sandal, rose-water, camphor, musk, ambergris* and *butter* as the ingredients); John T. Platts, *A Dictionary of Urdu, Classical Hindi and English* (London: W. H. Allen & Co., 1884), 41.
49 Saqi Must'ad Khan, *Maasir-I-Alamgiri*, trans. and annotated Sir Jadunath Sarkar (Kolkata: Asiatic Society, 2008), 21–2; Khan, *The Shahjahannama*, 62–3; 254.
50 Khan, *The Shahjahannama*, 500.
51 Ashin Das Gupta, 'Introduction II: The Story', in *India and the Indian Ocean, 1500–1800*, ed. Ashin Das Gupta and M. N. Pearson (Calcutta: Oxford University Press, 1987), 28; Michael Pearson, *The Indian Ocean* (London and New York: Routledge, 2003), 113.
52 Pius Malekandathil, 'Introduction', in *Maritime Trade: Trade, Religion and Polity in the Indian Ocean* (New Delhi: Primus Books, 2013), xiii.
53 S. Arasaratnam, 'India and the Indian Ocean in the Seventeenth Century', in *India and the Indian Ocean, 1500–1800*, ed. Ashin Das Gupta and M. N. Pearson (Calcutta: Oxford University Press, 1987), 97.
54 Ruth Barnes, ed., *Textiles in Indian Ocean Studies* (London and New York: Routledge, 2005).
55 Ghulam A. Nadri, *The Political Economy of Indigo in India, 1580–1930: A Global Perspective* (Leiden: Brill, 2016).
56 C. R. Boxer, 'A Note on Portuguese Reactions to the Revival of the Red Sea Spice Trade and the Rise of Atjeh, 1540–1600', *Journal of Southeast Asian History* 10, no. 3 (1969): 415–28.
57 Corbin, *The Foul and the Fragrant*.
58 K. N. Chaudhuri, *Trade and Civilisation in the Indian Ocean: An Economic History from the Rise of Islam to 1750* (Cambridge: Cambridge University Press, 1985), 189–90.
59 Genevieve Bouchon and Denys Lombard, 'The Indian Ocean in The Fifteenth Century', in *India and Indian Ocean 1500–1800*, ed. Ashin Das Gupta and M. N. Pearson (Calcutta: Oxford University Press, 1987), 53–4.
60 Ibid., 52.
61 Malekandathil, 'Introduction', xiii.
62 Bouchon and Lombard, 'The Indian Ocean in the Fifteenth Century', 52.
63 McHugh, *Sandalwood and Carrion*, 8.
64 Giovani Francesco Gemelli Careri, *Indian Travels of Thevenot and Careri*, ed. Surendranath Sen (New Delhi: National Archives of India, 1949), 205; Fazl, *The*

Ain-i-Akbari, 84–5; William Finch, *Early Travels in India 1583–1619*, ed. William Foster (New Delhi: Low Price Publications, 2007), 169.
65 Mundy, *The Travels of Peter Mundy*, 154.
66 Seer or ser is an Indic expression used to denote commodity-weight during this period.
67 Mundy, *The Travels of Peter Mundy*, 154.
68 An Indic term or unit of measurement used during this period denoting distance. It was originally signified 'a call', hence the distance at which a man's call can be heard. 'The *kos* as laid down in the *Ain* was of 5000 *gaz*. The official decision of the British Government has assigned the length of Akbar's *Ilāhī gaz* as 33 inches, and this would make Akbar's *kos* = 2m. 4f. 183⅓ yards.' See 'Coss' in Henry Yule and A. C. Burnell, *Hobson-Jobson: A Glossary of Colloquial Anglo-Indian Words and Phrases and of Kindred Terms, Etymological, Historical, Geographical and Discursive* ([1886] Cambridge University Press, 2010), 202.
69 Palsaert, *Jahangir's India*, 35–6.
70 John Marshall, *John Marshall in India: Notes and Observations in Bengal, 1668–1672*, ed. Shafaat Ahmad Khan (London: Oxford University Press, H. Milford, 1927), 413.
71 Ralph Fitch, *England's Pioneer to India and Burma: His Companions and Contemporaries*, trans. J. Horton Ryley (London: T. Fisher Unwin, 1899), 189.
72 Thakkura Pheru, *Dravya Pariksha aur Dhatutpatti*, ed. B. Nahta (Vaisali: Research Institute of Prakriti Jinalogy and Ahimsa, 1976), 17.
73 Named after an island in Ceylon; Fazl, *The Ain-i-Akbari*, 78–9.
74 Fitch, *England's Pioneer to India and Burma*, 161.
75 Bernier, *Travels in the Mogul Empire 1656–1668*, 135–7.
76 Ibid., 427.
77 Jean Baptiste Tavernier, *Travels in India*, Vol. *II*, trans. V. Ball (London: Macmillan & Co, 1889), 143.
78 Finch, *Early Travels in India 1583–1619*, 168–70.
79 Bernier, *Travels in the Mogul Empire 1656–1668*, 426–7.
80 Gagan D. S. Sood, 'Circulation and the Exchange in Islamicate Eurasia: A Regional Approach to the Early Modern World', *Past & Present* 212, no. 1 (2011): 113–62.
81 *The English Factories in India 1642–1645: A Calendar of Documents In The India Office, British Museum and the Public Records Office, ETC.*, ed. William Foster (Oxford: Clarendon Press, 1913), 7, 139.
82 Rila Mukherjee, 'Introduction: Bengal and the Northern Bay of Bengal', in *Pelagic Passageways: The Northern Bay of Bengal before Colonialism*, ed. Rila Mukherjee (Delhi: Primus Books, 2011), 27
83 Fitch, *England's Pioneer to India and Burma*, 59.
84 Careri, *Indian Travels of Thevenot and Careri*, 197.
85 Palsaert, *Jahangir's India*, 25.

86 *The English Factories in India 1630–1633: A Calendar Of Documents In The India Office, Bombay Record Office, ETC.*, ed. William Foster (Oxford: Clarendon Press, 1914), 111; *The English Factories in India 1634–1636: A Calendar Of Documents In The India Office, British Museum and The Public Record Office*, ed. William Foster (Oxford: Clarendon Press, 1911), 296; *The English Factories in India 1637–1641: A Calendar of Documents In The India Office, British Museum and The Public Record Office*, ed. William Foster (Oxford: Clarendon Press, 1911), 173.

87 *The English Factories in India 1646–1650: A Calendar of Documents In The India Office, Westminster*, ed. William Foster (Oxford: Clarendon Press, 1914), 111.

88 Even though Pires doesn't mention the exact currency in which profits were made, it can be assumed from his own description that in Bengal most of the transactions were carried out either in gold or silver coinage or *tanqat* or *taka*. The silver coinage was worth twenty *calains* (Malaccan tin currency) in Malacca and seven *cahon* in Bengal. And each *cahon* was worth 1,280 *kury* or cowries and a *tanqat* was worth 8,960 cowries. Cowries were valid throughout Bengal and accepted for a large number of commodities. Hence, considering these are valuable goods and these were voluminous overseas transactions, presumably, the profit made on one commodity in Bengal had a margin of two to three *tanqats*; Tomé Pires and Francisco Rodrigues, *The Suma Oriental of Tomé Pires: An Account of the East, from the Red Sea to Japan, written in Malacca and India, 1512–1525 and The Book of Francisco Rodrigues: Rutter of a Voyage in the Red Sea, Nautical Rules, Alamanack and Maps, written and drawn in the East Before 1515*, Vol. 1, trans. Armando Cortesao (London: Hakluyt Society, 1944), 93–4.

89 Pires and Rodrigues, *The Suma Oriental of Tomé Pires*, 93.

90 Rila Mukherjee, ed., *Vanguards of Globalization: Port-Cities from the Classical to the Modern* (Delhi: Primus Books, 2014).

91 Fitch, *England's Pioneer to India and Burma*, 165–6.

92 Pires and Rodrigues, *The Suma Oriental of Tomé Pires*, 96.

93 Musk was obtained from the goats of the mountainous tracts of Arakan by a group of local people; Ibid., 96.

94 Mundy, *The Travels of Peter Mundy*, 369.

95 Manucci, *Storio do Mogor*, Vol. II, 83–4.

96 Jean de Thevenot, *The Travels of Monsieur de Thevenot into the Levant Part III: The Relation of Indostan, the New Moguls and of other People and Countries of the Indies* (Booksellers: London, 1687), 17.

97 Ibid., 12.

98 Amar Zohar and Efraim Lev, 'Trends in the Use of Perfumes and Incense in the Near East after the Muslim Conquests', *Journal of the Royal Asiatic Society* 23, no. 1 (2013): 28–9.

99 Ibid., 27.
100 Kopytoff, 'The Cultural Biography of Things', 73.
101 'It was the trading world of the Indian Ocean that brought "people of different races – English, Portuguese, French, Dutch, Chinese, Bengalis, Burmese, Tamils and Malays" – into contact and into conflict.' Sunil S. Amrith, *Crossing the Bay of Bengal: The Furies of Nature and the Fortunes of Migrants* (Cambridge, MA: Harvard University Press, 2013), 283.
102 Fazl, *The Ain-i-Akbari*, 76.
103 Sumbul Halim Khan, *Art and Craft Workshop under the Mughals: A Study of Jaipur Karkhanas* (New Delhi: Primus Books, 2015), 2.
104 The two major thoroughfares in Shahjahanabad were called *bazaars*, streets lined on both sides with shops of merchants, artisans and others. The largest and richest stretched from the Lahori gate of the fort to the Fathpuri mosque, which later came to be known as Chandni Chowk or Moonlight square. Stephen Blake, *Shahjahanabad, The Sovereign City in Mughal India 1639–1739* (Cambridge: Cambridge University Press, 1991), 55–6.
105 Dargah Quli Khan, *Muraqqa e Dehli: The Mughal Capital In Muhammad Shah's Time*, trans. Chander Shekhar and Shama Mitra Chenoy (New Delhi: Deputy Publication, 1989), 21–3.
106 Even though the text remains a much-cited work, it is almost impossible to ignore its richness on the urban culture of the city in the eighteenth century.
107 Dargah Quli Khan, *Muraqqa i Dehli*, ed. and trans. Khaliq Anjum (New Delhi: Samsar Offset Printers, 1993, Persian text), 60–1; The translation of the phrases in this sentence has been done by me.
108 Perfume sellers.
109 Khan, trans. Shekhar and Chenoy, *Muraqqa e Dehli*, 24–5.
110 Farhat Hasan, 'Forms of Civility and Publicness in Pre-British India', in *Civil Society, Public Sphere, and Citizenship: Dialogues and Perceptions*, ed. Rajeev Bhargava and Helmut Reifeld (New Delhi: Sage Publications, 2005), 102–5; Farhat Hasan, *Paper, Performance and the State: Social Change and Political Culture in Mughal India* (Cambridge: Cambridge University Press, 2021), 92.
111 Hasan, 'Forms of civility and publicness in pre-British India'.
112 See Khan, trans. Shekhar and Chenoy, *Muraqqa e Dehli*, 25.
113 See Corbin, *The Foul and The Fragrant*.
114 Abhishek Kaicker, *The King and the People: Sovereignty and Popular Politics in Mughal India* (New York: Oxford University Press, 2020); He looks at the unpublished text *Tarikh i Shahadat Farrukhsiyar wa Julus i Muhammad Shah* by Muhammad Bakhsh 'Ashob'.
115 Kaicker, *The King and the People*, 45.
116 Ibid., 44–5.

117 Najaf Haider, 'Violence and Defiance of Authority in Mughal India: A Study of the Shoe Sellers' Riot of Shahjahanabad', *Studies in History* 36, no. 2 (2020): 163–77.

118 Abhishek Kaicker in his work mentions the common practice of men like Lutf Allah Khan (an important Mughal courtier who survived the Nadir Shah invasion but fell into disgrace for disloyalty; his son served the Mughals afterwards) visiting Mughal court in the eighteenth-century wearing clothes smelling of the 'stench of the tailor's urine'. This information also reflects on the foul smells of the period; See Kaicker, *The King and the People*, 24, 85.

119 Haider, 'Violence and Defiance of Authority in Mughal India', 164; Khan, trans. Shekhar and Chenoy, *Muraqqa e Dehli*, 4–5.

120 Blake, *Shahjahanabad*, 121.

121 Ibid., 118–19.

122 Stephen Blake, 'The Urban Economy in Premodern Muslim India: Shahjahanabad 1639–1739', *Modern Asian Studies* 21, no. 3 (1987): 470.

123 Aziz Ahmed's translation of *Mirzanama* shows that during the seventeenth century there was a persistent expectation from the *Mirzas* to conserve their class exclusivity by deliberately maintaining a segregation of their spaces from the space of *bazaars*, in terms of spatial aesthetics, material choices and habits. Ahmed, 'The British Museum Mirzanama and the Seventeenth-Century Mirza in India', 101–6.

124 Banarasidas, *The Ardhakathanaka (Half A Tale)*, ed. and trans. Mukund Lath (Jaipur: Prakriti Bharati Sanasthan, 1981), 71–7.

125 David Curley, '"Tribute Exchange" and the Liminality of Foreign Merchants in Mukunda's Candimangal', in his *Poetry and History: Bengali Mangal-kavya and Social Change in Precolonial Bengal* (New Delhi: Chronicle Books, 2008), 117.

126 Tilottama Mukherjee, *Political Culture and Economy in Eighteenth-Century Bengal: Networks of Exchange, Consumption and Communication* (New Delhi: Orient Black Swan, 2013), 67.

127 Manucci describes Ja'far Khan as a merchant who had the responsibility for providing a great amir's household with vegetables during a trip to Kashmir. Manucci, *Storio do Mogor*, Vol. III, 416. Stephen Blake also mentions him as one of the client merchants of the time. See Blake, 'The Urban Economy in Premodern Muslim India: Shahjahanabad. 1639–1739', 468.

128 Manucci, *Storio do Mogor*, Vol. III, 416–17.

129 Sanjay Subrahmanyam, ed., *Merchants, Markets and the State in Early Modern India* (New Delhi: Oxford University Press, 1990); Rajat Datta, *Society, Economy and the Market. Commercialization in Rural Bengal c. 1760–1800* (Delhi: Manohar Publishers, 2000), Kumkum Chatterjee, *Merchants, Politics and Society in Early Modern India, Bihar: 1733–1820* (Leiden: Brill, 1996).

130 Tilottama Mukherjee, 'Markets in Eighteenth Century Bengal Economy', *Indian Economic and Social History Review* 48, no. 2 (2011): 168.

131 Ibid., 144.
132 McHugh, *Sandalwood and Carrion,* 246.
133 Tilottama Mukherjee, 'The Co-Ordinating State and the Economy: The Nizamat in Eighteenth-Century Bengal', *Modern Asian Studies* 43, no. 2 (2009): 435.
134 Ibid., 435.

6

Letters to the Vaidyan

The circulation of Ayurvedic drugs and knowledge from Kottakkal Aryavaidyasala to South-east Asia

Burton Cleetus

Introduction

Therapeutic practices of the Indian subcontinent underwent considerable strain after the influence of Western medicine under British colonialism. As a response, the emerging elite within indigenous medicine sought to reposition contemporary medical practices of the late nineteenth and the twentieth centuries within the broad ambit of the classical Sanskrit textual tradition.[1] The modernization of Ayurveda was possible by establishing medical schools and clinics and standardizing drug production following the classical texts. Scholars identify this as 'revitalisation', a means of negotiating Indian medical traditions with the challenges posed by Western medicine and thereby crafting a distinct identity for Ayurveda that was capable of meeting the challenges of twentieth-century contemporary needs.[2] I argue that the negotiation between the practitioner and the patient in shaping twentieth-century Ayurveda remains an essential element in its transition to modernity. By engaging with the patient files at the Kottakkal Aryavaidyasala, a clinic in the south-western Indian state of Kerala, this chapter engages with the changing world of disease and cure under colonial contexts.

Migration, mobility and the changing world of disease

Reminiscing on his maternal uncle, who died of malaria in the 1930s in Assam, George Francis spoke of the pervasive intrusions of colonial modernity into a small hamlet in Kerala in the early decades of the twentieth century.

in those days, he says, the government recruited people from Kollam to clear the forest and make it suitable for tea cultivation. Each unit had 800 men and was hired from various parts of the district, promising to pay one rupee per day. To get rid of terrible poverty, he (his uncle) went to Assam. He was deeply attached to his mother, hence was tormented to leave her. Depressed and miserable of being away from home, he fell ill, like many others, of malaria and died.[3]

Colonialism for him was about migration, mobility, disease and death. By the early decades of the twentieth century, the colonial state had extended its reach to the remotest corners of the subcontinent. For the indigenous societies, it was about a passionate desire to change the material conditions of life, though accompanied by the painful separation from family and community in a different and challenging terrain, which in the last instance was felled by disease and sealed by death.

Located in the north-eastern frontier region of the Indian subcontinent, the British province of Assam had emerged as a global supplier of tea by the early decades of the twentieth century. Large-scale labour was necessary for clearing the woods and preparing the ground for tea plantations. Commercial cultivation of crops also opened up new opportunities for the educated as clerks and managers.[4] As commercial cultivation of tea, rubber and teak occurred across the eastern borders of the subcontinent, there was an intense dislocation of people to new geographical spaces. Migration brought about a sense of alienation, which had a profound effect on the bodies and minds of the people. Fear of physical and mental violation and attempts to regain the self profoundly impacted indigenous therapeutic imaginations.

Krishnan Vaidyan, an Ayurvedic physician from Mayyanad, a region in southern Kerala from where large-scale labour migration occurred, notes in his diary as follows: 'the balance of the bile and phlegm came to be disturbed in the new and alien environment of the tobacco plantations of Jaffna in Ceylon'. According to him, this was due to the higher temperature of Ceylon than in Kerala. He further argues that disease emerged when the migrant set foot in Jaffna, though it manifests only at a stage in which the body could no longer withstand the adversities of harsh climatic conditions. Such migration, he notes, had altered the bodily constitutions of migrant bodies. The migrant body was further disturbed by tobacco consumption and untimely food intake. Krishnan Vaidyan hopes that people, irrespective of their travel and work, have faith in the efficacy of Ayurveda as a means of rejuvenating the body.[5]

Colonialism and medicine

Scholarly thoughts on Indian modernization under colonialism were primarily concerned with the rise of political movements in India. The idea that health, bodies and medicine were integral to the state and its political practice was recognized, in academic writings, only by the closing decades of the twentieth century. Sivaramakrishnan argues that the desire among Ayurvedic physicians for power and prestige within indigenous societies shaped the movement towards institutionalization.[6] Thus, morbidity and cure were central to the changing ideological and social contexts of late nineteenth- and early twentieth-century India.

The emergence of bounded geography, a sanctified historical past shaped by its cultural traditions, defined the nation among the newly educated elite.[7] Yet beneath this enthusiasm for the nation and its historical and cultural pasts lay a desire to streamline Ayurveda by purging localized medicinal practices and moving towards a homogenous national therapeutic identity. Such centralizing tendencies also took regional forms, as linguistic differences gave Ayurveda a distinctly regional flavour. Nevertheless, as medicine was cultural and social, as much as bodily, multiple perceptions and practices of the body thrived among local communities and groups.

In the new context, the Malayalam-speaking region, which later formed the state of Kerala, united primarily by language, its climate and ecology were desired by the migrants as the panacea to bodily ailments in an age marked by constant fluctuations and displacements. Migrants conceived geographies outside their homeland as generating disease. Thus, neither the humoral imbalance depicted in the classical Sanskrit texts nor putrid geographies that predominated colonial concerns, rather alien terrains, were the primary cause of morbidity. Thus, in the new conception of disease causation, places themselves were not inherently diseased, but these unfamiliar spaces, not in tune with the bodies of the migrants, caused disease.

Disease in the new context resulted from geographical displacement, yet it was also a manifestation of moral, social and cultural compromises. As people migrated to new geographical zones, they felt that they had become vulnerable to the pleasures of the body and, therefore, the mind. To be dislocated from a geographical location meant alienation, a crisis that brought about long-term emotional and physical stress leading to the drain of vital energy. Yet dislocation and alienation were closely interlinked with the more significant ideological concerns generated under colonialism.[8] Migration only accentuated and manifested a reality emerging under colonialism as it brought to the fore a sense of being and the consciousness of loss.

Colonialism and migration

The British administration located places and people belonging to different regional, caste and linguistic spaces through an elaborate mapping network.[9] The framing of the tropics also shaped European understandings of morbidity within India. Miasmas, putrefaction and poisons shaped tropical climatic zones, an idea closely connected to the ideological necessities of colonialism in India. James Johnson, William Twining and others saw the human body as a microcosm of the environment, with social and environmental dissolution reflected in bodily decay.[10] British concerns with Indian medicine often preferred the classical texts over contemporary therapeutic practices. Arnold describes British interest in Indian medicine as primarily twofold. First, it was to understand the 'medicine' of the Hindus, as represented through the classical Sanskrit texts and, second, to locate plants and their medicinal uses to expand British pharmacopoeia.[11]

Contemporary medical traditions of the indigenous societies were localized and bounded within the social and religious world.[12] The *vaidyan* (physician) commanded authority within the locality as he was both the practitioner and priest moulded into one.[13] Within Kerala, multiple forms of practices existed which included *manthram* (sorcery), *tanthram* (methods of performing witchcraft), *ottamooli* (a single medicine with mystical powers), *kaipunyam* (medical powers inherent in a vaidyan), *vishachikitsa* (poison treatment), *kannuvaidyam* (treatment of the eyes) and *jyotisham* (astronomy). While some practised Chintamani treatment (widely prevalent in Tamil lands), some were proficient in medicine based on *Ashtangahridhayam*. Yet, they were all part of the constellation of contemporary medical practices of the nineteenth century. It was the mystic powers of the physician, which made him central to the therapeutic world of the locality.

In its twentieth-century manifestation, Ayurveda was both a generic term representing contemporary medical practices and a learned classical medical tradition derived from the Sanskrit texts, particularly *Charaka Samhita, Suśruta Samhitā, Ashtangahridhaya Samhita* and their latter-day commentaries.[14] Classical Ayurveda rests on a theory of cooking. The consumed food transforms into seven stages: *rasa, rakhta, mamsa, medas, asthi, majja* and *shukra*, loosely translated as chime, blood, flesh, fat, bone, marrow and sperm. Disease categorization follows the classification of places and people following the hot/cold binary primarily defined through the theory of *Tridoshas* or the three humours: *vata, pita* and *kapha*.

In the emergence of national consciousness, Ayurveda symbolized national science. Therefore, the consumption of Ayurvedic drugs became a cultural and therapeutic necessity. Institutionalized Ayurvedic medicines adhered to the Sanskrit textual tradition to conform to homogeneity and centrality essential for national identity.[15] Under nationalist revival, places within the Indian subcontinent, particularly those under princely rulers, took initiatives towards organizing traditional knowledge forms to formulate new identities. Ayurveda emerged as the principal site of Indian science, deemed necessary for a society reeling under the fears of physical and cultural loss under colonial dominance. The revival of the classical tradition in medicine, as a site of Indian science, was guided by a desire to locate contemporary Indian societies within stable foundations as states sought to reorder indigenous medical domains through state-centred regulatory practices.[16] Thus, the practice of healing is as social, cultural and ideological as it is bodily.

Ayurveda was no longer just a home-based remedy; instead, physicians started *vaidyasalas*, or clinics, near towns and bazaars. They maintained records of the patients, preserved drugs, raised botanical gardens and introduced new drugs. Such centres of Ayurvedic medicine were deemed necessary primarily to contain the spread of contagious diseases like cholera, malaria and plague, which had emerged as a matter of concern for the state. The princely state of Travancore, which later became part of the state of Kerala, introduced a financial aid system to those vaidyasalas who conformed to state norms. Thus, the priorities of the state systems significantly shaped the character of the practice and the nature of pharmaceutical innovation. As the production of drugs shifted from home to mass production for the needs of the wider public, the knowledge of drug preparation became elaborate and centralized.

Thus, in late nineteenth- and twentieth-century Kerala, a dominant centralized Ayurvedic practice supported and patronized by the ruling authority and legitimized through a consensus of the social elites emerged. The classical tradition was mapped onto the social and cultural domain of Kerala, by bringing in the classical as the medicine of the land, raising plants which were mentioned within the classical texts, and by establishing clinics and teaching hospitals in the state. While the state emerged to define itself as a medieval aristocracy defined by ancient knowledge forms within the idiom of colonial modernity, the classical came to be re-constituted. This was also done by outlawing a variety of localized practices as quackery that did not meet the changing ideologies of the state. These outlawed practices were the medical traditions of contemporary society, which were not in conformity with state-recognized medical practice.

Kottakkal Aryavaidyasala

The imaginations and therapeutic concerns of the migrants were positioned within the changing contexts of the desire for tradition. This led migrants to look to Kottakkal Aryavaidyasala for Ayurvedic medicine. Kottakkal by the early decades of the twentieth century had emerged as the epitome of the institutionalized form of Ayurveda, through the establishment of a formal clinical practice and through centralized pharmaceutical drug production.

While localized vaidyans in their capacities adapted to the changing concerns of Ayurvedic modernization, an Ayurvedic clinic established by Panayinpalli Shankunni Varier in 1903 at Kottakkal emerged as the most important centre for the production and distribution of Ayurvedic drugs in Kerala. P. S. Varier's attempts to reorder Ayurveda stems from his resolve to reposition Ayurveda as the science of the indigenous. Attempts to redefine Ayurveda following the challenges posed by Western medicine led to two broad trends. One was the standardization of the practice; the second was that physicians had to deal with new disease categories, aetiology and pharmaceutical methods. Varier made new mixtures and gave them his own names. *Agnideepa dravakam*, a carminative tonic, cured indigestion and quelled *agni*, the fire in the stomach. The *jvarahari dravam* contained quinine for fever.[17] He experimented with neem bark to create an alternative to cinchona. Varier speaks about the new drugs he produced in the Ayurvedic journal *Danvantri*, which he published:

> As the number of malaria patients increased, *Koina* (cinchona) became insufficient. Hence, I made a *Kashayam* (bark of the neem boiled in water) and distributed it. From my preliminary understanding I realise that it produced results. While two ounces of Koina can stop the fever, six ounces give the effect in the case of kashayam. Though this is my preliminary observation, I firmly believe that neem is an alternative for cinchona as it is more popular. It would be much easier to counter the spread of malaria effectively in the future.[18]

Varier often tried to revisit the humoral theory in light of Western medicine. He argued that *Charakasamhita* and *Ashtangahridhayam* or their later commentaries spoke of minute particles or organisms that cause diseases. For him, minute organisms caused smallpox and are not due to the influence of the *devi* as was popularly believed.[19] He thus tried to forge epistemic parallels between Western medicine and Ayurveda. As malaria spread, he wondered, 'how would diseases affect an entire society, since *doshic* principles differ from individual to individual?'.[20]

Varier and his co-practitioners nevertheless argued that sages of the past, who knew the plants of the subcontinent, the nature of human bodies, diseases and their cures, structured the humoral theory foundations.[21] According to him, the human body and the environment provide a natural balance. The disturbance in this synthesis causes ailments. He argued:

> Ordinary medical herbs around us can replace most of the medicines mentioned in British pharmacopoeia, and in most cases, these medicines are more effective. Hence, we do not need any medication other than the English medicine digitalis. And even for this, we can make medicine by mixing up two or more drugs.[22]

Thus, beyond the nationalist upsurge and the revival of Sanskrit-based textual traditions, the geography of Kerala and its biological wealth were seen to provide the primary defence against diseases. A distinct regional Ayurveda emerged within this growing sense of geo-cultural and linguistic identity. Plants encompassed the essences of the land. Its consumption was like a sacrament, ensuring an organic link between the self and the land. Plants and diseases were specific to the ecology, providing defence against diseases. This regional variant of Ayurveda finds reflection in the words of Varier. He writes:

> The Vaidya system of Kerala had many peculiarities, and our ancestors had identified and brought into practice many medicines over time. Though the Ayurveda treatment system has undergone substantial change, it is doubtful whether the practitioners are clear about the quality of these medicines. The reason is that there is no proper method to coordinate and monitor the system. At present, even the number of physicians who know those medicines are few, and those who are present are old. At this rate, the peculiarities of the Malayalam treatment would go into oblivion.[23]

Varier started a *patasala* (an Ayurveda school), a medical journal, *Danvantri*, and a *vaidyasala* (clinic) and engaged in the mass production of drugs. The possibility of communicating with the *vaidyasala* through the newly introduced postal system meant opportunities for expanding the market for drugs, underlining the fact that new concerns for what constitutes ailments were evolving from the network of communication.

Promiscuity, sin and disease

In this context of Ayurvedic modernization, people from far afield sought medical aid at the Kottakkal Aryavaidyasala. Varier kept careful records of the letters that reached him and dispensed medicines with the regimen. People often demanded medical care for sexual disorders, considered morally disgraceful. For them, sexual liaison with multiple women or masturbation led to the corruption of the *indriyam* (the senses) and finally to the loss of *ojas* (vitality). Mammad Koya writing from Bombay in 1936, says that he had been indulging in 'unwanted habits' in the past and hence could not get pleasure while engaging in sex with his wife. He had taken *Shathavarigulam* from Kottakkal, which did not give relief. Consequently, *Dasamoolarishtam* and *Swarnabhasmam* were prescribed.[24]

Similarly, one Nair writing from Colombo mentions taking *Firangahara* and *Gulgulathigridham* for his sexual illness. He states that he was suffering from sugar and albumin in urine and hence took six bottles of medicine for six months from the Venus Pharmacy, which caused stomach upset, headache and memory loss. He writes that 'unwanted habits' led to the blockage of ejaculation. He also feared that his kidney, liver and bladder might have been affected. As this disease persists, it might have led to *rakthadooshyam* (impure blood), leading to faulty blood circulation. He also doubts that blood in the urine might be due to wheat intake. He describes that he has less blood in the body, weak veins, phlegm in the throat and sores in the mouth. He also says that he has been ill for the last twenty years, and hence his body is weak yet interested in having sex. He further states that he is suffering from *shuklasthambham* (blockage of sperm) and *vaatarogam* (disturbance of bile).[25]

Disease, therefore, was caused by an alien and hostile climate and a promiscuous life. The resulting blockage of the sperms, which made the blood impure, adversely affected the circulation of blood, leading to the rise of *vatam*. Thus, in the imagination of the body and morbidity, elements of classical Ayurveda, tropical disease causation and Western medical understandings of the body coexisted. Here the humoral theory of disease causation came to be negotiated through physiology familiarized by Western medicine. Illness arose from guilt and the fear of sin inflicted on the individual's body. Disease, therefore, was the price that one had to pay for the violation of the self, an idea popularized within Kerala by the Christian missionaries, who, through a network of educational and health institutions, had argued that disease was synonymous with individual and social sins.[26]

Environment, food and fears of the bodily constitution

Within the changing contexts of colonialism, the individual, both as a caregiver and as a patient, had to negotiate new notions of morbidity and cure. The challenge was to explain morbidity following disease categories according to Ayurveda. Intense displacement brought about by migration led to the separation from the homeland was also from the self. The body becomes an object of enquiry, not just for the practitioner but for the patient himself. He is no longer an object within the cosmological world of the patient; instead, he was increasingly placed outside of it. Thus, as Charles Rosenberg argues, disease incidence and outcomes and even the provisions of care were subject matters that reflected an understanding of medicine far broader than that bounded by the activities of the physicians.[27]

The fear that the foreign land corrupted their bodily composition led people to write to Kottakkal for drugs. The physician made his diagnoses on the basis of the descriptions given by the patient. Chathappan, for example, writes that 'for the last six months he was suffering from swelling and pain in the right leg. His hands were aching with pain in the back and hips followed by constipation'.[28] Similarly, U. A. Raman writes from Pollachi that a 26-year-old lady was suffering from an irregular menstrual cycle. She took allopathic medicine, but it did not work. Varier prescribed *Shatavari Kashayam*, a decoction of the *Asparagus racemosus*.[29] Irregular bowel movements and menstrual cycles regularly featured in the letters asking for medical help.

For menstrual irregularity, the patient was given *Valiyamadhu sneheerasayanam*, 1/2 kathukkam and 1/2 panamida (1/6th of a gram) of *rasasindhooram*. These were to be taken in the morning and afternoon at 3:30, along with a lot of milk and 1/4th ounce *gulgulati kashayam* was to be mixed with ten drops of *ksheerabala101* along with 1/2 ounce of castor oil, to be taken twice before food. For head *balam*, *Guguchyakki* for body. Apply *pindathailam* and then take a bath.

The patient was advised to take medicines with dietary restrictions and report regularly about progress. The patient was advised not to take tamarind, salt and chilli. Dietary restrictions became an essential constituent in the regime of medical therapy. Over the years, the letters became more descriptive and elaborate, with details of the ailments explained. The combinations of medicines became extensive and the restrictions on diet also became elaborate so as to make the drugs effective. The intention was to isolate the bodies from an alien environment. The extensive regimen that followed the consumption of the drug created a new regimen around the migrant lives to make the drugs effective. It was not just the drugs but a regimented cultural world that was exported to regulate the patient's life.

By the 1950s elaborate restrictions on diet and regimen came to be prescribed. There was a shift from simple dietary restrictions to increasing control over the dietary habits of the patient. The total number of drugs prescribed ranged from two or three in the 1930s to six or seven by the 1950s. Similarly, the number of medicines to be combined also increased. This meant that Ayurveda was subjected to considerable reordering consequent to the expansion of the pharmaceutical industry. Migrants were also consuming food supplements and nutraceuticals that were familiarized by European drug manufacturers. For instance, one Menon writing from Malaysia mentions that a six-month-old child does not have any strength in her hands and legs, does not look straight and has difficulty breathing. He mentions that the child was also taken to an allopathic doctor and was also given Allenbury's milk and Lactogen as supplements.[30]

One Nair from Ceylon writes that a child was given Ayurvedic drugs for regular bowel movements. The child is now seven years old, and still the problem of excretion prevails. The child was given cows milk and Lactogen for some months, but this was stopped and given orange juice instead. He was delivered to the hospital. The doctors advised not to give oil because of the cold climate.[31]

Patients were constantly engaging with different kinds of medical practices, including allopathy and homeopathy. A. K. G. Iyer writes from Madras, that his daughter has swellings in the eye and also has small pimples. She took a Bismuth injection and then took treatment from Doraiswami Iyer for two years and is now undergoing homeopathic treatment. He writes that 'my neighbor has taken your *asanavilvadhi* oil and has got some respite. But my daughter is not getting any respite from this oil and she is suffering for more than five years'.[32]

Daniel, writing from Cuttack in Orissa, notes that the Diwan of the Raja of Cuttak was suffering from pain and numbness. He was advised to take *Dhanwantharam 101, Pindathailam, Dhanwanthram* and *Navarakizhi*. E. K. Nair from Myanmar writes that a Telugu native aged roughly fifty, is suffering from scrotal swelling and pain. It goes up until it becomes difficult for him to breathe. When it occurs, he will have to be in bed for ten days and endure severe pain. *Sukumarakritham, dhanwantharam101, dasamoolarishtam* and *Ashwanthadhikridham* were prescribed.

Those who wrote to Kottakkal were largely concerned about *ojas*, or vital energy, being drained through urine, which was seen as the primary cause of disease. Kunjappu writing from Pollachi writes that he is having white discharge, which is causing dizziness and pain in the eye.[33] While the symptoms in general pointed to the drain of vital energy in a foreign land, which had to be addressed through the consumption of drugs, building defences of the body. Some drugs gained prominence over time; *Sukumaralehyam, ksheerabalathailam* and *dhanwantharam101* emerged as important drugs towards building the vitality of the body. This was a new development as the element of purging, which was central to Ayurveda was increasingly giving way to the idea of building bodily strength and resistance.

In tune with the current sensibilities, Kottakkal advertised their drugs as follows:

Ajamamsarasayanam: it cures all kinds of vata, kshaya and helps in rejuvenating health;

Chinchilaadhi lehyam: lot of iron is included;

Chyavanaprasham: people whose bodies have become tired, those affected with tuberculosis, old and they will become like young. Those ailments connected with urine and ailments connected with sperm (Shukla) will be cured;

dhaatupushti (muscle strength): it prevents memory loss, mind becomes alert, hence it is best for students. Longevity, strength to the *indreeyam* (the senses), beauty to the body, digestion, throat, diseases connected to the heart, and lungs, and anyone can consume it, irrespective of the sexes.[34]

Varier writes that the medicines produced by the *vaidyasala* became so popular that people have started forgetting the way in which *kashayams* are made. He also states that even though the cost of medicines produced by Kottakal is relatively higher it reduced the burden of producing medicines and even established physicians either buy medicines from the *vaidyasala* or advices patients to buy medicines, rather than produce medicines on their own.[35] Six months after the *vaidyasala* was established there was an outbreak of cholera in the vicinity of Kottakal and Varier visited the houses of the people around and distributed medicines.

When pharmaceutical industrial methods were introduced the Kottakal claimed that they have not moved away from the classical texts. The basic argument was that:

the equipment (mechanization) is not for changing the *kalpana* principle of the medicine but for maximizing the speed of processing. Kalpana is the basic form in which a medicine is conceived according to the shastric texts. . . . to begin with, the mechanization of medicine manufacture at the Aryavaidyasala was mainly to augment the speed of processing and not to replace the traditional process as such.[36]

Matters that enter and exist in the body: Spirits, food and sex

Movement of people to new geographies made them to imagine that new climatic zones had heated the body, generated yearnings, both for food and sex, and disturbed the internal composition of the body. Uncontrolled desire in a new context was a disease; as it was an aberration to the norm. The return to the norm was possible only by returning to the homeland, which was not possible given the nature of migration that made displacement a reality, to the point of no return. It is in this context that migrants feared the displacement of the mind and the body. While it was prudent for migrants to locate the cause of their ailments in a variety of ecological, dietary and moral dislocations, it became increasingly difficult to come to terms with the bodily changes and ailments that they had to encounter. People wrote in detail about what was visible in the body and what they felt to the Kottakal Aryavaidyasala.

One of the major concerns that dominated the letters that reached the *vaidyasala* was the fear of the supernatural. Shankararaman from Nungambakkom writes that 'his brother was suffering from an unfamiliar disease for the last ten months where he takes his hand and turns and twists and hit his head and chest and turns his head on both sides'. In traditional society, mental ailments were largely believed to be caused both by the derangement of the humors or due to the possession of evil spirits.[37] One of the major concerns of the revival movement in Ayurveda was to create a rational medical tradition that saw evil spirits and possessions as deviation from the classical Sanskrit textual tradition, which was seen as scientific. Yet the new medical movement led by Varier responded to patient concerns on spirits and possessions and incorporated local beliefs on diseases and drugs. People increasingly wrote to Kottakkal for drugs for mental ailments for which Varier produced a new medicine, *Bhootasaharadravakom*, signifying that epilepsy continued to be seen as resulting from possession. Thus, the notion of disease itself depends rather on the decision of the society than on objective facts. This is particularly obvious in, but not limited to, the field of mental illness.[38]

The consumption of new products like tobacco, alcohol and at times even wheat was seen to disturb bodily composition and caused ailments. The exposure to foreign climates and lands weakened the body as the blood became impure and disturbed the regular flow of blood. This weakened the body through blockages of the vitals leading to the discharge of pus in the urine, phlegm, regular coughing and the improper discharge of the stool. The bodies transform in accordance with what you consume. Things that enter the bodies, transform and exit. The contact with other places and other bodies had made people ill. It was not about having sexual contact, but about having sexual contact in a different locale that was considered a violation of the body. Being spoilt and violated by the temptations of the foreign land, that had brought about a guilt that had drained the bodies of the vital energy.

One was not only outside the geographical boundaries of Kerala but outside the cultural boundaries, even when living within the domestic society. This fear of the body was central to the social reform movement across the subcontinent. Within Kerala, this was witnessed among the Ezhavas, a lower-caste social group, who had transformed much of their contemporary practices as a means of social mobility. Narayana, who spearheaded the movement, was a social reformer and an Ayurvedic practitioner. He argued that social backwardness resulted primarily from physical and mental backwardness. His attempt therefore was to regain the morbid selves. Even when he challenged social hierarchies based on caste, he advised his followers to desist from the consumption of fish, meat and alcohol as they were thought to cause internal purification and therefore morbid bodies. He too considered diseases to be caused by internal blockages, impure blood and leading to the collapse of bodily composition. However, for Narayana, such bodily weakness did not result from the concerns of external migration as is witnessed in the patient records at Kottakal; rather morbidity was a condition of his community, which he desired to change. The disease was therefore not individual but rather social in character, which had engulfed the bodies of his community, primarily due to what they consumed, across generations, underlining that disease was primarily historical in nature and not contemporary as was the case with the migrants. Social morbidity was to be ensured by building moral courage, possible only through overcoming desire. The consumption of fish, meat and alcohol, widely prevalent among the Ezhavas, was considered as visible expressions of desire. On a visit to the house of his disciple, Krishnan, Narayana urged the family to desist from the consumption of meat and fish.[39] Animal matter and alcohol were deemed to generate heat in the blood that transformed bodily composition and transformed the mind. For him, the practice of consuming animal matter led to the collapse of the internal composition of the body. This affected the *datus* and drained the body of its *ojas*. For him *ojas*, or vital energy, had to be regained through the consumption of plant matter, and therefore the organic link between Ezhava bodies and nature had to be repositioned. The failure to control desire was seen to be the cause of individual and social failure. Thus, while migrants considered that disease was an aberration and the disruption of the order, for lower-caste social reformers, the present provided the opportunity to disrupt the traditional order, which was morbid and had acquired a certain permanence historically.

The healthy ideal aimed to create moral and therapeutic resistance. It resisted desires, both in terms of food and sex. An environmental ethic of the body had been the central element in the discourse on bodies in the tropics. The emergence of Ayurveda was negotiated through the new ideas of the bodies and ailments that were framed through the notion of dirt and impurity. It is from the unstable past, from the binaries between the pure and the impure structured through moral and physical boundaries, that Ayurveda emerged in the late nineteenth and twentieth century. The concept of tropical disease familiarized a new concept of environmental ethic of disease causation that underlined sensuality as the primary cause of disease. The missionary ethic of overcoming the diseased environment through regulation, moderation and through resistance of desire became important in shaping the struggle towards regulating the influence of the environment.

Conclusion

The value of the thing is decided in accordance with the context in which it is located. Neither medicine nor ailments have universal meaning.[40] Ayurveda as we understand it in the present context therefore is shaped by multiple factors including ideological and institutional structures that were constituted in an age of British colonialism. Ayurveda came to be viewed largely as preventive medicine by retaining the health and vitality of the body. The strength of this medical tradition was identified as a home-grown medical practice, where human bodies and their existences were seen to be part of the same ecological and cultural contexts within which plants were located. They were seen to be part of the same cultural and environmental contexts. Thus, bodies were seen to be corrupted, weak and disorganized as has been seen from the irregular flow of the menstrual blood or the uncontrolled discharge of the semen, or the inability of men to effectively partake in sexual relations. Illness as conceived by the patient became an important element in shaping indigenous medical knowledge in twentieth-century Kerala. However, illness is contextual and cultural and hence beyond the structural changes witnessed within Indian medical practice. Changing perceptions of the body under colonial contexts had an important bearing on Ayurveda.

Notes

1. Charles Leslie, *Asian Medical Systems: A Comparative Study* (Delhi: Motilal Banarsidass, 1998).
2. K. N. Panikkar, *Culture, Ideology, Hegemony: Intellectuals and Social Consciousness in Colonial India* (New Delhi: Tulika, 1995), 145–75; *Disease and Medicine in India: A Historical Overview*, ed. Deepak Kumar (New Delhi: Tulika, 2001).
3. Oral testimony of George Francis on 21 December 2005, at Kollam, Kerala.
4. Rana P. Behal, 'Power Structure, Discipline, and Labour in Assam Tea Plantations under Colonial Rule', *International Review of Social History* 51 (2006): 143–72.
5. *Danvantri (Malayalam)* 1932.
6. Kavita Sivaramakrishnan, *Old Potions, New bottles: Recasting Indigenous Medicine in Colonial Punjab (1850–1945)* (New Delhi: Orient Longman, 2006).
7. Partha Chatterjee, *The Nation and Its Fragments: Colonial and Postcolonial Histories* (Princeton: Princeton University Press, 1994).
8. *Psychiatry and Empire*, ed. Sloan Mahone and Megan Vaughan (Basingstoke: Palgrave Macmillan, 2007), 7.
9. Bernard S. Cohn, *Colonialisms and its Forms of Knowledge: The British in India* (Princeton: Princeton University Press, 1996).
10. Mark Harrison, 'Racial Pathologies: Morbid Anatomy in British India, 1770–1850', in *The Social History of Health and Medicine in Colonial India*, ed. Biswamoy Pati and Mark Harrison (Abingdon: Routledge, 2008), 174.
11. David Arnold, *Colonising the Body: State Medicine and Epidemic Disease in Nineteenth-Century India* (Berkeley: University of California Press, 1993).
12. Steven Engler, '"Science" vs. "Religion" in Classical Ayurveda', *Numen: International Review for the History of Religions* 50, no. 4 (2003): 416–63; Harish Naraindas, 'Care, Welfare, and Treason: The Advent of Vaccination in the 19th Century', *Contributions to Indian Sociology* 32, no.1 (1998): 67–96.
13. Ayurvedic Patasala: Opening of Ayurvedic Botanical Garden, Proceedings of His Highness the Maharajah of Travancore. From Rao Bahadur M.C. Koman, Honorary Physician, General Hospital, and Officer, in charge of investigation into indigenous drugs. To the Honorable Surgeon General, Government of Madras, I.G.O. No. E. 1282, Dated 18 April 1918, Kerala State Archives, Thiruvananthapuram.
14. Dominic Wujastyk, *The Roots of Ayurveda: Selections from Sanskrit Medical Writings* (London: Penguin Books, 2003).
15. Charles Leslie, 'The Professionalising Ideology of Medical Revivalism', in *Entrepreneurship and Modernisation of Occupational Cultures in South Asia*, ed. Milton Singer (Durham: Duke University Press, 1973), 217.
16. Mr Kunjan Thirumulpad in his application for the award of a grant-in-aid for the conduct of Vaidyasala writes that he, 'after undergoing a course of study of the

science of Ayurveda under the late Ananthapurathu Mootha Koil Thampuran had also passed the Government Ayurveda Examination in the year 1076 (1900) as second in the first class. *Continuance of the Vaidyasala at Edapally with Mr. Kunjan Thirumulpad as the grant-in-aid Vaidyan*, Kerala State Archives, Thiruvananthapuram.

17 Gita Krishnankutty, *A Life of Healing: A Biography of Vaidyaratnam P. S. Varier* (New Delhi: Viking, 2001), 118.
18 *Danvantri* 1914.
19 *Danvantri* 1921.
20 *Danvantri* 1919.
21 *Danvantri* 1921.
22 *Danvantri* 1914.
23 *Danvantri* 1917.
24 Aryavaidyasala, Kottakkal, Patient files. Case No 4747.
25 Aryavaidyasala, Kottakkal, Patient files. Case No 4886.
26 Sundararaj Manickam, *The Social Setting of Christian Conversion in South India: The Impact of the Wesleyan Methodist Missionaries on the Trichy-Tanjore Diocese with Special Reference to the Harijan Communities of the Mass Movement Area 1820–1947* (Wiesbaden: Steiner, 1977).
27 Charles E. Rosenberg, 'Erwin H. Ackerknecht, Social Medicine, and the History of Medicine', *Bulletin of the History of Medicine* 81, no. 3 (2007): 511–32.
28 Aryavaidyasala, Kottakkal, Patient files. Case No 4311.
29 Aryavaidyasala, Kottakkal, Patient files. Case No 4416.
30 Aryavaidyasala, Kottakkal, Patient files. Case No. 4860.
31 Aryavaidyasala, Kottakkal, Patient files. Case No. 4182.
32 Aryavaidyasala, Kottakkal, Patient files. Case No. 4210.
33 Aryavaidyasala Kottakkal. Patient files. Case No. 7425.
34 The Golden Jubilee souvenir. 1954 Vaidyarathnam P Varier's Aryavaidya Sala, Kottakkal.
35 Danvantri.
36 Krishnankutty, *A Life of Healing*.
37 Wujastyk, *The Roots of Ayurveda*.
38 Rosenberg, 'Erwin H. Ackerknecht'.
39 *Who's who in Sree Narayana Dharma Paripalana Yogam* (Kollam, 1956), 72.
40 Arjun Appadurai, *The Social Life of Things: Commodities in Cultural Perspective* (Cambridge: Cambridge University Press, 1986).

7

Toxic trading

Poisons and medicines in British India

David Arnold

Studies of the Indian Ocean world have increasingly reflected on this vast maritime region as a zone for the transmission of disease and an arena within (and across) which medicinal substances and therapeutic practices have long been traded.[1] Unlike the Atlantic, in the Indian Ocean this network of medical connections and exchanges dates back many centuries, to well before the beginning of European intervention in the region from 1498 onwards. It does, though, seem plausible to argue that, through the expansion of sea-borne trade, the increased movement of goods and people, the opening up of maritime highways to areas beyond the ocean's own perimeters, and the introduction of new diseases and innovative therapeutic practices, the advent of European power substantially changed or greatly accentuated pre-existing patterns of trading and transaction.

While recognizing the major contribution made by the existing literature on the Indian Ocean world, this chapter follows a somewhat different trajectory from earlier narratives of pathogens, trade and therapeutics. It focuses specifically on India in the nineteenth and early twentieth centuries, at the height of British rule in the subcontinent, and, in keeping with this volume's material culture remit, it examines the historical nature and cultural significance of three substances, all of which had some medicinal uses.[2] But each of those 'peculiar', border-crossing ingredients had a dual identity, as commodities that could poison, incapacitate and kill as well as substances that could serve medicinal and public health purposes.[3] This chapter engages with the concept of the pharmakon, that is, the idea that the same substance could both poison *and* cure, depending on the dosage given, the manner in which it was used, or even how it was culturally understood.[4] While singling out three specific commodities for discussion – nux vomica, arsenic and kerosene – the chapter seeks to illustrate the circulation more generally of medicinally and toxicologically ambiguous substances within, and beyond, the Indian Ocean world. It offers a 'connected history' both in the sense, first, that it connects medicines to poisons and, second, that it links the sites of production of these toxic/therapeutic substances to their ultimate point of consumption. The substances discussed here illuminate a wider connectivity as, in their various forms and incarnations, they crossed and re-crossed the Indian Ocean and its outer peripheries. But the chapter seeks, too, to enlarge on the existing understanding of the nature and function of medicinal drugs and related objects in the Indian Ocean world by suggesting that the ocean served not just passively to transport substances, but also functioned, more actively, as a transformative space that facilitated the conversion of substances from one physical or epistemic form (say, as a poison) into another (such as a medicine). The ocean did not in itself materially change the substances (except in the sense that long sea voyages made them stale and less fit for their intended purpose), but it often marked a radical transformation in meaning and use as a commodity travelled from one transoceanic location to another.

This chapter makes no apologies for coupling the idea of medicines with that of poisons, for this duality was present in many substances and their social uses. The history of medicine as an academic discipline can be understood as the struggle between two competing teleologies. On the one hand there is the whiggish idea that, despite setbacks and false leads, things generally get better and that the history of modern medical science is a history of progress and improvement, articulated through the discovery of new drugs (or new uses for known substances), through innovative therapeutic procedures and through an evolving understanding of how medicines operate on the human body. On the other hand, there is the contrary view that medicinal substances are always apt to be hazardous, can have dangerous side effects, are in effect poisons or are part of processes of industrial and pharmaceutical production that release toxic substances into the environment and into human bodies. In aspiring to make things better, medicine (especially, but not exclusively, modern medicine) can make matters worse or substitute one kind of evil for another. The history of medicine is inherently – not just accidentally or occasionally – also a history of toxicity.

Attention to the physical and cultural mobility of medicinal/toxic substances challenges many of our received ideas about 'medical systems' and the tendency to over-compartmentalize colonial and indigenous medicine as if they were entirely separate sets of knowledge.[5] If substances like arsenic and nux vomica could shuffle not just between the toxic and the therapeutic but also between Western biomedicine and Ayurveda or Unani in India, and move thus with surprising freedom, then the supposed integrity and uniqueness of those systems come into question. Or perhaps such evidence of substance mobility gives fresh impetus to our thinking about systems not as rigid entities but as culturally constructed spaces allowing the very same substance to be judged poisonous in one medical tradition while appearing in another as a tonic, aphrodisiac or febrifuge.

Nux vomica

The history of medicine in India has seldom looked to the forest as the ultimate provider of the subcontinent's cornucopia of medicinal drugs and toxic substances, or indeed enquired very deeply into where such substances came from at all.[6] Some were clearly the products of overland or overseas trade; others are associated (for religious as well as ecological reasons) with the Himalaya, or were the common botanicals of gardens, fields and wastes.[7] Nux vomica was one of many forest products to be given medicinal use; but, in its simultaneous toxicity, it also aptly captures the principle of the pharmakon. The range of its properties was succinctly described in a pharmacological text published in Calcutta in 1901: 'In small doses tonic; in large doses a nervous and general stimulant; larger doses are poisonous.'[8] The substance originated as the small, shiny, disc-shaped nut of a deciduous tree, *Strychnos nux-vomica*, native to certain wooded tracts in the Madras Presidency and neighbouring Travancore. It was harvested by forest tribes (*adivasis*) who collected the fallen nuts and who were cognizant of the poisonous and/or therapeutic properties of several parts of the tree (its roots and bark), and not just its more commercially and therapeutically sought-after nuts.[9]

Among these tribal nut-gatherers were the Yanadis of Nellore district (formerly in the Madras Presidency, now part of Andhra Pradesh). Characterized ethnographically as among the most 'primitive' communities in South India, largely nomadic and making fire with sticks, the Yanadis' knowledge of forest flora and fauna was extensive: apart from nux vomica, they also collected honey, tamarinds, rattans and other forest produce with medicinal uses such as myrobalan fruits, soap nuts and sarsaparilla root.[10] Although the long history of the drug's use is impossible to trace, it is possible to intercept its modern history through colonial materia medica, ethnography, administrative reports and newspaper entries. Nux vomica appears to be one of a large number of plant drugs found across India that originated with tribal societies before they were incorporated into Ayurveda (and its regional variants) and later entered the Western pharmacopoeia.[11] The tribal gatherers formed part of a larger transactional system: they supplied the nux vomica nuts to the traders who ventured into the forests or gathered on their margins during the harvest season, and this then made the nuts available to *vaids* (medical practitioners) and their apothecaries for use in Ayurvedic tonics and therapeutic prescriptions. As part of the extension of their political authority and quest for additional revenue sources, in the 1830s the British took control of the forests of Nellore and made direct contact with the Yanadis. Although classed only as 'minor forest produce' (compared to the wholesale extraction of timber and firewood from state-run forests), nux vomica seeds and similar forest commodities usefully augmented the Madras government's revenues. Operating either through their own agents or via Indian contractors, the British took over the existing system of extraction, receiving the harvested nuts from 'Government Yanadis', along with other forest produce, in return for grain, tobacco, cloth and small sums of cash. They also tried, with limited success, to induct them into the colonial educational system and to encourage them in settled agriculture.[12] At the same time, therefore, that the extreme 'primitiveness' of the nomadic Yanadis, and indeed their criminality (some groups becoming subject to the Criminal Tribes Act of 1911) were being stressed, their role as gatherers of forest produce was valued and profitably annexed to the colonial structure of commodity and revenue extraction.

The tree and its nut had various local names, such as *kanjiram* in Malayalam and *kuchila* in Hindi.[13] These vernacular names were sometimes used by colonial writers, especially when considering Indian materia medica from the 'standpoint of local knowledge',[14] and this in part reflected their engagement both with the forest collectors and with the physicians (*vaids* or *vythians*) from whom they learned of the nut's properties. In the main, however, nux vomica was referred to by botanists, ethnographers, traders and pharmacists by its Latin nomenclature. Knowledge of the 'poison-nut' tree reached Europe through pioneering botanical surveys like Van Rheede's *Hortus Malabaricus* in the mid-sixteenth century.[15] It received its botanical name *Strychnos nux-vomica* a century later from Linnaeus, who clearly recognized the nuts' less pleasant properties. But the tree did not grow in Europe (or almost anywhere else in Asia apart from South India) and the nuts were not much discussed in the medical literature before the early nineteenth century; at that point, however, nux vomica and its medicinal/toxic properties began to attract extensive comment from chemists and pharmacologists in Europe and from botanists and physicians in India. A transformative moment came in 1818 when the French chemists J.-B. Caventou and P.-J. Pelletier identified the bitter alkaloids strychnine and brucine contained in the nuts: both substances were quickly recognized as exceptionally potent and deadly poisons.[16] East India Company physicians, like W. B. O'Shaughnessy and J. F. Royle, themselves representative of a mobile medical culture that moved (over the course of their careers and through their published works) from Britain to India and back to Britain again, were further instrumental in the 1830s and 1840s in bringing the drug to Western attention. They, too, formed a link in the extended knowledge and commodity chain that now stretched from forest India and its tribal inhabitants to Western laboratories and industrial pharmacists.[17] But O'Shaughnessy and Royle did more than simply gather and pass on vernacular medical knowledge. They also radically rewrote it by identifying nux vomica as one of the many highly toxic vegetable substances originating in India that was (in their view) recklessly employed by local practitioners, the *vaids* and *hakims*. Generalizing from this and other toxic/therapeutic plant substances like croton, aconitum and datura, colonial botanists and physicians used nux vomica as a discursive tool to epitomize what they saw as the inherently dangerous and irresponsible nature of Indian therapeutic practice.[18] In this censorious view, nux vomica and similar drugs were more appropriately categorized as poisons than as medicines – until such time, that is, that their toxic wildness was tamed and, refined through modern chemistry and industrial pharmacology, became of wide medicinal value.

Despite their administrative status as 'minor forest produce', the 'poison-tree' nuts were not commercially insignificant. In 1912–13, 2,076 tonnes of them were shipped from India with a value of £14,408. By the mid-1920s between 2,000 and 2,500 tonnes were exported annually, worth from £15,000 to 25,000.[19] It is important to note that the Indian agency was present at this stage too: Parsi and Muslim trading houses were leading figures in the export trade. However, nothing materially happened to the nuts when they left Indian ports – Madras, Bombay, Calicut and Cochin – and entered the Indian Ocean on their voyage westward. But, on arrival in London, Liverpool and Hamburg they became one of the countless raw materials from 'the colonies' to be auctioned and re-sold for commercial use. In Liverpool's produce market, for example, in the 1870s the nuts sold for £11 a tonne.[20] Even though the Indian provenance of the drug was seldom highlighted, in nineteenth- and early twentieth-century Europe strychnine gained great notoriety as a deadly homicidal poison, difficult to trace even with the latest forensic testing.[21] But in the imperial metropole strychnine was reinstated as a medicinal drug and authorized for use, like a large number of other Indian plant substances, by the *British Pharmacopoeia*.[22] It was incorporated into various patent medicines, tonics and laxatives and as such exported to, among other places, British India. A commodity that departed India as a raw, unprocessed material returned, transformed, bottled and packaged, into a modern medicine.

While for the Yanadis of Nellore and for many indigenous practitioners in India several parts of the 'poison nut' tree had therapeutic properties, Western manufacturers were only interested in the nuts and the tiny quantities of chemically active material extracted from them: strychnine and brucine constituted less than 2 per cent of the nuts' total volume. By the time the active ingredients made their return journey, through the Red Sea or around the Cape of Good Hope, the bright, metallic-looking nuts had been metamorphosed into something very different. Strychnine was the principal ingredient, for instance, in Easton's Syrup, marketed as a cure for boils, nervousness, debility and 'poverty of the blood', and marketed in Bombay in the 1870s for Rs 2 and Rs 3–8 a bottle.[23] Nux vomica was an ingredient, too, in pills sold by Kirby & Co. of London as a remedy for constipation, nervous depression, gout, neuralgia and 'lowness of spirits, arising from overwork'.[24] The Indian Ocean has rightly been viewed as a subaltern lake,[25] but here were the fruits of the labour of one of the most subaltern communities imaginable in the ocean's littoral returning as a tonic to soothe the nervous debility of the colonial (and conceivably Indian) middle-classes. At the same time the processed and imported strychnine and brucine derived from the nuts also appeared in textbooks of toxicology and medical jurisprudence in India as being among the most dangerous of all known alkaloid poisons,[26] even though strychnine was far less commonly used for homicidal or suicidal purposes in India than opium and arsenic.[27]

Nux vomica thus helped to describe and define a whole circuit of imperial knowledge, resource extraction and commodity exchange that stretched from the forests of Nellore and Travancore to centres of processing and manufacture in Britain, Germany and elsewhere in the West, and then back, in greatly modified form, to India. But such valuable materia medica was not immune to a form of cultural and political re-appropriation. From early in the nineteenth century the British administration in India had encouraged the use of local plant drugs that might provide cheaper, fresher and more efficacious medicines for colonial use. That ambition ran up against the predisposition of physicians trained in Britain to look to drugs already familiar to them, such as digitalis and belladonna, which also had both toxic and therapeutic properties, rather than

Indian plant drugs whose qualities were less well known to them. By the 1920s, however, some medicinal plant drugs of European origin were themselves being grown and processed in India, while, conversely, with the revival of Ayurveda and a new nationalist pride in India's own natural products, the identification and use of indigenous plant drugs were given fresh stimulus.[28] A catalogue of drugs, prepared by the Calcutta firm of B. K. Paul & Co. in 1924, listed eighty-five plants or plant-based substances, approved by the *British Pharmacopoeia*, that either grew wild or were cultivated in India. Reinstated as an ingredient in modern India's patriotic pharmacopoeia, nux vomica was one of these.[29] It had, in a cultural and geographic sense, returned home.

Arsenic

Vital though field and forest were to the provision of Indian medicines and poisons, plants were not the only available source. In the nineteenth century, India's pharmacology was represented by colonial botanists and Ayurvedic practitioners as a largely plant-based system, tapping into the natural abundance and healing powers (as well as the poisonous potentialities) of the plant wealth of India, in contrast to the chemical concoctions seen to characterize both medicine and poisoning in the modern West. In reality, inorganic substances, minerals and chemicals of various descriptions, had long been part of the Indian, as well as the Western, pharmacopoeia, and this traditional use or its ongoing adaptation was encouraged by the greater availability of many such inorganic substances as international trade, mining and manufacture burgeoned in the late nineteenth and early twentieth centuries. In 1904 Collis Barry, a chemical analyser for the Bombay government, noted that there was perhaps 'no country in the world more richly supplied with lethal material in the shape of vegetable poisons than India', and yet in recent times, it was a largely imported mineral poison, arsenic, to which the criminally inclined 'native' most commonly turned for homicidal or cattle-killing purposes.[30]

Arsenic had long held a recognized place in Indian medicine and in wider social and industrial use. Like the renowned inhabitants of Styria in southern Austria, India, too, had its 'arsenic eaters', men who believed that the substance was a powerful aphrodisiac or an aid to physical prowess and corporeal well-being.[31] While colonial opprobrium was principally directed at plant substances like nux vomica and aconitum, arsenic did not escape hostile comment – at least as it was reputedly used by Indian physicians.[32] It seems likely, however, that arsenic was less commonly used medicinally and in various trades before the colonial era in its pure form (white arsenic, known locally as *sanchya*) so much as the sulphides of arsenic, orpiment (yellow arsenic, *hurtal*) and realgar (red arsenic, *mansil*), which contained only 60–70 per cent arsenic. As well as an aphrodisiac, arsenic was taken as a nerve tonic, stimulant and febrifuge; it was also used as an abortifacient.[33] In medical prescriptions it was treated with extreme caution, administered orally in very small quantities, and 'cooked' or combined with other drugs in order to enhance its therapeutic properties or constrain its latent toxicity.[34]

Arsenic did not to any great extent occur naturally in India. In the nineteenth and early twentieth centuries, it was imported by sea from the West or brought overland from China (via Yunnan and Burma). One source mentions the Persian Gulf as supplying large quantities for India, without giving further details as to its exact geographical origin.[35] Thus, while some medicinal/toxic plant drugs, like nux vomica, exited India, arsenic was one of the many mineral commodities that entered India from outside. Ship manifests from the late nineteenth and early twentieth centuries indicate that as well as occasional large shipments, much of the arsenic entering Indian ports came in small quantities, probably of white arsenic in crude crystalline form, and from a few bags to two dozen crates at a time. These consignments formed part of miscellaneous cargoes, arriving anywhere from Basra and Yokohama to London, Antwerp and Hamburg, along with other chemicals, glassware, rope and wire. Again, like the outgoing nux vomica, such cargoes were commonly handled on arrival in Indian ports by Muslim or Parsi trading houses.[36]

As a commercial and industrial commodity, arsenic had, by the second half of the nineteenth century, an extraordinarily wide range of uses in India and elsewhere. It was incorporated in paints and dyes, used in papermaking, as a colourant, flavour-enhancer or preservative in food and drink (including beer) and as a depilatory and skin-whitener. Arsenic was also an insecticide, used to kill rats and vermin, and in the form of the arseno-copper compound Paris Green was sprayed on stagnant pools to kill malarial mosquitoes and their larvae.[37] One of its main commercial uses was in the leather industry to preserve hides and skins, and as India's leather export trade boomed from the 1870s, so did the wholesale importation of arsenic. Between the 1870s and 1920s, 100 to 150 tonnes of white arsenic were imported annually.[38] Perhaps not surprisingly, given its cheapness and availability in almost every bazaar, arsenic featured prominently in the poison culture of nineteenth-century India. Poisoning by arsenic became far more common than previously.[39] Throughout India, it was said, 'arsenic is the poison almost invariably selected by the poisoner'.[40] Of the 4,719 suspected cases of poisoning investigated by Punjab's chemical examiner between 1861 and 1887, 1,286 were attributed to arsenic and only 350 to opium and 180 datura. In the Bombay Presidency from 1875 to 1884, 947 deaths were attributed to poison: of these 507 were said to be due to arsenic and only 151 to opium and 74 to datura.[41]

While opium, a common household item, was often taken for suicidal purposes, the user drifting relatively painlessly into stupor and death, arsenic was a more obviously violent and homicidal substance. Sometimes used as an aggressive instrument of revenge or in fractious disputes, one of its more prevalent uses was by young wives to rid themselves of their vexatious older husbands or sexually predatory in-laws. But the claim could always be made that the arsenic had been intended (as vernacular use suggested) as a tonic or a love potion, and the courts seem to view such cases (especially when the accused was young and no death had actually resulted) with some leniency.[42] In addition, arsenic was extensively used to kill cattle, especially by low-caste Chamars who, having the customary right to remove and dispose of such carcases, collected the hides and sold them to the traders who had provided them with arsenic in the first place.[43] Given the importance of the leather industry to colonial India's export economy, it was this spate of cattle-poisoning that finally persuaded the government to support calls for an Indian Poisons Act.[44]

However, we might note two further aspects of the use of arsenic in its dual role as poison and/or medicine. Unlike many of India's plant poisons, arsenic became fairly easy to identify and trace. The raw substance had a physical appearance and chemical composition that could readily be analysed in the laboratory and observed under the microscope – one of the many forensic tasks assigned to provincial chemical examiners from the 1860s onwards. It was claimed that ultimately the homicidal use of arsenic in India declined precisely because its use could be so easily detected, though this claim might be treated with some scepticism given that most Hindu bodies were cremated within hours of death, leaving no detectable trace of poisoning, and recourse to post-mortems was widely opposed.[45] And a question was often raised as to how much arsenic was necessary to kill a given individual and how could it be proved that the intention behind its administration was criminal when perhaps the prescriber had been a qualified physician or a nursing relative intending a dose of arsenic, or a medicine containing the drug, to cure a complaint rather than to kill the recipient.[46] Since arsenic was a naturally occurring element, as well as one widely used in preservatives including food and drink, tiny quantities could be chemically detected in hair and other parts of the human body. Were these miniscule anatomical traces sufficient to prove criminal intent or to distinguish murder from accidental death?

Apart from sales through leading import firms and distributors in Calcutta, Bombay and other cities, arsenic was widely sold in Indian bazaars, whether in crude crystalline lumps or as a refined powder. The fear that such casual and unregulated merchandizing could lead to the contamination of other substances (especially salt and sugar, from which it might be visually indistinguishable) was one of several considerations that lay behind calls for India to follow Britain in passing an act to regulate the sale of poisons. This long-standing concern eventually resulted in the Indian Poisons Act of 1904, in which arsenic was named in the schedule of poisonous substances: indeed, the act was principally an act for the regulation of the sale of arsenic, so widespread had alarm become about its use as a homicidal and cattle-killing poison.[47] The act did not, however, prohibit or even restrict the importation of arsenic, nor limit its industrial use: business interests had strongly opposed any move that would prevent the sale and use of so useful a commodity. Rather the act targeted what was seen as its criminal misuse, including its allegedly wide and indiscriminate employment as an ingredient in vernacular medicine.

But therapeutically as well as physically, arsenic remains a highly mobile substance. For all its criminal associations, arsenic was written into the narrative of India's medical progress. It was an active ingredient in several widely recommended tonics, including Fowler's Solution and Donovan's Solution, both of which were supplied to Indian dispensaries.[48] It was also the principal element in Paul Ehrlich's wonder-drug salvarsan discovered in 1909. This was a drug of global significance and one of the first to use the known toxicity of a substance as an agent in modern chemotherapy. But it had a particular significance for India where the hospitalization (and occasional death) of British soldiers from venereal disease had for decades been a major concern for the colonial health authorities. This story of discovery and progress had, however, a darker side. The administration of salvarsan could have severe toxic side effects and a number of cases of this nature were reported from Indian hospitals and clinics, even with follow-up drugs, such as neo-salvarsan, which were intended to be less toxic. India was certainly not alone in this, but the adverse effect of arsenic-based drugs does provide a further local illustration of the pharmakon medicine/poison conundrum and the paradox of condemning in indigenous medicine a therapeutic strategy contemporaneously employed in Western chemotherapeutic technique.[49]

Kerosene

Kerosene further extends the arguments already made about the transoceanic trafficking of substances and their toxic/therapeutic transformation. Nux vomica and arsenic fit with ease into the conventions and ambiguities of the pharmakon: in India their use as both poisonous substances and as medical ingredients was ancient, if greatly accentuated, at both extremes, as both poison and medicine, in colonial times. Rather different was the case of kerosene, which had no immediate precedents in either capacity, but was a by-product of the modern petroleum industry. Indeed, kerosene attests to the many rapid changes occurring in India's material culture in the late nineteenth and early twentieth centuries, as much in relation to its everyday technologies as to its medicinal culture and public health regime.[50]

In the late nineteenth century, India's kerosene came mostly from the United States and southern Russia. In 1887, 30 million gallons entered Indian ports, with a value of Rs 12 million.[51] Six years later, in 1893, 64 million gallons were imported. By 1911 this had risen to over 75 million gallons, with a value of over £2 million, though by that date India's supply increasingly came from the oilfields of British Burma: already a major supplier of rice, Burma now added a second essential commodity – kerosene.[52] One of kerosene's principal uses was as 'lamp oil', to provide lighting for streets and homes, and in this role foreign oil rapidly displaced indigenous sources of illumination such as coconut and vegetable oil. It is indicative of its growing popularity and wide distribution that in 1882 Bombay municipality issued twenty-three licences to wholesale kerosene vendors and 672 to retail outlets.[53] In 1888 one visitor remarked that kerosene was 'now almost universally used for lighting by the native population'.[54] As a means of street lighting, kerosene was soon superseded by gas and electricity, but at the peak of their popularity, around 1900, there had been more 2,000 kerosene street lamps in Calcutta alone.[55] Kerosene also found a place in the kitchen, the *Times of India* declaring in 1897: 'We seem to be approaching the time when kerosene will displace every other fuel for cooking by sheer force of economy.'[56] Even the tins in which kerosene was sold entered everyday use, for carrying water or and as cladding for slum dwellings.[57] As liquid paraffin, kerosene also entered the *British Pharmacopoeia* and was incorporated into a variety of medicinal ointments.[58] It was extensively used in India (as elsewhere) as a disinfectant and, as a highly inflammable substance, it was used in the 1890s and 1900s to incinerate dead rats and burn plague-infected clothing and property. By the 1900s, as the role of anopheles mosquitoes in the transmission of malaria came to be understood, it was sprayed (like the arsenical Paris Green) on pools and watercourses to kill their larvae.[59] Kerosene thus had an impressively wide range of medical and sanitary uses.

It was not, in any conventional sense, a poison, but its capacity to harm or kill was enormous. A highly volatile fuel, kerosene presented new dangers, particularly to the city and its residents. As elsewhere in the world, urban India had long been prone to fierce conflagrations in which lives were lost and property destroyed. But the arrival of kerosene and its sale, storage and home use greatly increased the fire risk. Just as arsenic was becoming subject to new regulatory controls, so municipal authorities responded to the urban fire hazard by prohibiting the storage of large quantities of kerosene or by restricting it to locations where it posed less of a danger.[60] Nevertheless, house fires and accidental deaths due to burning kerosene proliferated from the early 1870s onwards. For instance, in 1875 at a wedding in Meerut, a case of kerosene left near a burning wick exploded, killing two people and injuring five others. Such deaths were certainly not confined to India: when the *Times of India* remarked in 1876 that kerosene-related accidents were 'daily becoming more numerous' it was referring to recent fatalities in London as well as in Cawnpore (Kanpur).[61] At work and in the home, men, women and children were all vulnerable, but across India a growing number of domestic fires and accidents caused by burning kerosene involved women. In lighting a kerosene stove or lamp or in sprinkling on kerosene to rouse a reluctant fire, women accidentally ignited their clothing – a sari or shawl caught fire and they suffered serious burns or fatal injuries.[62]

Most of these domestic incidents were recorded as accidental, but many of them were not. Quite a few kerosene-related deaths were shown on investigation by the police to be cases of wife-murder and the husband or in-laws were charged with causing the wife's death.[63] In 1906 there were eighty-nine reported deaths from burns in Calcutta alone, the great majority concerning women. But alongside these supposedly accidental deaths, or in reality murders, there were many other incidents ascribed to self-immolation and suicide. In Calcutta in 1918–19 there were twenty recorded deaths or serious injuries due to burns: some were of men but most involved women, who poured kerosene over their clothes and, in a manner that replicated the outlawed practice of sati, deliberately set themselves alight.[64] Under the headline 'Suttee in Calcutta', the *Times of India* carried a report in March 1913 about a widow who was left 'inconsolable' by her husband's death, and, while preparations were being made for his cremation, she 'quietly went on to the terrace of the house and after saturating her body with kerosene oil set fire to herself'. The building was 'practically burnt to a cinder before the inmates ... became aware of her terrible fate'.[65]

In 1929 the same newspaper reported a 'grave suspicion' in 'semi-official circles' in Poona (Pune) about the alarming number of cases in which young girls and widows had burnt to death, supposedly while lighting or trimming kerosene lamps. The connection with sati was again noted, for these were evidently not accidents but domestic murders or sati-like suicides. The reporter observed that anyone 'acquainted with the religious customs of the country' would be aware that 'the victims have either voluntarily or at the persuasion of others adopted a variation of the now illegal custom of suttee'.[66] A few years earlier Margaret Sinclair Stevenson vividly described the fate of many young widows in Gujarat. 'We English', she wrote, 'believe *sati* to be extinct; [Indian] reformers in certain districts of India will tell us differently.' Some widows were poisoned, others burnt to death. 'It is quite simple to soak a heavy wadded quilt in paraffin, to tie a young widow up in it, pour more oil over her, set fire to it and lock her up in a room.' The neighbours were told that the woman's clothing had accidentally caught fire while cooking or, 'like a faithful wife', she had committed sati. A simple but chilling phrase was used to allude to this widow-murder: 'paraffin is cheap ... '[67]

There was no question of banning so widely traded and extensively utilized a commodity as kerosene, still less of regulating and restricting its sale as had been the case with arsenic, strychnine and other potentially lethal poisons. Kerosene was not in a formal sense a poison, and yet it too found a place in the annals of Indian murder, suicide and accidental death.

Conclusion

Three substances – nux vomica/strychnine, arsenic and kerosene – have been highlighted in this discussion to describe the phenomenon of the pharmakon, in which, according to situation, perception and use, substances moved, often erratically, between the seemingly discrete but only superficially distinct spheres of the toxic and the therapeutic. The cases discussed suggest the importance of the Indian Ocean as a maritime region from which, and through which, a great number of drugs constantly travelled, sometimes in bulk, often in relatively small quantities, first as raw materials and then in a highly processed, refined and manufactured form. But these examples surely suggest more. They illuminate the ways in which the same substance (or material derived from it) might move into and out of British India, through the ports of the Indian Ocean, and in the process undergo very substantial changes, not through any action of the sea itself but in relation to the meanings and usages assigned to such toxic/therapeutic commodities. Arsenic might be a poison and a medicament anywhere in the world, kerosene might have its medicinal and public health applications; but the uses to which these substances were put, not least in their toxic rather than their therapeutic roles, might vary enormously, according to the cultural and political context in which they operated. In India arsenic could find use as an aphrodisiac and a nerve tonic; nux vomica could symbolize the emergence of a revitalized indigenous medicine and a patriotic pharmacopoeia. Kerosene could be a healing substance, an antiseptic; but it could also be deployed, in a fire-and-gender idiom peculiar to India, for killing wives and widows and for sati-like acts of self-immolation.

These cases further suggest the latent power such mineral or biochemical substances possessed. In themselves, we might argue, they had no intrinsic capacity to heal or to harm, until, that is, they were pressed into the human service, until they became instrumental in human activities and the power relations those activities entailed. Who, then, gave agency to these substances, to these organic or inorganic materials? The nux vomica nuts collected by the Yanadis of Nellore became enfolded within a complex system of resource and revenue extraction and an expanding network of political authority and global economic activity, in which Indians and non-British Europeans were also to varying degrees involved – as traders, shippers, manufacturers and chemists. Imported arsenic served the growing needs of Indian industry and commerce, but it might also be said to have empowered, however temporarily, subaltern communities of unhappy wives and low-caste cow-killers – until, that is, the power of the colonial state intervened to curb such practices and sought to prohibit or curtail them under the Poisons Act of 1904. The ambiguity inherent in such traded substances contributed to this potency: were they poisons or were they medicines? It left room for those who used them or opposed their use to determine whether they stood for good or evil, for preserving and improving human life or, on the contrary, for causing its imminent and treacherous destruction.

Notes

1 David Arnold, 'The Indian Ocean as a Disease Zone, 1500–1950', *South Asia* 14, no. 2 (1991): 1–21; Michael Pearson, 'Medical Connections and Exchanges in the

Early Modern World', *PORTAL* 8, no. 2 (2011): 1–15; *Histories of Medicine and Healing in the Indian Ocean World*, ed. Anna Winterbottom and Facil Tesfaye, 2 vols (Basingstoke: Palgrave Macmillan, 2016); *Disease Dispersion and Impact in the Indian Ocean World*, ed. Gwyn Campbell and Eva-Maria Knoll (Basingstoke: Palgrave Macmillan, 2020).

2 A methodology employed, for a much earlier period, in Elizabeth A. Lambourn, *Abraham's Luggage: A Social Life of Things in the Medieval Indian Ocean World* (Cambridge: Cambridge University Press, 2018), especially chapter 8.

3 Andrew Sherratt, 'Introduction: Peculiar Substances', in *Consuming Habits: Drugs in History and Anthropology*, ed. Jordan Goodman, Paul E. Lovejoy, and Andrew Sherratt (London: Routledge, 1995), 1–10.

4 This chapter extends and develops the discussion in David Arnold, *Toxic Histories: Poison and Pollution in Modern India* (Cambridge: Cambridge University Press, 2016), 41–77.

5 On 'medical systems', see T. A. Wise, *Commentary on the Hindu System of Medicine* (London: Smith, Elder, 1845); *Asian Medical Systems: A Comparative Study*, ed. Charles Leslie (Berkeley: University of California Press, 1976); Guy Attewell, *Refiguring Unani Tibb: Plural Healing in Late Colonial India* (Hyderabad: Orient Blackswan, 2007).

6 A significant exception being Francis Zimmermann, *The Jungle and the Aroma of Meats: An Ecological Theme in Hindu Medicine* (Berkeley: University of California Press, 1987).

7 The diverse geographical and material sources of Indian medicine are, however, clear from such works as W. Ainslie, *Materia Indica*, 2 vols (London: Longman, Rees, Orme, Brown and Green, 1826). For nux vomica, see ibid., 1: 317–22.

8 C. F. Ponder and D. Hooper, *An Introduction to Materia Medica for India* (Calcutta: Thacker, Spink, 1901), 115.

9 The bark, however, was sold in Calcutta as a febrifuge: *Royle's Manual of Materia Medica*, ed. John Harley, 6th ed. (London: J. and A. Churchill, 1876), 513. The roots were said to cure snakebite: Ainslie, *Materia Indica*, 1: 319.

10 Edgar Thurston with K. Rangachari, *Castes and Tribes of Southern India*, 7 vols (Madras: Government Press, 1909), 7: 416–34.

11 Known in Sanskrit as *Culcka* or *Kataka*, nux vomica was the Koochla (Kuchla) of the Hindus 'by whom it has long been used as medicine': *Royle's Manual of Materia Medica*, 511. On tribal ethnobotany, see S. K. Varma, D. K. Sriwastawa, and A. K. Pandey, *Ethnobotany of Santhal Pargana* (Delhi: Narenda, 1999).

12 Thurston and Rangachari, *Castes and Tribes*, 7: 418, 430. This reflects a more general use of India's 'wild tribes' as gatherers of 'minor produce' for the colonial state: see *Report of the Bombay Forest Commission*, 4 vols (Bombay: Government Central Press, 1887), 1: 104–8.

13 J. S. Gamble, *A Manual of Indian Timbers*, 2nd edn (London: Sampson Low, Marston, 1920), 497; Ainslie, *Materia Indica*, 1: 317.
14 Ponder and Hooper, *An Introduction to Materia Medica*, i.
15 Ainslie, *Materia Indica*, 1: 318–19; Kapil Raj, *Relocating Modern Science: Circulation and the Construction of Knowledge in South Asia and Europe, 1650–1900* (London: Palgrave Macmillan, 2007), 48–9.
16 Robert Christison, *A Treatise on Poisons* (Philadelphia: Edward Barrington and George D. Haswell, 1845), 686–91.
17 W. B. O'Shaughnessy, *Bengal Dispensatory and Pharmacopoeia* (Calcutta: Bishop's College Press, 1841), 438–9.
18 For datura and its uses, see Arnold, *Toxic Histories*, 63–7.
19 J. J. Sudborough and J. L. Simonsen, 'Chemical Industries', in *Industrial Handbook* (Calcutta: Indian Munitions Board, 1919), 96; E. A. Smythies, *India's Forest Wealth*, 2nd ed. (London: Oxford University Press, 1925), 107.
20 *Times of India* (hereafter *ToI*) 27 October 1870, 4.
21 J. E. De Vry and E. A. Van der Burg, 'On the Detection of Strychnine in Cases of Poisoning', *Pharmaceutical Journal*, March 1857, 1–4.
22 Listed as both nux vomica and strychnine in the *British Pharmacopoeia* (London: Spottiswoode, 1898), 222, 314. In 1913 the *Pharmacopoeia* listed at least twenty-one drugs of Indian origin: David Hooper, 'Drug Culture in British India', *Indian Forester* 39, no. 9 (1913): 440–6.
23 *ToI*, 21 September 1874, 1. Easton's contained quinine, iron phosphate and 1/32 of a grain of strychnine: R. Wright, 'Note on Easton's Syrup', *American Journal of Pharmacy*, November 1893, 538. Due to its potency and the danger of overdosage, it was not considered suitable for children.
24 *ToI*, 29 April 1879; ibid., 4 April 1885, 8.
25 Clare Anderson, *Subaltern Lives: Biographies of Colonialism in the Indian Ocean World, 1790–1920* (Cambridge: Cambridge University Press, 2012).
26 For instance, Collis Barry, *Legal Medicine (in India) and Toxicology*, 2nd ed., 2 vols (Bombay: Thacker, 1904), 1: 447–57.
27 In 1926 there were fifty-two reported cases of poisoning by strychnine in India out of 3,281: this compared to more than a thousand deaths from both opium and arsenic: 'Statistical Abstract for British India, 1917–1918 to 1926–1927', *Parliamentary Papers*, Cmd 3291, 1927, table 189, 402.
28 B. D. Basu, 'On the Study of Indigenous Drugs', *Indian Medical Gazette* 26, no. 7 (1891): 199–203; K. M. Nadkarni, *Indian Plants and Drugs with their Medical Properties and Uses* (Madras: Norton, 1908).
29 *Representative Drugs of India* (Calcutta: B. K. Paul, 1924), 8.
30 Barry, *Legal Medicine*, 1: 294.
31 P. Hehir and J. D. B. Gribble, *Outlines of Medical Jurisprudence for India*, 5th ed. (Madras: Higginbotham, 1908), 533.

32 J. Forbes Royle, *Illustrations of the Botany and Other Branches of the Natural History of the Himalayan Mountains*, 2 vols (London: W. H. Allen, 1839), 1: 48; James Ranald Martin, *The Influence of Tropical Climates on European Constitutions* (London: John Churchill, 1856), 167–8. For the adoption and then rejection of Indian arsenic pills by Western physicians, see Pratik Chakrabarti, *Materials and Medicine: Trade, Conquest and Therapeutics in the Eighteenth Century* (Manchester: Manchester University Press, 2010), 182–7.

33 *Royle's Manual of Materia Medica*, 287–92; Barry, *Legal Medicine*, 1: 362–6.

34 Ainslie, *Materia Indica*, 1: 501–2.

35 Hehir and Gribble, *Outlines of Medical Jurisprudence*, 532.

36 E.g., *Bombay Times* (hereafter *BT*), 24 November 1856, 4782; *ToI*, 2 September 1892, 3; ibid., 6 December 1928, 9; ibid., 15 July 1929, 9.

37 Malcolm Morris, 'Arsenic', in *Dangerous Trades: The Historical, Social, and Legal Aspects of Industrial Occupations as Affecting Health*, ed. Thomas Oliver (London: John Murray, 1902), 378–81.

38 V. Ball, *Manual of the Geology of India, Part III* (Calcutta: Office of the Geological Survey of India, 1881), 572–3.

39 For a discussion of India's poison culture, see Arnold, *Toxic Histories*.

40 Hehir and Gribble, *Outlines of Medical Jurisprudence*, 532.

41 T. E. B. Brown, *Punjab Poisons*, 3rd ed. (Lahore: Civil and Military Gazette Press, 1888), 19; 'Poisoning in India', *British Medical Journal*, 17 September 1892, 642.

42 See, for instance, *BT*, 1 February 1853, 213; ibid., 21 February 1853, 350; *ToI*, 18 July 1901, 3; ibid., 21 August 1920, 18.

43 *ToI*, 17 May 1893, 4; Hehir and Gribble, *Outlines of Medical Jurisprudence*, 545–6.

44 Arnold, *Toxic Histories*, 151–6.

45 *ToI*, 27 April 1893, 4.

46 A 'medicinal dose' of arsenic might be an eighth of a grain; anywhere between two and twenty grains might kill an adult. See the Nagpada poisoning case in Bombay: *ToI*, 3 February 1888, 3.

47 On the Indian Poisons Act, see Arnold, *Toxic Histories*, 156–62.

48 Hehir and Gribble, *Outlines of Medical Jurisprudence*, 532.

49 Arnold, *Toxic Histories*, 170.

50 David Arnold, *Everyday Technology: Machines and the Making of India's Modernity* (Chicago: University of Chicago Press, 2013).

51 *Accounts Relating to the Sea-Borne Trade and Navigation of British India, March 1890*, 20–1.

52 *ToI*, 25 August 1894, 4, ibid., 23 April 1910, 11; *Accounts Relating to the Sea-Borne Trade and Navigation of British India, 1913*, 27.

53 *Annual Report of the Municipal Commissioner, Bombay, 1882*, 369.

54 Robert Wallace, *India in 1887* (Edinburgh: Oliver and Boyd, 1888), 221.

55 *Report on the Municipal Administration of Calcutta, 1901–1902*, 54; ibid., *1910–1911*, xviii.
56 *ToI*, 17 July 1897, 4.
57 Sidney Low, *A Vision of India*, 2nd ed. (London: Smith, Elder, 1907), 80, and photograph facing 84; *ToI*, 2 February 1897, 5.
58 *British Pharmacopoeia*, 239–40.
59 *Report on the Municipal Administration of Calcutta, 1906–1907*, 69.
60 *Report on the Municipal Administration of Calcutta, 1911–1912*, 95.
61 *ToI*, 9 May 1875, 3; ibid., 10 June 1876, 3.
62 *ToI*, 25 January 1892, 3; *Bombay Chronicle*, 22 January 1927, 4.
63 *Report and Statistical Tables of the Calcutta Fire Brigade, 1916*, xi.
64 *Report on the Municipal Administration of Calcutta, 1906–1907*, appx. J, 92; *Report and Statistical Tables of the Calcutta Fire Brigade, 1919*, appx. 12, xii.
65 *ToI*, 3 March 1913, 10. Also see *ToI*, 19 March 1918, 9; ibid., 25 April 1931, 14.
66 *ToI*, 28 May 1929, 10.
67 [Margaret] Sinclair Stevenson, *Rites of the Twice-Born* (London: Oxford University Press, 1920), 207–8.

8

'The all-cleansing soap'? History of soap in Keralam c. 1880–1950

Greeshma Justin John

Introduction

K. R. Gowriyamma (1919–2021), one of Keralam's[1] pre-eminent political leaders of the twentieth century, writes in her 2010 autobiography, entitled *Aathmakatha*:

> Today, Kerala(m) is celebrated for hygiene and cleanliness of attire. The land that consumes the largest quantity of soap. However, some of my earliest memories are of poor men and women in dirty, soiled clothes. Men would wrap themselves in modest loincloths. A decent piece of clothing was beyond the means of the masses.[2]

Gowriyamma's claim of Kerala's supposedly high soap consumption encapsulates the story of soap's transition into an everyday object in the region over approximately a century. Under the influence of the manifold shifts brought about by colonial modernity, communities and groups in Keralam in the late nineteenth and early twentieth centuries had sought to transform their social condition by initiating changes in material life. The human body became a critical site around which social change was concretized. These transitions were more pertinent to social groups that were considered lower in the caste hierarchy. Reform leaders from these sections identified the new material practices of hygiene as one avenue for social mobility. Bodily cleanliness, therefore, came to be negotiated through the use of the object: soap. By placing soap at the juncture of the material-discursive shifts around cleanliness, this chapter attempts to understand the meanings it acquired in Keralam between the late nineteenth and mid-twentieth centuries. I argue that soap became a thing of power, with which different communities and groups in Keralam negotiated their social position.

The chapter opens by making a case for the emphasis on Keralam. It then identifies the developing soap manufacturing networks in the early twentieth century that took soap to a broader swathe of the Malayali populace. The often-fraught relationship between different production networks resulted in the colonial classification of soap into 'standard' and 'spurious'. The subsequent section narrates how dominant social groups in Keralam appropriated this classification to articulate anxieties about soap's subversive effects on 'Malayaliness', notably when middle-class women and lower classes (and by extension, 'lower castes') used it. Finally, the chapter will show how soap assumed therapeutic properties, not just as the *oushadham*/medicine that preserves the physical body but also as a curative for the illness of caste that affected the social body of Keralam. I begin by elaborating why a focus on Keralam is of value by highlighting certain departures in soap production and consumption in early twentieth-century Keralam vis-à-vis that of the subcontinent.

Soap's regional trajectory

Modern, industrially produced soap made inroads into Keralam from the late nineteenth century. This was when soap, imported primarily from England, was introduced into the subcontinent. At the turn of the twentieth century, soap was more of a luxury good consumed along with flannels and hats, clocks and oyster plates, tea biscuits and cocoa.[3] Given the unique social geography of Keralam in the late nineteenth century,[4] the modernizing social groups, drawn mainly from the upper echelons of caste hierarchy, formed the biggest consumers of soap.[5] Their association with colonial administration and ready access to modern education, overseas travel/migration, commodity market and the emerging print public sphere had facilitated the exchange of ideas and materials across spaces.[6] These exchanges brought the dominant social groups into contact with novel habits like the use of soap. While this early trajectory of soap in Keralam fits with that of the subcontinent, some regional factors altered its production and consumption subsequently.

Keralam's physical geography, for example, which supported extensive coconut cultivations and a robust, local oil industry developing since the late nineteenth century, was one. With the global shift from tallow to vegetable oils as the chief ingredient of soap by the early twentieth century,[7] Keralam's abundant coconut oil supply attracted subcontinental and international trade, simultaneously nurturing a regional soap industry.[8] In the aftermath of the First World War, the decline in copra price spurred an emerging group of entrepreneurs who aspired to manoeuvre such global trends.[9] Coupled with technological and financial backing by the colonial and princely governments, soap manufacturers increased in the opening decades of the twentieth century;[10] and large-scale soap factories like Kerala Soap Institute (hereafter KSI), established in Kozhikode by the Madras government in 1917, captured markets in Keralam and beyond.[11] By the early 1930s, soap manufacturing units seemed to have clustered around 'important towns' across Keralam, such as Kozhikode (Malabar), Thrissur (Cochin) and Kollam (Travancore).[12]

In terms of consumption, imported soaps had commanded a steady market in the subcontinent until the intensification of the Swadeshi movement around 1915,[13] whenceforth locally manufactured soaps began to expand their market. The response to Pears', an English brand, shows the impact of Swadeshi in Keralam. Even as Keralam embraced the Swadeshi call for soap manufacturing early on,[14] the penchant for Bilathi (English) brands lingered among the modernizing middle-classes.[15] Of these, Pears' Glycerine was regarded as a soap of superior quality.[16] When Pears' was disparaged elsewhere in India in the 1930s,[17] a 1933 school textbook from Cochin carried an image of a Pears' cake in a chapter on soap.[18] Adherence to colonial notions of quality had resulted in the continuing popularity of *Bilathi* soaps among the modernized middle-classes. In contrast, factors like affordability and sensorial appeal seemed to have determined soap consumption among 'the poor'.[19] Be it the locally produced, so-called spurious imitations of well-known brands or imported Japanese soaps that flooded markets in the Madras Presidency in the early twentieth century, this consumer strata had a range of low-priced options.[20] Japanese soaps of attractive colours, perfumes and packaging, but allegedly of substandard quality particularly fit the often-pejorative portrayals of 'mass taste'.[21] We thus see the crystallization of a set of values shaping consumer preferences around class, which existed separately from the nationalist impulses animating the Swadeshi movement, and probably subduing them too. Even if such consumption patterns existed elsewhere in the subcontinent, we could still find instances of a region-specific interpretation of the meaning of *swadeshi* in Keralam. When KSI's soaps, including its *swadeshi*-labelled, vegetable-oil brands, faced a boycott in Tamil and Telugu-speaking regions in the 1920s for their association with the British government, Malayalis continued to patronize the company.[22] Malabar remained KSI's principal market for decades. KSI soaps registered a boost in sales in the 1930s in the princely state of Cochin as well.[23] Staffed predominantly by Malayalis and maintaining multiple social ties with the regional milieu, KSI was practically a *swadeshi* company in Keralam. This might explain the sale of the 'government' soaps (as KSI soaps were known locally) in *swadeshi* goods stores in Cochin and securing gold medals in the All India Khadi and Swadeshi Exhibition: an annual exhibition organized in Kozhikode by Malabar-based activists in the 1930s.[24] In this period, KSI products were also showcased on several regional platforms, including *melas* (fairs) and community-specific events like the Keraliya Nayar Samajam Conference in Chavara (Travancore).[25]

This response to soaps with tallow content further illustrates the peculiarity of Keralam's soap consumption in the early twentieth century. By the early 1920s, large-scale companies like Godrej, headquartered in colonial cities like Bombay, began to market vegetable-oil-based soaps through intense advertising campaigns against tallow-based soaps.[26] Such strategies sought to tap into the cultural sentiments of people, rooted chiefly in caste, against soaps with animal fat content.[27] However, sources allude to the relatively slow percolation and limited influence of anti-tallow discourses in Keralam. The imported, tallow-based soaps posed a strong competition for vegetable-oil-based soaps, and the putrefying effect of the local climate on vegetable-oil-based products led to animal fat being seen as an essential ingredient in soap manufacture in Keralam. KSI, for instance, found that its vegetable-oil-based soaps rarely 'approach either in colour, feeling or smell, the usual quality imported from England' and that without tallow, the soaps turned rancid in the monsoon season.[28] Between 1930 and 1950, KSI used imported Australian tallow and 'country tallow' procured from suppliers based in Alappuzha (Travancore) and Kozhikode.[29] KSI was not an exception, though; companies like Techno Chemical Industries, established in 1930 in Kozhikode by dominant caste Swadeshi entrepreneurs, produced soaps using 'indigenously sourced' tallow.[30]

As regards consumers, the tallow content of soap was widely known, certainly among literate sections in Keralam, as hinted by an array of sources ranging from late nineteenth-century school textbooks to advice literature appearing in the 1910s.[31] At this point, opposition to soap by traditionalists was couched in arguments about the evils of consumerist vanity or the practical difficulties in using soap, and made no mention of its tallow content.[32] Culturally, the abhorrence for animal fat including tallow was of limited purchase in Keralam as most Malayalis, who belonged to subjugated castes and non-Hindu communities,[33] did not share the aversion as much as the dominant castes. Consequently, matters with animal ingredients, be it food, medicine, cosmetic agents or artisanal materials, were part of the everyday life of Keralam. This context perhaps explains the Cochin school textbook's nonchalant reference to soap's *kozhuppu* (animal fat) content.[34] But anti-tallow discourses seeped into Keralam eventually, as suggested by a review of soap advertisements in *Mathrubhumi Weekly* between 1932 and 1953. Accordingly, very few companies emphasized the vegetable content of soaps until the early 1940s. As a host of companies from Bombay, including TOMCO and Swastik Oil Mills, began to advertise their animal-fat-free soaps extensively in Keralam, regional soap brands including the *oushadha* (medicinal) soaps fashioned from *nattuvaidya* traditions, began to emulate the trend.[35]

To summarize, the geographical advantage in production and consumption trends shaped by region-specific interpretations of soap's *swadeshi* character, centred on the identification of manufacturers as 'foreign' or 'local' and purity, based on soap's tallow or vegetable-oil content, plotted a different trajectory for soap in Keralam compared to rest of the subcontinent. The following section will look at the emerging soap industry in the early twentieth century.

Networks of soap production

The coexistence of soap makers of diverse scales, employing varied production techniques, ingredients and marketing strategies, characterized the soap production landscape of early twentieth-century Keralam. A network of manufacturers developed around the institutional initiatives of colonial and princely governments, as aspiring soap makers received support through information disseminated in print media by government chemists, public demonstrations of manufacturing processes, rewards and financial assistance.[36] Moreover, the governments offered training either by offering overseas scholarships or through its agencies, such as Travancore's Industrial Research Laboratory and KSI, the Madras government concern.[37] KSI became a node for training in soap manufacture in Keralam, and trainees from the Institute launched soap companies across the region.[38] However, the formal soap production networks catered primarily to entrepreneurs from dominant social groups, who possessed adequately modern, scientific knowledge to acquire training and sufficient capital to launch businesses of scale and sophistication.[39]

Simultaneously, cottage-scale soap manufacturing units started to develop, drawing on alternate, informal nodes of knowledge transfer and located mainly outside the domain of institutional networks.[40] Compared to formal networks, soap makers of such alternate networks hailed from diverse socio-economic backgrounds. In colonial descriptions, a cottage-scale unit consisted of 'a small room or two or some backspace behind the kitchen'.[41] Sometimes, they functioned alongside oil mills, like the Lazar Rice-Oil-Soap Mills based in Irinjalakkuda (Cochin).[42] These soap manufacturers utilized diverse ingredients and techniques. Consider V. K. Kunju Muhammad, a merchant from Kodungallur (Cochin), who launched one of the earliest modern soap companies around 1900: the firm's Camel-brand laundry soaps, produced through the cold-process method and using materials like *neettu kakka* (quicklime obtained by heating locally sourced clamshells), found a steady market in Malabar.[43] Similarly, a Namboothiri Brahmin in Tiruvalla (Travancore) reportedly ran a concern around 1919 'based entirely on old books', employing locally sourced ingredients like *cadjan* ashes for alkali.[44] However, smaller firms drew on the name, labelling, colouring and/or packaging techniques of established companies. See, for example, the Kozhikode-based 'Garland' soap company, which sounded like 'Government' in local parlance, or the 'Sarkar' Vegetable Soap from Palakkad, which sounded like 'Sirkar' (government), as KSI brands were known.[45]

While large-scale firms maintained extensive marketing and distribution mechanisms, cottage companies relied on informal, local channels and networks of distribution. For instance, writer-reformer V. T. Bhattathiripad (1896–1982) mentions the itinerant Chetty women vendors who sold soap and cosmetics across households; the figure of the hawker, who announces his/her arrival by calling out 'soapu . . . cheepu . . . kannaadi . . . ' (soap, comb, mirror), is etched in Malayalam popular culture as well.[46] While large-scale firms attempted to entice customers with 'gifts' like extra soap, perfumes and towels, small-scale companies resorted to strategies like the 'credit system': an arrangement based on trust wherein consumers could purchase soap and settle their payment later.[47] The rootedness of cottage soap firms in the local social milieu enabled flexibility in distribution, something that was difficult for large-scale companies with formalized distribution systems.

In the 1920s, only about six factories in India, including KSI, could afford the more sophisticated boiled-process method appropriate for the production of milled toilet soaps.[48] Most soap makers in Keralam, irrespective of scale, employed the cold-process method, which allows soaps to be manufactured at room temperature with rudimentary equipment and readily available oils like coconut oil.[49] The production process of cottage-scale soap makers was termed crude and unscientific by colonial experts, who portrayed these soaps as inferior. A standard manufacturing formula unavailable till 1924,[50] most soaps came with excessive oil and/or alkali content. By colonial standards, several local brands would be listed as 'adulterated'.[51] Firms accused of imitating KSI's Vegetol brand were said to be misleading 'the ignorant public'.[52] Contentions around soap quality between the formal and alternate soap production networks gave rise to the classification of soaps into 'standard' and 'spurious' in the 1920s. Despite this labelling, cottage soap makers flourished in the subsequent decades, impacting the business of large-scale companies.[53] When a crop of soap makers who could adopt sophisticated production techniques emerged in Keralam in the subsequent decades, they came to share the colonial concern with adulteration and quality. Thus, the South-Indian Soap Manufacturer's Association, an alliance of some of the well-heeled, regional soap firms, raised concerns about the quality and 'purity' of soaps and called for regulation and control in 1947.[54]

While the colonial government used the discourse of adulteration to control the emerging local soap industry, concern for the quality of soaps among Malayalis transformed into exercises in social hegemony. We see, for example, that the seemingly damaging effects of soap on skin and clothes supplied ammunition for censure of its consumption by women and 'the poor'. The following section will elucidate the sociological implications of the discourse on adulteration in Keralam.

Purity and danger

In a 1907 article on *sthreedharmam* (women's duties) in a women's magazine, writer Karat Achyutha Menon (1866–1913) stated:

> The application of soap on the body – sometimes even laundry soaps – has become common by the erroneous notion of its goodness or due to its modern aura or simply for its ephemeral effect on body odour. Most toilet soaps are harmful to the skin. After all, the *ennathechukuli* suits *us* (my emphasis) best. The treatment prescribed in *Arogya Chinthamani* for body odour is preferable to soap.[55]

The appearance of this subtle admonishment of toilet soap consumption coincided with the reconfigurations of gender relations and the moulding of a domestic realm in early twentieth-century Keralam.[56] In this period, writings by/for middle-class, dominant caste women appearing in Malayalam magazines began to associate female domestic labour with laundry/household soaps and peculiar notions of femininity, toilet soaps.[57] This gendered deployment of soap, which would be reinforced through advertisements, simultaneously reflected and shaped its consumption by middle-class women, instantaneously attracting patriarchal antagonism. For example, novelist Thakazhi Sivasankara Pillai's (1912–99) childhood memoir reveals how laundry soap triggered 'domestic instability' in his house and village in early twentieth-century Travancore, pitting 'housewives' against men. For women, *soapukaram* (soap-powder) was a convenient substitute for *cadjan* ashes, the preparation of which was a labourious process. At the same time, men dismissed soap as an abrasive detergent that spoiled the cloth.[58] A greater risk, however, was the possible damage that toilet soaps, with its potentially transgressive ideas of convenience, female beauty and agency, inflicted on the fabric of Malayali culture. The discourse of adulteration fitted neatly with the resultant need to discredit and discourage the consumption culture emerging around soap. As we saw, Karat Achyutha Menon considered the use of toilet soaps as driven by vain, superficial concerns to the extent that consumers seemingly disregarded its detrimental effects.[59] The alternative to modern soap was 'tradition', embodied in *ennathechukuli* and the deodorizing method prescribed in *Arogya Chinthamani*: smearing the body with a mixture of (the ritually significant) cow-urine and buffalo-dung and washing it off with a herbal concoction.[60] This criticism of soap, while not entirely directed at women, entrusts housewives with the duty of preserving Malayali culture and tradition represented by conventional bathing techniques against the onslaught of *parishkaram* (reform/modernisation) embodied by soap. Menon's advice, in effect, sought to curb women's participation, real or potential, in the consumption of soap.

The juxtaposition of tradition as the remedy for the supposed dangers of modern soap did not spare men either: in a 1917 article, for example, Chengalath Kunhirama Menon (1857–1935), a prominent Nair journalist, satirized the vanity of modern consumerism that objects like soap epitomized, and specifically, the Nair proclivity for *parishkaram*.[61] The article featured the caricature of a modernized, male Menon lawyer who, among other things, used Pears' and Cuticura soap and his rustic, traditional-minded wife, struggling to keep up with her *parishkari* husband's exotic tastes.[62] For the author, the frivolity also stemmed from the perceived illogicality in soap, which had oil content, replacing oil-bathing besides being a time-consuming habit.[63] The article's publication in *Mangalodayam*, the mouthpiece of Yogakshema Sabha, which was a Namboothiri organization, also suggests the divergent approaches of Namboothiri Brahmins and Nairs on the question of *parishkaram* in the early twentieth century. While most modernized Nairs had cultivated novel corporeal habits from at least the late nineteenth century, Namboothiris, by and large, remained rigidly protective of their ritual practices and what they understood as tradition, even decades into the twentieth century.[64] Such aversion to matters modern meant that while Nairs had come to access soap from the late nineteenth century, its entry into the Brahmin households was delayed by a few decades. Namboothiri writer Devaki Nilayangodu's (born 1928) evocative recollection of her first experience of soap in the mid-1930s illustrates this. That Nilayangodu's first cake of soap was a gift from her modernized Nair cousins was far from a coincidence, and she treasured the object for a long time, using it only minimally.[65]

The contrasting attitudes to soap notwithstanding, most middle-class, dominant caste critics and advocates of soap shared notions of the inferior quality of cottage-produced soaps. Combined with the judgement on the taste (or lack of it) of those beneath them emerged the criticism of soap consumption of 'the poorer classes' in the early twentieth century. A dip in prices of locally produced soaps in the 1920s had widened the product's consumer base across Keralam. In 1924, an industry watcher, N. K. Krishna Pilla, observed that 'white soaps' (i.e. probably laundry soaps) that cost two *chakram* per cake earlier were available in the local bazaars of Travancore for two *anna* per dozen.[66] But Pilla's jubilation about the replacement of *videshi* by the *swadeshi* white soaps was marked by reservations about the quality of the local product. Apprehensions of soap's quality with respect to its consumption by the lower classes were commonly expressed in the early twentieth-century Malayalam periodicals. As early as 1905, a commentator observed that, of the different kinds of soaps available in the bazaar, *saadhaarana janangal* (ordinary people) purchased soaps by their scents and price, unmindful of their quality.[67] The article, therefore, requested the Malabar-based medical journal *Dhanwantari* to publish information about the composition and types of soaps for the benefit of 'non-chemists'. The *saadharana janangal*, however, continued to use soaps deemed substandard by colonial and middle-class elites, regardless of the many cautionary tales directed at them. The frequent references to the losses incurred by the popularity of 'ridiculously low-priced' coloured imitations and Japanese soaps in KSI documents between the 1920s and 1930s indicate this. Correspondingly, observations hinting at the recalcitrance of the masses persisted: a 1937 article opined that *sadhukkal* (the poor) chose to risk their well-being by using cheap, substandard soaps.[68] Compared to the more expensive flower-mark (*poo chaappa*) and scented toilet (*vaasana/mana*) soap brands available in the market, cheaper soaps that came in attractive flavours and wrappers provided affordable choices for lower classes while also addressing their consumer tastes. Sometimes, laundry soaps doubled up as toilet soaps for the poorer classes.[69] However, this consumer segment gained value for large-scale companies, and a bevy of strategies was devised to absorb them. The production of multipurpose (i.e. laundry-cum-toilet) soaps and the sale of soaps in various dimensions such as half/quarter cake, scraps, and loose chips[70] by companies furnished make-do options for lower middle-classes and those beneath them. Already by the 1920s, a shift in trend favouring 'durable', scented soaps over lathering, 'wasteful' soaps was observed.[71] While thrift is not an exclusively lower-middle-class value/practice, it nevertheless points to the emergence of an alternate perception of soap as a mass commodity, at least by soap companies.

Consumption of soap by 'the poor' in the first half of the twentieth century happened despite the grave socio-economic conditions in Keralam, caused by the successive waves of epidemics, famines, natural disasters like the flood of 1924, the aftereffects of the Great Depression and social-political upheavals.[72] The durability of this culture of soap, while derided by dominant social groups, therefore played a crucial role in transforming soap into an affordable commodity in early twentieth-century Keralam. In contrast, dominant castes maintained an ambiguous relationship with soap, exemplified by responses ranging from explicit opposition and selective acceptance to appreciating soap as a *nirantharopakari* (constant benefactor) and an indispensable everyday object that assured its users a place in the civilizational ladder of modernity.[73] This equivocal approach to soap must be placed in the context of the appropriation of modern, European sensibilities of cleanliness in India in the late nineteenth and early twentieth centuries.[74] In Keralam, the public health and educational interventions of colonial and princely governments,[75] missionary mediations[76] and social reform movements[77] were crucial disseminators of modern ideas of cleanliness. And meanings of ablutions, concerned exclusively with the maintenance of *shudham* (the ritual purity associated with caste),[78] began to be challenged from the framework of *shuchithvam/vrithi* (hygiene/cleanliness).[79] This contestation, however, hardly caused the erasure of the premodern by the modern. Rather, *shudham* was 'transcoded' as hygiene, a manoeuvre Pandian relates to the pan-Indian process of 'secularisation of caste', by which dominant social groups rationalized caste by using modern discourses like hygiene.[80] In Keralam, as elsewhere, the construction of the binary of 'cleanly upper caste' versus 'filthy lower caste' accompanied the secularization of caste.[81] However, the generalization of grooming practices chiefly associated with dominant castes as Keralam's and the associated claims-making was a particular development; so much so that in transferring bathing, including practices like *thechukuli* from their caste locations to hygiene, its daily/regular practice was generalized as a quintessential Malayali habit.[82] Such discursive moves also pitted Malayalis as superior to other linguistic communities in the subcontinent, like Tamilians[83] as well as Europeans.[84] These positions were self-characterizations at best, considering that only dominant castes possessed the leisure and resources necessary for elaborate bathing practices like *thechukuli*.

To some extent, the recasting of dominant caste bathing practices as everyday Malayali habits created an opposition against soap, marking it off as an alien, impure object. Thus, Karat Achyutha Menon's claim that Malayali meticulousness in bodily cleanliness was unparalleled on earth appears in his defence of *thechukuli* against modern soap.[85] Chengalath Kunhirama Menon's criticism of the use of soap as an oil-wasting, time-consuming practice derives more from an acquaintance with *thechukuli* than anything else.[86] Modern soap, therefore, embodied different kinds of threats to dominant social groups: to health, social order and ultimately, their status. Their anxieties, in turn, dovetailed into perceived threat to what might be termed 'Malayaliness': the region's values and ways of life. Curiously, the antidote to the danger was soap itself, 'indigenized' as vegetable-oil-based soaps.[87] Neutralized of the risk of caste pollution posed by tallow, vegetable-oil-based soaps became incorporated into the framework of *shudham*. An incident writer-poet Madhavikutty (1934–2009) describes from her childhood in Cochin is illuminative of how soap was employed to cleanse caste pollution or *theendal*: as a child, Madhavikutty was bathed with (the vegetable-oil-based) Godrej soap, for playing with another girl, a lower-class Christian, because 'they' (*avattakal*, the abject other) reeked of fish, their staple diet.[88] By the 1930s, advertisers began to draw on the recently minted notion of Malayali fastidiousness in cleanliness (Figure 8.1).[89]

From being viewed as an object irreconcilable with Malayaliness, soap began to be projected as a commodity that could preserve the regional distinctiveness of cleanliness. In this context, a region-specific, therapeutic refashioning of soap as *oushadha* soaps occurring in early twentieth-century Keralam could bolster the predominantly caste Hindu claims of Malayali cleanliness of the time. Already by the 1940s, *oushadha* soaps came to be represented as vegetable-oil-based soaps. However, *oushadha* brands, and soap in general, accommodated a wider social constituency, when it assumed significance as a curative for the ills afflicting the social body of Keralam, especially caste. The following section analyses this layer of meaning forming around soap.

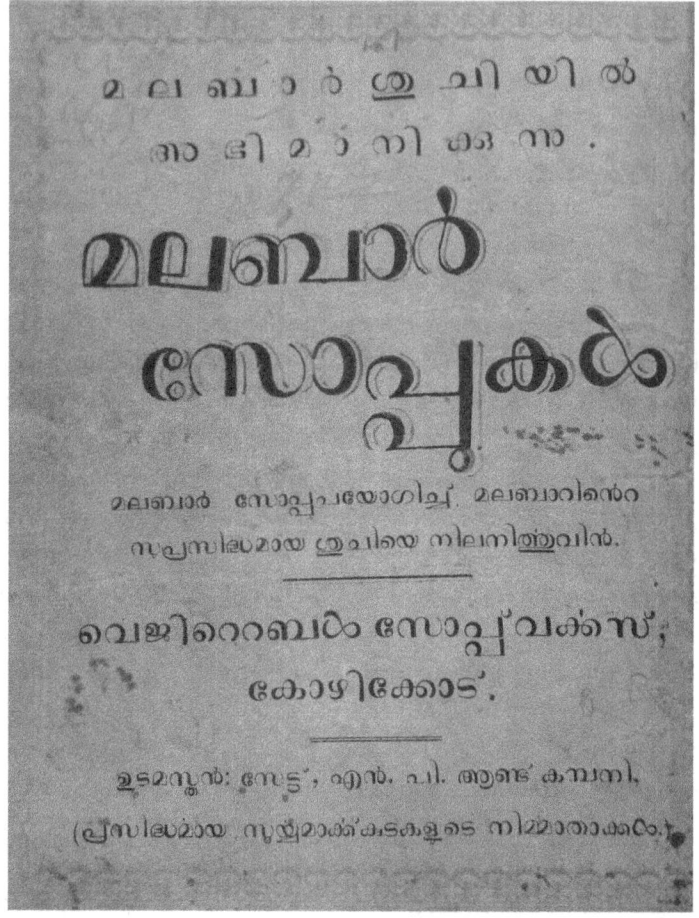

Figure 8.1 *Malabar takes pride in hygiene. Use Malabar Soaps, uphold Malabar's celebrated hygiene.* 'Malabar Soaps', Vegetable Soap Works, Kozhikode: (*Murali* 1, no. 7–8, April 1934). The name 'Malabar', meaning 'mountainous land', was historically applied to describe Keralam as well.

Cleansing the social body

In the backdrop waves of epidemics afflicting Keralam in the late nineteenth and early twentieth centuries, soap's intrinsic cleansing and germicidal properties converted it into an indispensable therapeutic object. Modern medical practitioners began to champion soaps, especially the carbolic and coal tar varieties,[90] and Malayali soap companies began to produce them. While medicated soaps were becoming a worldwide phenomenon in the period,[91] soap acquired a distinct regional spin in being recast as *oushadha* soaps by incorporating elements from the varied *nattuvaidyam* traditions in Keralam such as Ayurvedam, Siddhavaidyam and Vishavaidyam.⁹² *Oushadha* soaps claimed to cater to commonly reported skin ailments in Keralam such as leprosy, scabies, eczema and other conditions like arthritis, impure blood and envenomation. Such prescriptions were consistent with the humoral conception of the human body followed by some of the *nattuvaidya* traditions.⁹³ As the blend of *nattuvaidya* medicines and novel techniques that enhanced their shelf life, *oushadha* soaps exemplified the modernization of regional medical traditions.⁹⁴

Advertisements in Malayalam magazines and secondary literature suggest that *nattuvaidya* practitioners entered the commercial production of *oushadha* soaps from the early twentieth century. One of the first companies to manufacture *oushadha* soaps in Keralam was the Sadananda Soap Works in Kottarakkara (Travancore). Established alongside the Sadananda Avadhootha Asramam, a monastery-cum-clinic, around 1900 by the seer and *vaidya* (medical practitioner) Sadananda Swami (1877–1924), the company claimed to be the pioneer soap maker in Keralam.⁹⁵ Sadananda produced soaps infused with Ayurvedic and Siddha *oushadhas* to treat skin diseases, arthritis and other maladies. The company claimed that its soaps were best-suited for the constitution of *ee naatukaar* (the people of this land/region).⁹⁶ By the 1930s, *oushadha* soap brands proliferated in Keralam. The Malabar Shakti Oushadhasala, established in Kozhikode in 1930, produced Nalpamara Soap (*nalpamara* being a blend of medicinal herbs). Around the same time, Ramananda Swami (1896–1957), a seer and renowned Siddha *vaidya*, developed Saseendra Soap from the medical potion he had conceived to treat skin diseases at his Sidhavaidya Asramam in Thrissur. However, C. R. Kesavan Vaidyar created the more successful Chandrika Ayurvedic Soap based on the recipe developed by his *guru*, Ramananda Swami.⁹⁷ Launched in the early 1940s as a cottage-scale firm at Vaidyar's Siddha Ashramam in Irinjalakkuda (Cochin), Chandrika grew from an *oushadha* to a top vegetable-oil-based toilet soap brand in and outside Keralam within a few decades.⁹⁸ In 1938, KSI prepared *oushadha* soaps for an ayurvedic *vaidya* in Travancore; and soap for snakebite for a member of the Cochin royal house who purportedly testified to its efficacy.⁹⁹ Udaya Oushadha Soap was another well-known brand in the 1950s, produced by Thottungal Vaidya Niketanam (Thrissur).

Soap, however, became more than an *oushadham* of the physical body as it came to be absorbed into struggles for social change by subjugated castes in Kerala. *Nattuvaidyam* being an assortment of diverse social-material practices, *vaidyas* came from all castes, including those at the margins of caste society. Scholars have foregrounded the critical role played by Ezhavas/Thiyyas, who possessed a rich heritage of *nattuvaidyam*, in the reconceptualization of regional medical traditions. Cleetus, for example, links the active participation of Ezhavas in the therapeutic culture of the late nineteenth and early twentieth century Keralam to the community's quests for social mobility, whereby *vaidya* practices became entangled with the body-politic of society.[100] Early twentieth-century Keralam had witnessed a steady process of social mobilization by Ezhavas, steered by individuals like Sree Narayana Guru (1855–1928), a seer, *vaidya* and anti-caste philosopher; and organizations like Sree Narayana Dharma Paripalana (SNDP) Yogam, founded in 1903 for the material and spiritual uplift of the community. The interventions of *oushadha* soap entrepreneurs like Ramananda Swami and Kesavan Vaidyar must also be located within this broader societal process. From its inception, Ramananda Swami was a member of the Sree Narayana Dharma Sangham, a community of monks founded by Narayana Guru in 1928. Kesavan Vaidyar was a dedicated follower of Guru who propagated his messages through literary and cultural interventions, besides serving as the long-time president of SNDP.

In the early-twentieth century, Ezhavas ventured into the production of non-*oushadha* soaps as well. For instance, Puthiyara Chaathu set up the Puthiyara Soap Works in the 1940s in Kozhikode, drawing on his experience as a labour and salesperson in other soap companies in Malabar.[101] The company's laundry brands 'Prabha' and '315' were marketed in Malabar throughout the 1950s. However, soap's role as a curative for the maladies afflicting society went beyond the *vaidya* and entrepreneurial practices of Ezhavas. In Malabar, the Basel Evangelical Missionary Society (BEMS) missionaries trained Dalits and other subjugated castes, who formed a significant section of Christian converts, in soap manufacturing. The German missionaries offered training to enable converted Christians to cope with the socio-economic boycott the latter faced after conversion.[102] Soap's therapeutic effects on society became particularly animated in consumption, when the use of different kinds of soaps became part of several early-twentieth century social movements, especially Dalit movements that challenged caste oppression.

Modern notions of bodily cleanliness were central to the anti-caste movements of late nineteenth and early twentieth-century Keralam.[103] Given the rigid social-spatial restrictions of caste, most Dalits could access soap only by the early twentieth century, in ways distinctly different from that of the dominant social groups. More importantly, soap and hygiene were part of the training in domesticity, which the European missionary ladies imparted to converted Christian women in the region. For example, there are references to the use of soap ('carbolic bath') by inmates of the women's boarding home in Attingal, Travancore, run by the English matrons of London Missionary Society in the 1940s.[104] While soap and hygiene may have been an agent of gendering (as in the case of middle-class, dominant caste women), installing Dalit women into the modern domestic order, domesticity and modern cleanliness occasioned the possibility of improved quality of life for them.[105] Here, it is pertinent to consider a 1928 petition by the Cheramar Sthree Samajam (a women's organization of Cheramars, a community of Pulaya people), which argued that compared to the arduous labour Dalit women are forced to perform in harsh conditions outdoor, they yearned to spend time resting at home.[106] Given the new ideas and practices of the body that hygiene presented, soap opened the possibility of a radically new embodiment to Dalits, one promising social mobility. The propagation of soap by Dalit anti-caste leaders in their constituencies in the early twentieth century can be seen from this angle. For example, Poikayil Yohannan (1879–1939), a social reformer from the Paraya community, took his followers to riverbanks in places such as Maniyattumukku, Kalluppara, Nakkada and Maraman in Travancore and taught them the use of oil and soap for bathing.[107] Yohannan also encouraged and demonstrated the use of soap to wash clothes.[108] Similarly, K. P. Vallon (1894–1940), who hailed from the Pulaya community in Cochin, distributed soap and oil among them, besides instructing them on its use.[109] Infused with meanings of aspiration and liberation from caste oppression, soap assumed revolutionary powers in the emerging modern social order. The radical, therapeutic meaning of soap in society could also partly explain its relatively stable patronage by 'the poor masses', most of whom occupied the lower tiers of caste society as well. This potential of soap prompted dominant social groups to obstruct the access of soap by castes beneath them. An example is the restriction against the sale of superior-quality toilet soaps to subjugated castes (even when it was affordable to them) that existed in Malabar; a local shop owner would not risk the prospect of earning the ire of the affluent, dominant communities by breaking this unwritten rule.[110] Critics of the use of 'substandard' soap by *sadhukkal* overlooked the role such social sanctions played in perpetrating the consumer behaviour they decried.

At the same time, dominant castes formed the key driving force behind the Gandhian 'Harijan upliftment' programme,[111] as part of which, soap and oil were distributed to Dalits in places like Pakkanarpuram and Guruvayoor in Malabar[112] and Vadakkancherry in Cochin in the 1930s.[113] In 1935, volunteers of the Kerala State Harijana Sangham reportedly bathed about 5,320 Dalit children and supplied them with oil and soap as part of the Harijan Day-Gandhi Jayanthi celebrations.[114] An award-winning play serialized in the *Matrhubhumi Weekly* offers some clues on the deployment of soap by Malayali Gandhians.[115] The plot revolves around the Harijan upliftment initiatives undertaken in a village by four educated, unemployed, young men, hailing from Namboothiri, Ambalavasi, Nair and Ezhava castes each (in turn, representing the regional caste Hindu configuration). The reformers distribute soap and oil among the Pulayas and attempt to impress upon them the importance of bathing with soap.[116] While the older Pulaya men are apprehensive about soap, a younger man named Vellon exults that 'The *thambrans* got us oil and *chop* for our own good'.[117] The protagonists mark the success of their programme with the observation, 'the Harijans *look* (my emphasis) exactly like the *savarna* ['upper-caste'] Hindus now'.[118] *Harijanodharanam* locates the cleansing endeavours of the four Gandhian reformers on the pan-Indian discourse that attributed caste pollution to the supposed intrinsic filthiness of Dalits who performed unclean spatial-corporeal practices. In this imagination, Dalit bodies, *purified* with soap, made a conspicuous case for reform efforts seeking to facilitate the entry of Dalits into caste spaces such as temples.[119]

However, Dalit narratives from the early twentieth century critiqued attempts to secularize caste through hygiene. For example, in unambiguously declaring that caste deprived them of 'clean and healthful surroundings' to live and work,[120] the Cheramar Sthree Samajam pointed out the correlation between caste oppression and lack of hygiene. We can interpret this argument as implicit in the anti-caste interventions of Dalit reformers like Yohannan, who urged their peers to embrace modern corporeal practices, including soap, often at the risk of social sanctions by dominant social groups. For Gandhian reformers, the cultivation of soap and hygiene among Dalits was essentially a strategic move that enabled them to bargain/negotiate incremental reforms from their caste-class cohorts. In such a framework, soap was more of a cosmetic object that made Dalits agreeable in physical appearance to dominant castes than be treated as their social equals. Applied in such a manner, the efficacy of the Gandhian soap on the body social was only skin-deep. In comparison, Poikayil Yohannan and other Dalit reformers appropriated soap as a therapeutic object, a thing that could potentially liberate their bodies and minds from the malaise of caste. Such therapeutic deployments of soap by Dalits stripped caste of *some* of its power. Soap was thus becoming a vital constituent in the fashioning of a new bodily order in Keralam, that was as much a new sociopolitical order. It is perhaps this wider web of meanings woven around the object that Malayalam playwright, Thikkodiyan (1916–2001) invoked when he compared art to a soap that 'whitens' (cleanses) all social evils.[121] In its metamorphosis from the *oushadham* of the human body to that of the social body, soap floated seamlessly between the material and the metaphorical, the corporeal and the social, if not blurring the boundaries between them.

Conclusion

This chapter has shown the development of a distinct culture of soap in Keralam characterized by the complex interweaving of social, spatial and material realms between the late nineteenth and early twentieth centuries. Modern, industrially produced soap was an imported, luxury commodity in late nineteenth-century Keralam, consumed primarily by modernizing, dominant social groups. With the development of the regional soap industry in the early twentieth century, and the dip in prices, the consumer base of soap expanded to embrace a larger section of the Malayali populace. In this period, soap came to be imagined and appropriated in multiple ways, galvanizing diverse spaces, objects and bodies.

As soap became affordable, classes (and castes) at the bottom of social hierarchy readily incorporated it into their corporeal practices, fashioning a consumption culture different from that of dominant social groups. For Dalits specifically, soap embodied a radically novel corporeality that promised liberation from caste oppression and offered social mobility in the emerging modern social order. Even as soap became an instrument of gendering, middle-class women embraced the transgressive meanings of convenience and beauty woven around it, often eliciting patriarchal scrutiny. While critical of the alleged dangers soap presented to the (social) body, especially at the hands of the lower classes(-castes) and middle-class women, dominant castes also refashioned the artefact as per caste Hindu sensibilities. Through these different employments, soap segued from the material to the social, becoming an *oushadham*/curative of the physical body and the social body.

Modern soap marked its entry into Keralam at a time of intense social churning. In the late nineteenth and early twentieth centuries, the norms and practices of the region underwent significant shifts as a consequence of the multifarious societal transformations emerging from Keralam's encounter with colonial modernity. A vital impetus of this flux was the unsettling of existing social hierarchies by social groups that imbibed modern ideas and practices. The body emerged as a key site of this contestation, and novel concepts and practices of hygiene and cleanliness, including soap, began to connote a new social-material order. Soap, thus, metamorphosed into a thing of power through the many spaces it navigated and myriad meanings woven around it in its course in Keralam between the late nineteenth and mid-twentieth centuries.

Notes

1 Located in the southwest of the subcontinent of India, Keralam comprises Malabar, a district under the Madras Presidency in British India, and the princely states of Cochin and Travancore. Following India's independence, the three regions merged to form the state of Kerala in 1956. The varied social-spatial experiences of the groups that constitute it render a homogenous portrayal of Keralam impossible. However, factors like Malayalam, the common language spoken by people and the shared history of European colonialism bind the regions together. See G. Aloysius, *Interpreting Kerala's Social Development* (New Delhi: Critical Quest, 2005).

2 K. R. Gowriyamma was born in an affluent yet subjugated caste (Ezhava) background. *Aathmakatha* locates Gowriyamma's early life within the current of the sociopolitical transformations sweeping early-twentieth-century Keralam. Quotation from *Aathmakatha*, 3rd ed. (Kozhikode: Mathrubhumi Books, 2011), 34. Unless otherwise indicated, all translations are mine.

3 See the advertisement by A. T. S. Menon, a merchant from Palakkad (Malabar): 'Notice', *Rasikaranjini* 2, no. 4 (1903): 262 (i).

4 Caste offered the primary grid of social differentiation in nineteenth-century Keralam. See Udaya Kumar, 'Self, Body and Inner Sense: Some Reflections on Sree Narayana Guru and Kumaran Asan', *Studies in History* 13, no. 2 (1997): 248. Historians have described Keralam's unique social geography of caste, *contra*, the normative, fourfold Brahmin–Kshatriya–Vysya–Sudra classificatory scheme applied to India. See Rajan Gurukkal, *Social Formations of Early South India* (New Delhi: Oxford University Press, 2010), 312–14. Accordingly, at the apex of the caste pyramid was the Namboothiri Brahmins followed by the intermediary, Ambalavasi/temple-castes. Although ranked Sudras, Nairs came next in hierarchy, and were proximate to Brahmins in status and farther from other Sudra communities, including Ezhavas/Thiyyas who occupied the tier beneath the Nairs. The group of 'outcastes' including Pulayas and Parayas, whom I refer to as Dalits, existed outside the varna scheme and faced extreme forms of oppression, including slavery. Caste or 'caste-like' features characterised the region's sizeable Christian and Muslim population as well.

5 Here, I primarily refer to Nairs/Nayars. By the early twentieth century, upwardly mobile classes of Thiyyas/Ezhavas would also join this consumer segment as

indicated by the recollections of writer Murkoth Kunhappa (1905-93): 'Soap', *Mathrubhumi Weekly* 28, no. 3 (1950): 15.

6 By the late nineteenth century, a print culture that became available in the public domain had come into existence. For an account of this history, see G. Arunima, 'Imagining Communities-Differently: Print, Language and the (Public Sphere) in Colonial Kerala', *The Indian Economic and Social History Review* 43, no. 1 (2006): 63-76.

7 In this period, 'tallow' primarily applied to cattle and sheep fat: Carl L. Alsberg and Alonzo E. Taylor, *Fats and Oils: A General View* (Stanford: Food Research Institute, 1928), 24.

8 A. K. Menon, *The Manufacture of Soap in India* (Simla: Government of India Press, 1938), 63.

9 The economic journal's exhortation to soap makers to take advantage of the post-First World War slump in coconut prices suggests the newfound entrepreneurial enthusiasm: 'Nammude Kaithozhilukal', *Lakshmeevilasam* 10, no. 3 (1915): 73-6.

10 For example, Travancore and Malabar registered a rise in the number of soap manufacturers: see S. G. Barker, *Report of the Industrial Survey of Travancore* (Trivandrum: Government Press, 1919), 13; and sections on Kerala Soap Institute in *Report of the Department of Industries, Madras* from 1928 to 1930.

11 Founded as Government Soap Factory, the laboratory-cum-factory was renamed around 1920 as Kerala Soap Institute (KSI). KSI expanded beyond Malabar, establishing 'important markets' in Cochin and Travancore. See sections on KSI in Madras industrial reports from 1932 to 1939.

12 *Fourth Reader*, Ramavarmapadaavali, 1933, 31.

13 'Swadeshi' literally translates to 'of one's own country'. Launched in 1905 to protest the partition of Bengal, the movement urged people to eschew *videshi* (foreign/British) goods and embrace local products. In 1906, the Indian National Congress that spearheaded the movement administered 'the Swadeshi vow' to soap, and foreign soap trade dropped from Rs 2 crores in 1920-1 to Rs 18 lakhs in 1940-1. See B. K. Karanjia, *Godrej: A Hundred Years (1897-1997)* (New Delhi and New York: Penguin Books, 1997), 48.

14 Swadeshi soap manufacturing units were reportedly established in Kannur (1907) and Kozhikode (1909): 'Editor's Notes - 1. Local News', *Lakshmeevilasam* 2, no. 8 (1907): 184 and *Lakshmeevilasam* 4, no. 2 (1909): 71.

15 See Kunhappa, 'Soap', 15.

16 T. Narayana Nambi, 'Thechukuli allenkil Abhyanga Snanam', *Dhanwantari* 4, no. 12 (1907): 243.

17 Douglas E. Haynes, 'Creating the Consumer? Advertising, Capitalism, and the Middle Class in Urban Western India, 1914-1940', in *Towards a History of Consumption in South Asia*, ed. Douglas E. Haynes et al. (New Delhi: Oxford University Press, 2010), 211 and footnote 89.

18 See chapter XI, 'Soap' in *Fourth Reader*, 30.
19 M. N. P. K., 'Orapeksha', *Dhanwantari* 2, no. 12 (1905): 236–7. I will elaborate on this point subsequently.
20 *Report of the Department of Industries* (Madras: Government Press, 1934), 26, 33.
21 'Industries – Kerala Soap Institute – Report – Analysis of Different Kinds of Soap – Regarding', 1924, para. 13.
22 In 1922, KSI's Vegetol brand soap consumption in Malabar amounted to over Rs 1 lakh, while Madras sales district purchased soaps worth Rs 60,000 and 'very little sales' were achieved in 'Telugu districts'. See C. W. E. Cotton, *Report of the Department of Industries* (Madras: Government Press, 1922), 22.
23 See *Report of the Department of Industries* (1934), 34.
24 *Report of the Department of Industries* (1934), 34; L. B. Green, *Report of the Department of Industries* (Madras: Government Press, 1938), 54.
25 V. Ramakrishna, *Report of the Department of Industries* (Madras: Government Press, 1932), 23.
26 Karanjia, *Godrej*, 49. See also Haynes, 'Creating the Consumer?', 211–12.
27 Considering the role of sentiments against animal fat in the Revolt of 1857, feelings against tallow could not have been distant in collective memory.
28 'Kerala Soap Institute, Calicut and Leather Traders Institute – Tallow Purchase from Australia – Sanctioned', 1927, 2.
29 'Purchase of Tallow during 1935–1936 – Regarding', 1935; 'Tallow Required for Manufacture of Soap – Import from Australia', 1943; 'Audit Report and Accounts for 1950–1951 – Orders Passed', 1952, 4.
30 See 'Application from M/S Techno Chemical Industries Ltd, Kozhikode – Loan – Reg' (1949), 13. In fact, Techno would advertise its (tallow-based) soaps by appealing to *parishkaram* (modernisation). See advertisement of Techno Toilet Soap: *Mathrubhumi Weekly* 26, no. 4 (1948): 18.
31 For textbooks, see C. V. Sankaranarayana Aiyar, 'Chapter 36: Soap', in *A Manual of Object Lessons* (Thiruvananthapuram: Shanmukhavilasam Press, 1896), 40–1. In familiarising soap and its manufacture through school curriculum, study tours to soap factories were organised. KSI, for instance, encouraged visits by school and college students to its factory in Kozhikode. See Cotton, *Report of the Department of Industries*, 24. For advice literature, see M. T. Narayanan, 'Shuchithvam', *Dhanwantari* 9, no. 12 (1912): 283.
32 See Chengalath Kunhirama Menon, 'Kaalam Poya Pokku', *Mangalodayam* 9, no. 9 (1916): 203.
33 In 1931, Keralam's population consisted of 63.4 per cent Hindus, 19.5 per cent Christians and 17.1 per cent Muslims. See Table I in K. C. Zachariah, 'Religious Denominations of Kerala', *Centre for Development Studies Working Papers* 468 (2016): 28. According to the 1931 census report, Travancore's population comprised 61.5 per cent Hindus, 31.5 per cent Christians and 6.9 per cent Muslims. The 'Depressed Classes' constituted 57 per cent of the total Hindu

population of Travancore and 35 per cent of the state's aggregate population. See *Census of India, 1931–Travancore* (Trivandrum: Government Press, 1932), 514, 516. This pattern of caste distribution more or less applied to the rest of Keralam.
34 See *Fourth Reader*, 30.
35 *Nattuvaidyam* is defined as an 'umbrella term under which a range of indigenous [medical] practices were represented'. See K. P. Girija, 'Interface with Media and Institutions: The Reordering of Indigenous Medical Practitioners in Twentieth-Century Kerala', *History and Sociology of South Asia* 11, no. 1 (2017): 2. Curiously, advertisements of edible medicines and unguents like *pothindravakam* (buffalo-broth), *karinkurangu rasayanam* (black-langur-tonic) and *neyyu* (fats) of animals including bear, jackal, lion and elephant graced the pages of *Mathrubhumi Weekly* along with that of vegetable-oil-based soaps in the 1940s and 1950s.
36 For government chemists, see C. Keralavarma Thirumulpad, 'Thelimayulla Soapukal/Transparent Soaps', *Thiruvithamkoor Krishivyavasaya Masika* 3, no. 11 (1922): 406–9. On public demonstrations of manufacturing processes, see 'Oachira Pradarshanam', *Vyavasaya Chandrika* 1, no. 4 (1909). On rewards, see the call for locally produced soaps with promises of reward for outstanding products in this announcement of an industrial exhibition: 'Thiruvananthapurathe Pradarshanam', *Thiruvithamkoor Krishivyavasaya Masika* 4, no. 11 (1924): 132. On financial assistance, see *Travancore Administration Report (1931–1932)* (Trivandrum: Government Press, 1933), 127.
37 Barker, *Report of the Industrial Survey of Travancore*, 3–4; *Travancore Administration Report (1931–1932)*, 127.
38 Although informal training was provided earlier, KSI began to offer a formal course in soap manufacture from 1927. See Muhammad Bazl-Ul-Lah, *Report of the Department of Industries* (Madras: Government Press, 1927), 28, 80. See also Cotton, *Report of the Department of Industries*, 23.
39 See discussions on the syllabus and other particulars of training in 'Training of Apprentices – Regarding', 1927.
40 The process of 'translation' of knowledge possessed by local communities like washers and dyers who produced pre-industrial soap into a modern industrial framework awaits investigation.
41 See paragraph 2 of the 1926 letter by KSI Superintendent to Director of Industries, Madras in 'Training of Apprentices', 7.
42 See advertisement by Kallikkadan Lonappan (John) in *Kadha Kouthukom* 1, no. 8 (1934): 17.
43 Beeyumma, Personal Interview, 2018 Tirur, Malappuram District, Kerala. Beeyumma is the wife of Kunju Muhammad's nephew, who expanded the business after the founder had passed away.
44 Barker, *Report of the Industrial Survey of Travancore*, 325–6.
45 See 'Interference by Rival Firms – Director's Reports – Regarding' (1929): 3.

46 'Chetty' denotes a trading caste. V. T. Bhattathirippad, *Kanneerum Kinavum* (Kottayam: D. C. Books, 2017), 43; Jayaprakash Kuloor, 'Soapu, Cheepu, Kannaadi', in *Jayaprakash Kuloorinte Pathinettu Nadakangal* (Thrissur: Nalanda Publications, 2016), 7–16.

47 L. B. Green, *Report of the Department of Industries* (Madras: Government Press, 1936), 41. KSI described the credit system as 'great obstacle to the development of business'. See L. B. Green, *Report of the Department of Industries* (Madras: Government Press, 1935), 33.

48 'Analysis of Different Kinds of Soap', 11.

49 Ibid., 7.

50 The Madras government issued a standard for soap manufacture in 1924. Accordingly, a good laundry soap contains 60 per cent fatty acids. Its moisture and free caustic alkali content must not exceed 32 per cent and 0.5 per cent, respectively. A standard toilet soap must have at least 60 per cent fatty acids, zero free caustic alkali, and no fillings except those enhancing soap's properties. See 'Analysis of Different Kinds of Soap', 35–6.

51 Examples include local brands such as Leelavathi Brown Soap, New Bar Soap, K. M. R. Soap, A. M. Soap and Pushpakanthi Soaps from Kozhikode and Tiger brand soap from Kannur. See 'Analysis of Different Kinds of Soap', 3–5.

52 While companies that mimicked KSI's logo faced legal suits from the Madras Government, there is no indication of punitive measures against adulterated soaps. 'Analysis of Different Kinds of Soap', 36.

53 Ramakrishna, *Report of the Department of Industries*, 22–3.

54 Formed in 1947, the association's members included the Vegetable Soap Works, Techno Chemical Industries, Victory Chemical & Pharmaceutical Works, Tirur Oil Mills (Malabar), Kalpaka Oil Mills Ltd (Cochin), Imperial Soap Factory and Islamia Soap Works (Travancore). See 'Permission to Enrol as Member of South Indian Soap Manufacturer's Association', 1947.

55 *Ennathechukuli/thechukuli* is an elaborate form of bathing involving oil massage and herbal scrubs. See Karat Achyutha Menon, 'Sthreedharmam', *Lakshmibai* 2, no. 8 (1907): 344.

56 See J. Devika, *En-Gendering Individuals: The Language of Re-Forming in Early Twentieth Century Keralam* (New Delhi: Orient Longman Private Limited, 2007) for an account of the reconstitution of gender in Keralam.

57 See for example, 'Grihakrithyangal', *The Sarada* 4, no. 4 (1909): 108; 'Ormikkendava', *The Sarada* 4, no. 5 (1909): 134; C. D. D., 'Grihabharanam', *Lakshmibai* 1, no. 7 (1906): 277–80; K. Narayana Menon, 'Soundaryam', *Sarada* 2, no. 6 (1907): 124.

58 Thakazhi Sivasankara Pillai, *Ente Balyakalakadha* (Thrissur: Mangalodayam, 1967), 44.

59 McGowan's work on the gendered politics of consumption in Western India mentions similar criticism of the frivolous consumption of women: Abigail McGowan, 'An All-Consuming Subject? Women and Consumption in Late-Nineteenth and Early-Twentieth-Century Western India', *Journal of Women's History* 18, no. 4 (2006): 44.

60 See Vallathol Narayana Menon, *Arogya Chinthamani*, 3rd ed. (Thrissur: Vallathol Press, 1976), 498–9. The text, first compiled in 1904, is a compendium of *nattuvaidya* treatment protocols.
61 See Menon, 'Kaalam Poya Pokku', 203. McGowan discusses similar narratives made by Europeans that implied the failure of Indian masculinity to fit Western norms of gender; Indian reformers, who subsequently took up this criticism, advised men and women to embrace *swadeshi* products. See 'An All-Consuming Subject?', 44.
62 'Menon' is a Nair sub-group.
63 Menon, 'Kaalam Poya Pokku'.
64 In note 58, we see exceptions like the Namboothiri entrepreneur who ventured into soap production, but such instances were very few.
65 Devaki Nilayangodu, *Kalappakarchakal* (Kozhikode: Mathrubhumi, 2008), 22.
66 N. K. Krishna Pilla, 'Thiruvithamkoorile Vividha Vyavasaaya Saukaryam II', *Thiruvithamkoor Krishivyavasaya Masika* 5, no. 11/12 (1924): 431; one *chakram* roughly equals 1/28.5 of a British rupee and one *anna* roughly equals 1/16 of a British rupee.
67 M. N. P. K., 'Orapeksha', 236–7.
68 P. V. Krishna Warrier, 'Abhyanga Snanam Allenkil Enna Thechukuli', *Mathrubhumi Weekly* 15, no. 6 (1937): 8.
69 'Training of Apprentices', 21.
70 Examples include Washwell soap (KSI's 'chief product' in the 1920s) and the 'twelve-ounce Swadeshi Golden Bar' marketed by South Malabar Soap Works in Thiruvananthapuram in the 1930s. See 'Training of Apprentices', 21; 'Advertisement "Smandi Borax Soap"', *Srimathi Special Issue* (1935): 112. Soap companies also began to market their products as catering to all classes of consumers. For instance, Techno Chemical Industries declared that its soaps were preferred across the class divide, while the Thrissur-based Iyyappen Soap Works used the stereotypes of 'the parsimonious poor' and 'the tasteful rich' in claiming the same. See 'Techno Soaps', *Mathrubhumi Weekly* 27, no. 9 (1949): 17; 'Iyyappen Soap Works, *Prabhatham* 1, no. 35 (1938): 20.
71 In the 1920s, KSI, with its elite clientele who patronized its 'high-class' soaps, noted a 'growing desire on the part of the public' to purchase 'economical' soaps. See Muhammad Bazl-Ul-Lah, *Report of the Department of Industries* (Madras: Government Press, 1926), 24.
72 The Indian Industrial Commission of 1916–1918 noted that although poverty and lack of education subdued the impact of imported, factory-made commodities in rural life, a host of commodities including soap had significantly improved the quality of life in the subcontinent. *Report of the Indian Industrial Commission 1916–1918* (London: Majesty's Stationery Office, 1919), 11. Consumption practices surrounding 'non-essential' items like soap by poorer classes must be read with the body of work that questions existing scholarship for side-lining consumption in

the colonial period. See Douglas E. Haynes and Abigail McGowan, 'Introduction', in *Towards a History of Consumption in South Asia*, 1–25.
73 K. Ramanmenon, 'Nirantharopakari [Soap]', *Lakshmeevilasam* 8, no. 1 (1913): 17.
74 See Haynes, 'Creating the Consumer?', 185–223; and Harminder Kaur, 'Of Soaps and Scents: Corporeal Cleanliness in Urban Colonial India', in *Towards a History of Consumption in South Asia*, 246–67.
75 Aparna Nair, 'Magic Lanterns, Mother-Craft and School Medical Inspections: Fashioning Modern Bodies and Identities in Travancore', *Tapasam* 8, no. 1–4 (2013): 62–87.
76 P. Sanal Mohan, *Modernity of Slavery: Struggles against Caste Inequality in Colonial India* (New Delhi: Oxford University Press, 2015), 176–7.
77 P. K. Michael Tharakan, 'A Note on Sree Narayana Guru's Teachings and Health in Rural Kerala', *Review of Agrarian Studies* 8, no. 1 (2018).
78 Texts like 'Sankarasmriti' prescribe elaborate injunctions for daily ablutions to remove *ashudham* (ritual impurity) emerging from one's bodily processes and through contact with other bodies/matter. See T. C. Parameshwaran Moosathu, *Sankarasmriti* (Thrissur: Bharatha Vilasam Press, 1906).
79 For examples of early-twentieth-century critiques that employed hygiene to contest *shudham*, see 'Shudham', *Vidyavinodini* 3, no. 10 (1892): 223–4; 'Our Letter Box', *The Mitavadi* 3, no. 5 (1915): 29–30.
80 M. S. S. Pandian, 'One Step Outside Modernity: Caste, Identity Politics and Public Sphere', *Economic & Political Weekly* 37, no. 18 (2002): 1737.
81 *Report on Native Papers in the Madras Presidency (March 1881)*, 6 provides an example of such narratives as appearing in *Kerala Mitram* (19 March 1881).
82 'Snaanam', *Vidyavinodini* 2, no. 7 (1891): 159.
83 Vidvan P. R. Warrier portrays Tamilians as a group disinclined to bathe or wash clothes in 'Malayaliyum Thamizhanum', *Mathrubhumi Weekly* 15, no. 22 (1944): 4.
84 Arguing for caste pollution, the Malayalam newspaper *Kerala Mitram* mocked the 'insufferable' stink of the Europeans and their futile attempts to conceal it with perfumes. See *Report on Native Papers in the Madras Presidency (March 1881)*, 6. Freedom fighter K. P. Kesava Menon (1886–1978), who studied law in London, recorded that while the English upper classes washed themselves occasionally, the poor did not bathe at all; in comparison, the Pulayas and other lower castes in Keralam were better off than England's poor. *Bilathi Visesham* (Calicut: Empress Victoria Press, 1916), 102, 117.
85 Menon, 'Sthreedharmam', 344.
86 Menon, 'Kaalam Poya Pokku', 203.
87 Kaur, 'Of Soaps and Scents', 262–3.
88 Fish is ritually polluting for caste elites. See Madhavikkutty, 'Balyakalasmaranakal', in *Madhavikkuttiyude Krithikal Sampoornam*, vol. 2 (Kottayam: D. C. Books, 2009), 591.
89 Studies have shown that while advertisements create knowledge, they simultaneously draw from the larger web of understandings, values and discourses of consumers. See Haynes, 'Creating the Consumer?', 186–7.

90 P. K. Warrier, 'Samkramika Rogangalum Avayude Nivaarana Margangalum', *Dhanwantari* 10, no. 1 (1912): 21–3; P. K. Warrier, 'Kshaurakkathiyum Pakarcha Vyadhikalum', *Dhanwantari* 10, no. 1 (1914): 261; T. P. Tiwari, 'Eettillam', *Arogyam* 10/11, no. 12 (1936): 279–83.

91 Brian Lewis, *'So Clean': Lord Leverhulme, Soap and Civilisation* (Manchester: Manchester University Press, 2012), 80–1.

92 Although Ayurvedam assumed the role of a 'professional classical tradition' in the colonial period, varied *vaidya* practices were alive in Keralam. *Vishavaidyam* refers to 'indigenous toxicology'; *Siddhavaidyam*, although of Tamil origin, was widely practised in Malayalam. See Girija, 'Interface with Media and Institutions', 2 and footnote 4.

93 See Burton Cleetus, 'Subaltern Medicine and Social Mobility: The Experience of the Ezhava in Kerala', *Indian Anthropologist* 37, no. 1 (2007): 153.

94 M. S. Harilal, '"Commercialising Traditional Medicine": Ayurvedic Manufacturing in Kerala', *Economic & Political Weekly* 44, no. 16 (2009): 44–51.

95 See advertisement in Vayaskara N. S. Mooss, ed., *The All India Ayurvedic Directory 1949* (Kottayam: The Vaidya Sarathy Press, 1949), 46. This recent biography of Sadananda Swami repeats the claim: Swami Chidananda Bharati, *Srimad Sadanandaswamikal* (Kollam: Sadananda Press, 2005), 15.

96 See 'Advertisement "Sadananda Ayurvedic Medicals and Soap Works"', *Lakshmibai* 9, no. 7 (1914).

97 B. V. Pavanan, 'Jeevitha Sugandhathinte Shilpi', in *C. R. Kesavan Vaidyar Navathi Smaranika* (Irinjalakkuda, 1994); See C. R. Kesavan Vaidyar's writings: *Vichara Darppanam*, 1st edn (Iringalakkuda: Vivekodayam Printing & Publishing Company, 1976), 157; *Gurucharanangalil*, 2nd edn (Kottayam: Current Books, 1993), 122–3.

98 I. M. Velayudhan and Velayudhan Panikkassery, *Vaidyarude Katha* (Kottayam: Current Books, 1999), 84–5.

99 Green, *Report of the Department of Industries* (1938), 52.

100 See Cleetus, 'Subaltern Medicine and Social Mobility', 147–72.

101 Gopinath K (son of Chaathu) *Personal Interview* (Kozhikode, 2018).

102 See *Brief History of Malayala Basel Mission Church: 1834–1934* (Calicut: Vintage Books, 1989), 186. Sources suggest that BEMS, which had established various industries in Malabar, sought to enter large-scale soap manufacturing as well. See 'Editor's Notes', *Lakshmeevilasam* 10, no. 4 (1915): 140. However, these efforts seemed to have stalled after the German missionaries left the British-administered Malabar during the First World War.

103 Kumar, 'Self, Body and Inner Sense', 247–70; Mohan, *Modernity of Slavery,* 176–80.

104 *Women's Work, Northern District*, London Missionary Society, Travancore, Report for 1945–1946 (Travancore, 1946), 8.

105 For Dalit articulations on the benefits of domesticity, see P. K., 'Arangathuninnu Adukkalayilekku: Avasha Samudayangalile Sthreekalodu Orabhyarthana', *Mathrubhumi Weekly* 11, no. 31 (1933): 24–6.

106 See C. Mariamma Cherammal, 'Petition from the Cheramar Sthree Samajam to Elizabeth Kuruvila, Member, Travancore Sree Mulam Praja Sabha', trans. by J Devika (1928). See https://swatantryavaadini.in/2021/09/07/petition-from-the-cheramar-sthree-samajam-to-elizabeth-kuruvila-member-travancore-sree-mulam-praja-sabha/ (accessed 8 September 2021). For a comparative perspective, see Victoria Kelley, '"The Virtues of a Drop of Cleansing Water": Domestic Work and Cleanliness in the British Working Classes, 1880–1914', *Women's History Review* 18, no. 5 (2009): 719–35.

107 Mohan, *Modernity of Slavery*, 177.

108 Satheesh Kidarakkuzhy, *Poikayil Sree Kumara Gurudevan* (Thiruvananthapuram: Kerala Bhasha Institute, 2016), 79.

109 P. Govindapillai, *Kerala Navodhanam: Yugasanthathikal Yugashilppikal*, Kerala Navodhanam (Trivandrum: Chintha Publishers, 2014), 238.

110 B. P. Sidiuque Haji, *Personal Interview* (Kozhikode, 2018). Haji, a second-generation soap manufacturer, was an office-bearer of the Kerala Small-scale Soap Manufacturers Association when interviewed in 2018.

111 In the Poona Pact of 1932, Dalits represented by B. R. Ambedkar, upon pressure from M. K. Gandhi, gave up their demand with the British government for a separate electorate. Subsequently, Gandhi launched a series of programmes to uplift 'Harijans' (a neologism meaning 'children of God' used to address Dalits) and eradicate untouchability. Cleanliness and hygiene formed a major thrust of this movement. See Bipan Chandra, *India's Struggle for Independence, 1857–1947* (New Delhi: Penguin, 1989), 290–5.

112 See 'Kerala Varthakal', *Mathrubhumi Weekly* 11, no. 7 (1933): 13.

113 'Kerala Varthakal', *Mathrubhumi Weekly* 14, no. 24 (1936): 16.

114 Gandhi Jayanthi means the birthday of Gandhi, 2nd of October. See 'Keralam', *Mathrubhumi Weekly* 13, no. 32 (1935): 16–17.

115 See 'Harijanodharanam adhava "Udyogam Kitti"' by Nambiaruveetil Narayana Menon, published between 23 October and 25 November 1935.

116 Menon, 'Harijanodharanam III', *Mathrubhumi Weekly* 13, no. 35 (1935): 28–30.

117 Ibid., 30. *Thambran* or 'lord' was the term used by Dalits to address Nairs and Namboothiris. *Chop* is a corruption of 'soap', an instance of the linguistic inferiority of the Pulayas, considering that by 1897, 'soap' was recognized as a loanword from English to Malayalam. See C. D. D., 'Malayala Bhasha', *Vidyavinodini* 7, no. 11 (1896): 449.

118 Menon, 'Harijanodharanam V', *Mathrubhumi Weekly* 13, no. 37 (1935): 31.

119 Menon, 'Harijanodharanam I', 33.

120 See Cherammal, 'Petition from the Cheramar Sthree Samajam'.

121 Thikkodiyan, 'Ellam Veluppikkunna Soap', in *Arangu Kanatha Nadan* (Kottayam: Sahithya Pravarthaka Co-operative Society, 1991), 247–51.

9

Chaulmoogra: Indian Ocean world leprosy remedies in the South Pacific

Jane Buckingham

In the garden of the P. J. Twomey Hospital, Suva, Fiji, two chaulmoogra trees now grow adjacent to a bronze fountain in the shape of a kiwi, a small flightless bird, which has become the emblem of New Zealand. This tryptic represents the southernmost Pacific reach of chaulmoogra's complex migratory history which traverses at least 2,000 years, connecting ancient Chinese and Indian medical therapeutic traditions with nineteenth-century French and British colonial-medical trade networks and twentieth-century Western medical approaches to leprosy management. How did an ancient Asian treatment for leprosy become the treatment of choice in a twentieth-century leprosy hospital in Fiji largely funded by New Zealand donors? What does the history of chaulmoogra as a medical commodity say about the role of colonial scientific and medical networks in linking and transforming the premodern and modern Indian Ocean and Pacific worlds?

Chaulmoogra was a tree of inland Asian forest regions. Indigenous to the forests of India, Burma and other regions of Southeast Asia, chaulmoogra was embedded in the ancient material and scientific culture of the Indian Ocean world.[1] Integrated into high-culture Ayurvedic Indian medical tradition, chaulmoogra was also part of earlier Buddhist healing traditions. The legends of the healing power of chaulmoogra reflect its connection with the traditions of the forest as a sacred place. For those with leprosy, the forest was a place of banishment but also of healing and restoration. Indian and Burmese legends tell of King Rama and Princess Priya, banished to the forest because of leprosy yet healed and restored by eating the fruit of the Kalaw, later identified as the source of chaulmoogra.[2] Found in the extensive interior forests of South and South-east Asia, chaulmoogra connected indigenous forest dwellers and local traders with the maritime and overland movements of philosophers, healers, merchants, storytellers and religious specialists. Chaulmoogra and the people who gathered and traded it formed part of wider histories of botanical exchange in the Indian Ocean world.[3] The forest dwellers and silk road merchants enriched the ancient and medieval Indian Ocean world, providing commodities, philosophies and scientific knowledge which travelled overseas through trade and religious pilgrimage networks connecting the Indian subcontinent eastwards with the South China Sea and westwards through the Persian Gulf to the Mediterranean and the empires of Greece and Rome.[4] Described as 'southernisation' by Shaffer, this process dispersed to west and east the cultures, technology and medical knowledge of the Indian Ocean during the premodern period.[5] From the sixteenth century, European trade and exploration in the Indian Ocean world began to challenge the land-based Islamic empires of South Asia and the Maghreb, integrating the culture and commodities of the region into new networks of European colonial knowledge and governance.[6] Medical knowledge was part of these networks, and Indian therapeutics and healing traditions influenced the empires of Greece, Rome and the trans-continental Islamic world before becoming embedded in new forms of European tropical and colonial medicine in eighteenth- and nineteenth-century India.[7]

In the Indian Ocean world, chaulmoogra represented the fluid materiality of medical knowledge. First known as a forest therapeutic, the seeds became integrated into the high-culture Indian medical tradition of Ayurveda as it developed from the late centuries BCE into a formalized tradition expressed in texts such as the *Caraka Samhita* and *Suśruta Samhitā*.[8] From at least the early centuries CE it was traded throughout Asia, its therapeutic powers communicated through Indian and Burmese healing legends. The integration of chaulmoogra into emerging Brahmanic high-culture medical systems of knowledge exchange, including written forms of medical knowledge in the early centuries CE, reflected the persistent authority of indigenous knowledge systems and local forest-healing cultures previously transmitted through oral tradition in early Indian culture.[9] Chaulmoogra was also part of the wider Asian pharmacopoeia, emerging in Chinese and Burmese compendia of medicinal substances as early as the sixth century CE.[10]

The reputation of chaulmoogra as a treatment for leprosy persisted in South and South-east Asia from these earliest traceable origins into the European colonial period. British colonial settlement of India brought British military and medical personnel into direct contact with endemic leprosy and a reigniting of the fear and horror of a disease which was still unmanageable except through isolation. The dominance of chaulmoogra in the Western global management of leprosy in the nineteenth and twentieth centuries resulted from a European recognition that traditional medicine in India might have something to offer the emerging 'scientific' medical culture of Britain and Europe. The transference of chaulmoogra into British medical practice in India and its status in the early twentieth century as the internationally preferred leprosy treatment was mediated by the networks of local medical knowledge and newly emerging forms of colonial medicine within the nineteenth-century Indian Ocean world. This chapter examines the contribution of chaulmoogra to the complex history of the medical and therapeutic culture of the Indian Ocean world and the role of imperial networks in bringing it from the Indian Ocean into Pacific medical practice.[11]

Chaulmoogra was introduced into Western medicine in 1854 by F. J. Moat, a medical doctor working in the Bengal Medical Service. He identified chaulmoogra as a remedy for leprosy, well known to 'native' practitioners and used in conjunction with dietary restrictions as part of Indian treatment for the disease.[12] Despite the uneasy transition between indigenous medicine, often dismissed as unscientific in European medical circles, and European medicine which, despite its claims to modernity, was still largely humoral in the nineteenth century, chaulmoogra became integrated into European colonial-medical networks. In the European medical context chaulmoogra as a therapeutic substance underwent a transformation. The ingestion of the oil and seeds which dated back to at least the early centuries CE persisted in Ayurvedic and other Indian medical practices into the British colonial period. Within the colonial-medical context, however, chaulmoogra was decoupled from its legendary association with the healing of kings in sacred forest groves and deconstructed to discover which chemical constituents could be isolated and stabilized as therapeutic measures against leprosy. Colonial-medical officers, medical and imperial research organizations such as the British Empire Leprosy Relief Association (BELRA)[13] and private companies such as Burroughs Wellcome invested in the integration of chaulmoogra as a medical commodity into tropical medicine. The therapeutic reach of chaulmoogra was no longer limited to the traditional medical systems of India and South-east Asia. During the nineteenth and twentieth centuries, chaulmoogra became embedded in the Western medical response to leprosy as a scientifically manipulated range of oils, esters and tinctures, traded as therapeutic commodities within imperial networks of scientific knowledge, trade, labour mobility and governance. By the nineteenth century these colonial networks and the impact of chaulmoogra stretched from the Indian Ocean to the South Pacific settler society of New Zealand and the British colony of Fiji. This chapter focuses on two aspects of the history of chaulmoogra as a therapeutic material traded within the networks established through British colonial connections between the Indian and Pacific Ocean worlds. First, it explores the integration of chaulmoogra into British colonial-medical knowledge systems in the nineteenth and twentieth centuries and emphasizes the scientific manipulation of the plant, a material transformation to suit it to distribution and trade beyond the Indian Ocean as a modern medical therapeutic substance. Second, this chapter considers the private individual therapeutic experience of chaulmoogra among leprosy-affected people in early twentieth-century New Zealand and Fiji and the transformation of the landscape and therapeutic economy of the Pacific world brought by its cultivation. Chaulmoogra not only affected the body of the person with leprosy but also shaped South Pacific landscapes. As a seed for cultivation promoted by BELRA throughout the British empire, chaulmoogra brought specific changes to the landscape and environment of Makogai Island where leprosy-affected people were sent for isolation and medical care at the Central Lepers' Hospital from 1911 to 1969.[14] On Makogai the forest fruit of ancient India became cultivated in this new place of banishment and healing, a new healing forest hemmed in by the waters of the Pacific.

Chaulmoogra as a British colonial therapeutic commodity

Just as its integration into the Hindu medical system of Ayurveda modified the cultural materiality of chaulmoogra from a healing seed associated with the mystery of tribe and forest legend into a textually endorsed therapeutic commodity, chaulmoogra was changed by its integration into emerging Western medical responses to the encounter with leprosy in the Indian Ocean world. By the late nineteenth century, chaulmoogra oil had become the standard treatment for leprosy in British colonies worldwide.[15] It was adopted also in French and Dutch colonial possessions in an effort to provide some therapeutic response to an illness that with the expansion of Europe into tropical zones had brought the disease back into European consciousness. Historically seen as a biblical and medieval disease in Europe, leprosy had reached endemic rates by the mid-nineteenth century in Norway.[16] In Britain, fear of leprosy was revived as an 'imperial danger'.[17] Memories of the lazar houses in England, largely closed since the sixteenth century, held a moral and symbolic resonance of a disease incurable and tainted by the stigma of sin.[18] Expansion into areas of the globe such as the East Indies where leprosy was endemic by the nineteenth century reignited a European fear of leprosy as an untreatable and intractable disease which put Europe at risk. Despite its long European history and the increase in cases in Norway, leprosy was reconfigured as a 'tropical disease'.[19] Increasingly from the eighteenth century, in the context of European colonial contact, the Indian Ocean world became part of a European colonial 'self-construction' which saw the 'tropics' as economically and territorially lucrative but a risk to the health and moral fibre of the white colonizers. Not only the climate and environment of the colonies was seen as dangerous, but the people who lived in these hot, febrile tropical regions were constituted as a risk, able to outnumber the Europeans who were unable to adapt to the conditions.[20] Despite their evident vulnerability, British and other European colonial therapeutic responses to leprosy within the Indian Ocean world were complicated by beliefs in the racial and cultural superiority of Western medicine over the medical systems of South and East Asia.[21]

Local British medical officers in India understood the limits of the Western medical tradition and, despite their assumptions of medical superiority, borrowed heavily from Indian therapeutic and treatment techniques. The integration of chaulmoogra into nineteenth-century British pharmacopoeia as a leprosy treatment has parallels with the integration of forest remedies into the high-culture Sanskrit traditions of Ayurvedic medicine by the sixth century CE. Both involved inclusion of local folk knowledge of therapeutic materials into medical systems associated with increasingly dominant newly emerging medical cultures. In the colonial context, the British medical response to leprosy in India was characterized by an assimilation of local Indian remedies to treat a disease intractable in the face of the mercury and arsenic therapies typically used in British medicine at the time.[22] By the mid-nineteenth century much of the premodern compatibility between Indian and British medical systems was being marginalized by British insistence locally and to the wider professional and scientific community that British medicine was scientific and evidence based, unlike Indian medical cultures identified as based in religious lore.[23] Even so, as late as the early twentieth century, both British colonial medicine and Western medicine as it emerged post-First World War still relied on the knowledge of jungle dwellers for the identification and collection of chaulmoogra seeds for processing and sale to local markets. Jungle dwellers remained the first step in bringing therapeutic materials from India's north-eastern interior forests into colonial-medical systems. The contribution of chaulmoogra to the Indian

Ocean world and the integration of that world into wider colonial therapeutic markets and scientific research networks relied on chains of human connection from the interior to the coastal colonial settlements. Some of the forest-sourced chaulmoogra was transferred from the interior to local markets and on to colonial towns and hospitals. Other chaulmoogra harvests were transported to rivers and sea ports for export throughout the British empire. Even the dealers in the Chittagong markets, closest to the north-eastern forest where the seeds were sourced had not seen them growing in the wild and were not familiar with their origin trees.[24]

Lack of connection between those who located and harvested chaulmoogra in forest areas and later steps in the supply chain directly impacted on the integration of the seed into British and other European colonial-medical knowledge systems. The botanical source of chaulmoogra oil was misidentified in 1815 by Dr William Roxburgh in *Hortus Bengalensis* as the seed of the *Chaulmoogra Odorata*, an error corrected only in 1900. Despite the error circulating through *Materia Medica*, medical journals and official publications, the correct therapeutic product derived from the seeds of *Taraktogenous kurzii* continued to be sold in the Calcutta bazaar and by the 'Paris and London drug dealers' as chaulmoogra oil.[25] F.J. Mouat introduced chaulmoogra into British colonial medicine in India, trialling it on patients in 1853 and publishing his results in the *Indian Annals of Medical Science*.[26] Mouat was cautiously optimistic about its therapeutic benefits. Chaulmoogra, along with other plant-based remedies, was extensively trialled in British colonial hospitals,[27] eliding the world of forest and tradition with the emerging construction of British colonial medicine as scientific and evidence based.

In the first decade of the twentieth century the materiality of chaulmoogra as a therapeutic agent was transformed. Building on nineteenth-century research, the London-based company Burroughs Wellcome was the first to comprehensively analyse the active chemical ingredients constituting an efficacious chaulmoogra oil. In 1904 Frederick B. Power, a research pharmacologist working in the Wellcome Chemical Research Laboratories, physically and chemically deconstructed *Taraktogenous kurzii* seeds bought from a London market to isolate the fatty acid 'chaulmoogric oil'. Power's research clearly distinguished the seeds of two additional trees as a source of this fatty acid, *Hydnocarpus Wightiana* and *Hydnocarpus Anthelmintica*, which produced an additional therapeutic substance named 'Hydnocarpus acid'. Applying chemical analysis to the seeds of *Gynocardia odorata*, Powers and his research colleagues confirmed that *Gynocardia odorata* was not a source of chaulmoogra or its therapeutic oils as Roxburgh had assumed in 1815.[28] Wellcome added a commercial arm to the manufacture and supply of chaulmoogra-based therapeutics supporting government research initiatives and distribution of the treatment throughout European and American territories. As late as 1938 the Cairo International Leprosy Congress declared that worldwide 'Hydnocarpus oil and its esters administered intramuscularly, subcutaneously and intradermally, remain, so far as our present knowledge goes, the most efficacious drugs for the special treatment of leprosy'.[29]

Chaulmoogra did not, however, destroy *Mycobacterium leprae*, which was discovered in Sweden in 1878 by Gerhard Armauer Hansen as the organism which caused leprosy. Recognizing that contagion rather than heredity was the principal cause of leprosy, the First International Leprosy Congress held in Berlin in 1897 recommended isolation as the principal leprosy management strategy.[30] Despite the range of treatments researched and trialled in colonial contexts during the nineteenth century and the identification of chaulmoogra as of therapeutic benefit, quarantine and isolation remained into the twentieth century the principal means of containing the spread of the disease. While affirming the therapeutic use of chaulmoogra, the 1931 International Leprology Congress cautioned against seeing the therapy as a cure for leprosy.[31] Outpatient treatment for leprosy would not become available until the development of sulphonamides (specifically Dapsone) in the 1940s and multi-drug therapy in the 1980s, necessitated by *M.leprae* becoming resistant. By the early twentieth century, chaulmoogra, once an ancient remedy for an exiled king, had become an internationally recognized and traded therapeutic substance, fully integrated into Western medical and scientific culture as the best available remedy for leprosy. By the early twentieth century, methods of consuming the seed and its oils or applying the oil or beaten flesh of the seeds to lesions initially adopted in colonial medicine from local Indian medical practice had been largely replaced by hypodermic injections of the oil with various carriers. Forest-gathered seeds had found their way into Western laboratories where specific chemical components of the oil had been isolated and used to develop formulations such as esters which had fewer side effects for patients already weakened by illness. In the leprosy isolation settlements and hospitals worldwide, chaulmoogra was administered orally and by injection by medical and nursing staff to patients isolated to contain the spread of their disease. In the absence of a cure, however, quarantine and isolation, modern medical versions of the tradition of banishment to the forest, remained a primary response to leprosy in colonial and independent territories.

Pacific islands of isolation and imperial networks of therapeutic commodities

When the British colonial government in Fiji established a leprosy hospital on the remote Fijian island of Makogai in 1911, chaulmoogra was sourced from India as the most efficacious remedy available. The commodity trade in Indian Ocean world chaulmoogra followed the movement of leprosy through the colonies with the colonial trade in labour. Leprosy-affected indentured labourers from India working on Fijian plantations were isolated on Makogai together with Fijians and others from the region.[32] As a British settler society, New Zealand mediated the colonial relationships between the Indian and Pacific oceans' trade and information networks supplying labour and medical commodities. P. J. Twomey's Lepers' Trust Board, funded by contributions from ordinary New Zealanders, supported the official networks relating to leprosy care with donated medical infrastructure.[33] The Fijian island of Makogai thus became a locus of colonial Indian and Pacific world networks of human migration, informal and formal medical knowledge, commodity and charitable exchange. In August 1925 a small group of people with leprosy were moved from the New Zealand quarantine station on Quail Island in Lyttelton Harbour to the new hospital and quarantine facilities developed on Makogai Island. Nine patients were moved by boat specially fitted out to enable isolation on board of leprosy-affected passengers from others who were not affected by the disease. Makogai Island thus became the space of isolation and banishment for leprosy sufferers of the British colonial South Pacific. Hidden within the sea and separated by currents and reefs from the ordinary movement of peoples, it functioned like the forest of the ancient Indian Ocean world where isolation offered the hope of healing. The movement of nine men to Makogai Island also marked the end of Quail Island's role as a leprosy isolation centre and coincided with a shift in the ideation of chaulmoogra as an imperially endorsed treatment for leprosy within the British colonial possessions abroad.

The movement of patients to Makogai Island in 1925 juxtaposed the private space of health experience with the global spaces of emerging imperial health organizations such as BELRA. On 16 July 1925, Frank Oldrieve, the secretary of BELRA, forwarded to the British Colonial Office, the 'Memorandum on the Prevalence and Prophylaxis against Leprosy in the British Empire' prepared by tropical medicine specialist, Dr Leonard Rogers.[34] The memorandum was developed after surveying all the leprosy institutions in British possessions including New Zealand's Quail Island. Central to this memorandum was the recommendation that the seeds of *Hydnocarpus Wightiana* be cultivated in all leprosy-affected countries. *Hydnocarpus Wightiana* was correctly identified through Power's work in the Wellcome laboratories as a source of the active ingredient found in chaulmoogra. Though BELRA's enquiry and recommendations focused on the British colonial possessions including Fiji, its members sought to include government, philanthropic and commercial interests in the effort to develop therapeutic remedies for leprosy with other colonial authorities. As Rogers noted with some chagrin, the Philippines, under United States authority, was well ahead of British research in the use of ethyl esters which had the advantage of fewer side effects than the oil.[35] BELRA's initiative also linked Makogai with the production of botanical treatments at Kew garden where Dr Hill, the director, was prepared to 'distribute the seed through the Colonial Agricultural departments to all our colonies'.[36] BELRA was willing to financially support the distribution of seed 'to those desiring to avail themselves of this offer'.[37] The intention was to spread the therapeutic opportunity throughout the British possessions in a way that reduced the cost of the oil and ethyl esters particularly since the trees fruited continuously from six or seven years of age. The goal was for all 'leper institutions and infected countries' to 'grow their own supplies' so that the 'full benefit of the recent advances will be generally available to those afflicted with leprosy'.[38]

This decision connected Makogai Island, where *Hydnocarpus* was planted at the Leprosy hospital to provide a source of chaulmoogra oil, with the wider network of specialist botanical and medical knowledge.[39] Rogers' recommendation also marked the severing of chaulmoogra from its ancient mooring in the forests of the Indian Ocean world. The traditional knowledge of the forest dweller, gathering seeds and introducing them into the market as raw materials for use in medicinal treatment was displaced by the changing expectations of a modern medical commodity. Chaulmoogra had been integrated into emerging modern ideas of therapeutic commodities. Dissected, analysed and described in terms of specific active ingredients which could be synthesized into different forms for therapeutic administration the materiality of its therapeutic value was changed. Volume and consistency in type, quality and efficacy of product were measured in the laboratory rather than identified and communicated through legend and tradition.[40] BELRA's global dispersal of chaulmoogra for growth as a plantation species reflected the movement towards standardized and industrial production of medicinal therapeutics both as part of commercial operations but also as part of emerging colonial interest in finding means to control 'tropical' diseases seen as a risk to European health. As the botanist and explorer Joseph F. Rock noted in 1922: 'no absolute statement of the source of commercial chaulmoogra oil can . . . be made so long as the seeds are gathered from wild-growing trees in different parts of Burma, Lower Bengal, and Assam'. The only guarantee of the 'source and purity' of the oil was the growing of *Taraktogenous kurzii* as a plantation crop.[41]

Therapeutic migration across ocean worlds

The movement of patients from Quail Island to Makogai was mirrored throughout the British colonial Pacific by the internal migration of leprosy-affected people from their home islands to Makogai as the colonial government expanded the network of dependencies permitted to send their patients there. The movement of people across the Pacific Ocean brings the materiality of the ocean, its quality as a space of constant movement into strong relief.[42] Movements from island to island by those with leprosy were by boat, often hazardous journeys of weeks through reefs and complex currents. The movement of medical commodities derived from chaulmoogra and seeds for planting was similarly part of these shifts through a fluid world, in which islands were but resting points in a restless sea. When the nine arrived from Quail Island there were already 300 people on Makogai which was established in 1911 not only to isolate leprosy-affected people but also to provide the best available treatment and care possible to those suffering the disease.[43] Among these were Indians, mostly indentured labourers or their descendants who had migrated from the Indian Ocean world to work on the sugar plantations of the Fijian islands.[44] Chaulmoogra followed this pattern of movement connecting the Indian Ocean and Pacific Ocean worlds. India remained the primary source of the raw material before BELRA encouraged plantations outside the Indian Ocean world. Chaulmoogra travelled along the same route as indentured labourers to the Pacific and was used to treat Indian labourers and their descendants with leprosy isolated on Makogai. Research laboratories funded by Wellcome, various governments and universities, developed chaulmoogra derivatives for therapeutic purposes using Indian-sourced seeds. Repatriation of Indians from Fiji to India was a priority, the Fijian colonial government not wishing to pay the cost of accommodation, food and treatment for Indians who could be sent home.[45] Even so, any Indian with leprosy who could not identify friends or family to care for them would be liable for confinement under the 1898 Lepers' Act if returned to India.[46] In many of these cases they preferred to remain on Makogai. Chaulmoogra remained too, an Indian Ocean world therapeutic remedy circulating through the

South Pacific which contributed to the transformation of the Fijian environment along with the other plants, seeds and spices carried by indentured workers in their *jahaji bandal* throughout the islands.[47] The need for chaulmoogra on Makogai was so great that in addition to the Central Leper Hospital cultivating the tree within hospital grounds, the medical superintendent requested that local planters grow the trees to supplement the Leprosy hospital's supply. The trees were also cultivated at the Fijian agricultural stations of Nasini and Sigatoka. The oils were extracted from the seeds and the various derivatives prepared at the pharmacy on Makogai for patient use.[48]

Chaulmoogra therapies on Quail Island, Lyttleton

In 1925, when the leprosy patients were moved from Quail Island to Makogai they were already familiar with chaulmoogra. Reflecting the interconnectedness of colonial health networks, Charles Upham, the Lyttelton Port Health Officer and General Practitioner who oversaw the leprosy patients on Quail Island had submitted a report as part of the New Zealand response to the BELRA survey. Though initially there was only one patient on the island, by the time of transfer to Makogai the population had risen to nine and Upham visited Quail Island at least monthly to attend to the leprosy-affected residents.[49] Upham was acutely aware of the physical and mental impact of the available leprosy treatments on the small number of patients on Quail Island. There was great optimism in New Zealand about the efficacy of chaulmoogra.[50] Leprosy was prevalent in Hawai'i and ethyl esters were obtained from Honolulu by the US Consul-General for use in treating leprosy patients in NZ. Optimism for their curative potential was reported by the Department of Health.[51] Upham was familiar with the various chaulmoogra derivatives and had worked closely with the patients on Quail Island to administer the substance in the form that would cause the least distress. In reply to the questions circulated by BELRA, Upham reported in 1924 on his own experience of using chaulmoogra oil, the physician's experience contributing to the complex private space of the patient's experience of treatment. Upham noted that he 'had been using Sodium Hydnodcarpate 2 gr in 4 c.c. intravenous, and the Ethyl Esters of the Chaulmoogra acid series for about 8 years . . . on nine lepers'.[52] He reported the devastating effects on the patients of the treatment at higher doses. All those treated had 'nodular leprosy' (Multibacilliary) which occurs when the patient has little resistance to the disease, a situation that Upham considered common among Pacific peoples.[53]

In Upham's experience, while the treatment tended to remove the appearance of the nodules so that the patient appeared recovered, massive and severe relapses occurred after a period of time causing intense suffering. After giving intravenous injections and four grains of Sodium Hydnocarpate per week to the patients on Quail Island, Upham reported: 'Two Chinamen did well, to all appearances recovered on intramuscular injections of the Ethyl Esters – but both together got a relapse . . . and have been very ill since.' Upham described the relapses in one case as taking the form 'of a very severe Nerve leprosy, and in the other of prolonged leprotic fever with successive crops of nodules'. Another patient described only as a Maori who arrived on the island 'very anaemic and feeble' and who had 'to all appearance recovered, also had a relapse and suffered much illness from sepsis resulting from extensive tarsal and metatarsal necrosis'.[54] If the patients were keen to avoid a repeat experience, so was Upham, who noted with feeling that: 'I shall never give so much again.' He considered chaulmoogra and its derivatives a 'potent' remedy 'but fearfully tricky like tuberculin, the slightest indiscretion of overdose reaps the whirlwind'. He had resolved before the patients left in 1925 that 'in future only those who I know can stand it will get more than 1 c.c. a week intramuscular injection of the Ethyl Esters'.[55] In the cold, windy, harsh conditions on Quail Island gaining the strength to bear the treatment would prove more difficult than on Makogai, where warmth, good food and daily hospital care were available. Upham was a local general practitioner with only nine very different patients to work with in his attempt to discover the limits and problems of using chaulmoogra. He also was aware of the limits of the patients' forbearance. Injection with Sodium Hydnocarpate risked causing thrombosis in the vein, something which had occurred in one case. Of greater concern for the patients, however, was the 'fulminating reactions that attend its use'. As Upham noted, this fear of the reactions made the patients 'kick against it, preferring the Ethyl Esters'.[56]

In the negotiations for the movement of the leprosy patients from Quail Island to Makogai, Thomas Fletcher Telford, Medical Office of Health for Christchurch, informed the director-general of Health that Upham's efforts with chaulmoogra treatment provided an incentive for at least three of the patients on Quail Island to leave for Makogai. Other patients on Quail Island were reluctant to leave and eager to be reassured that if they recovered on Makogai they could return to New Zealand. The two Chinese men referred to by Upham as Ah Pat and Ah Yip were, however, 'not doing well' and the Maori patient referred to by Upham, identified by Telford as Matawai, was 'suffering from a severe reaction'. Telford commented: 'The three of them are not at all pleased with Dr. Upham and his treatment, and for this reason I think they will be glad to get away.' In addition to the severe reactions from the treatment given, the next shipment of chaulmoogra received from Honolulu was 'green in colour instead of brown as formerly, and for this reason [Upham] cannot induce the two Chinamen to allow him to use it'.[57] Quail Island was connected to the worldwide trade in chaulmoogra but the patients taking the treatment were sensitive to variations in the remedy which in their experience might have severe and devastating repercussions. The standardization aspired to by Rogers and Rock was yet to occur. Chaulmoogra was still notorious for variation in quality and efficacy and was derived from a range of plant species. Further it was continually being altered to find ways of administering more easily what was a viscous and painful substance to inject. Dr Upham had changed suppliers and the appearance of the remedy was noticeably different. As Telford reported: 'It appears that Dr Upham previously added 2% iodine to a supply of Burrough & Wellcome's Moogrol which turned an identical colour to that now sent by the American Authorities, and the two Chinamen cannot be persuaded that this is not one and the same.'[58] This small event on a tiny isolation island in the South Pacific reflects the reach of the major drug companies of the period and the economic and therapeutic reach of chaulmoogra. In cases where laboratory facilities and the small number of patients made manufacturing derivative remedies for treatment impossible, Burroughs and Wellcome's trademarked esters were a valuable imported alternative.[59] Carville and other American facilities were developing the product as well and provided competition to the established Indian sources of the raw material and the commercial drug companies.

For all the patients' objections and hopes of a reprieve from the treatment, chaulmoogra was a fundamental aspect of the treatment regimen on Makogai Island. The treatment was repeatedly reported in the New Zealand press as evidence of the advanced medical care provided to the leprosy-affected people on the island. In 1925 the Wellington paper the *Evening Post* reported enthusiastically on the benefits of Makogai for those being moved from New Zealand:

> For the alleviation of the disease, experience shows that the chief factors are: Nutrition, fresh air, regulated exercise, amusement, and chaulmoogra oil. The leper's mind must be lifted by amusement and employment from the state of fatuity it is so liable to lapse into, and last but not least, chaulmoogra oil has a marked and beneficial effect on nearly all stages of leprosy. It is given at the asylum by the mouth daily in emulsion with lime water, and intra-muscularly weekly in the form of a mixture of chaulmoogra, resorcin, and camphor. The

surgical treatment is also of the greatest importance-the free removal of diseased bone and amputation of hopelessly septic limbs is of the greatest assistance in alleviating pain and improving the condition of the patient.[60]

Indian and Pacific world medical and trade networks

The establishment of the Leprosy hospital on Makogai created new sources, routes and networks for the movement of chaulmoogra within the Pacific. The hospital facilities were established with research laboratories, and the medical and nursing staff were deeply connected with international medical networks. In 1936, the import–export company, General Mercantile Corporation sent a form letter to the New Zealand Health Department offering to provide a supply of chaulmoogra oil from Cochin, 'packed in light steel drums of 40/44 gallons each at a rate of Sh.1/6 per pound for this medical oil'.[61] At the higher level of colonial trade relationships, encouragement of trade in therapeutics for leprosy treatment through the British Indian and Pacific colonial maritime networks also continued during the 1930s. The director-general of Commercial Intelligence and Statistics in Calcutta requested through the British trade Commissioner, the name of a New Zealand-based company who would act as local agents for the sale of both strychnine and 'leprosy preparations'. These were to be produced by an Indian-based firm.[62] The Indian Ocean trade in leprosy therapeutics coordinated through colonial government trade systems sought to extend their commercial reach into the antipodes. The offer was rejected on the grounds that New Zealand had few patients with leprosy and that those identified were sent to Makogai.[63] Similarly, the Burroughs Wellcome & Co trademarked 'Moogrol', described in the 1941 advertisement in *Leprosy Review* as 'a mixture of the ethyl esters of the acids of the chaulmoogric series to give the most satisfactory results' was little needed at the leprosaria.[64] Makogai had their own trees and were connected with the intercolonial research networks including those based at Carville, United States, where the efficacy of sulphones against leprosy was soon to be discovered.

Even as late as the 1940s, when leprosy treatment was on the brink of moving to sulphone therapy, leprosy-affected people in New Zealand were treated in hospital or at home with chaulmoogra until transport to Makogai could be arranged.[65] In 1944, a Niuean woman was diagnosed with leprosy in Palmerston Hospital. The director-general of Health, on the advice of two nursing sisters from Makogai requested that chaulmoogra oil with iodine for injection together with capsules for oral treatment be dispatched from Makogai which had developed its own supply.⁶⁶ When Makogai Island closed its hospital facilities in 1969, the impact of Dapsone making a large inpatient facility redundant, seeds from the trees grown on Makogai Island were brought to the new leprosy facility, P. J. Twomey Hospital in Suva to commemorate the importance of the oil in the history of leprosy in Fiji. These trees continue to produce fruit.

Conclusion

Chaulmoogra was a leprosy remedy with an ancient Chinese and Indian therapeutic history. Discovered in the context of British colonial engagement, misidentified and then integrated into colonial Materia Medica, chaulmoogra emerged from the nineteenth century as the only substance believed to have a genuinely therapeutic effect on leprosy. Its commercial importance is evident from the interest shown by drug companies and exporters in promoting the raw material and its derivatives. Administering the active ingredients in a way that did not produce acute nausea which inhibited absorption, severe drug reactions or vein thrombosis was the main challenge faced by those involved in the medical care of leprosy-affected people. Chaulmoogra spread from the Indian Ocean world to the Pacific world and became integrated into the landscapes of 'leprosy infested lands'.⁶⁷

As chaulmoogra was transformed from a folk remedy of the Indian Ocean world into a Western scientific medical commodity, the leprosy patient struggled with the contrast between the therapeutic promise of chaulmoogra and the risk of a catastrophic reaction to the treatment. For those isolated first on Quail Island in New Zealand, and then from 1911, on Makogai Island in Fiji, the sea was the medium for the transmission of medical culture from the Indian Ocean world to the Pacific. The sea also functioned like the forest of Indian tradition that sheltered King Rama exiled by his disease. The sea separated those on Quail and Makogai Islands from their communities. Travel to Makogai was particularly difficult with the lagoon protected by reefs and rough seas. But the sea also provided the means of bringing chaulmoogra to the islands and, until the 1940s, this Indian remedy which legend said had cured a king and a princess, was considered globally to be the best available for leprosy.

This discussion of the events of 1925, the transfer of patients within the South Pacific and the investigation and confirmation by BELRA of chaulmoogra as the principal therapy for leprosy on a global scale have shown that therapeutic value was never determined only by the medical, colonial or commercial authorities. The materiality of medical therapeutic commodities was fluid; chaulmoogra changed in both its physical form and its cultural resonance as it became integrated into nineteenth and twentieth-century networks of medical science and commodity trade. Through chaulmoogra the Indian Ocean world was connected to the landscapes and lives of people in New Zealand and Fiji. This therapeutic plant, originating in the Indian Ocean world became part of the landscapes of the South Pacific where, rather than exile to the forest to be healed with the fruit of the chaulmoogra tree, people with leprosy were exiled to islands where chaulmoogra plantations were established to secure local supply. Plantations of chaulmoogra-producing trees grown on the islands not only changed the landscape but also provided a therapeutic which promised if not a cure, then transformation of the leprous body into something unmarked by disease. Chaulmoogra transformed islands of isolation in the waters of the Pacific into places of healing where the chaulmoogra of ancient Indian forests grew in abundance.

Notes

1 Scott A. Norton, 'Useful Plants of Dermatology. I. Hydnocarpus and Chaulmoogra', *Journal of the American academy of Dermatology* 31, no. 4 (1994): 683–4; D. M. Thappa, 'History of Dermatology, Venereology and Leprology in India', *Journal of Postgraduate Medicine* 48 (2002): 160–5.
2 John Parascandola, 'Chaulmoogra Oil and the Treatment of Leprosy', *Pharmacy in History* 45, no. 2 (2003): 47–9.
3 Michael H. Fisher, *An Environmental History of India: From Earliest Times to the Twenty-First Century* (Cambridge: Cambridge University Press, 2018), 55–6; Haripriya Rangan, Judith Carney and Tim Denham, 'Environmental History of Botanical Exchanges in the Indian Ocean World', *Environment and History* 18 (2012): 311–42.
4 Xinru Liu, *Ancient India and Ancient China: Trade and Religious Exchanges AD 1-600* (New York: Oxford University Press, 1988); Raoul McLaughlin, *Rome and the Distant East: Trade Routes to the Ancient Lands of Arabia, India and China* (London: Bloomsbury Publishing, 2010).
5 Lynda Shaffer, 'Southernization', *Journal of World History* 5, no. 1 (1994): 1–21.
6 Gwyn Campbell, 'The Indian Ocean World Global Economy in the Context of Human-Environment Interaction, 300 BCE – 1750', *Global Environment* 13, no. 1 (2020): 30–66.

7 David Arnold, *Colonizing the Body: State Medicine and Epidemic Disease in Nineteenth – Century India* (Berkeley: University of California Press, 1993), 13–14; M. N. Pearson, 'Medical Connections and Exchanges in the Early Modern World', *PORTAL Journal of Multidisciplinary International Studies* 8, no. 2 (2011): 3–6.

8 Steven Engler, '"Science" vs. "Religion" in Classical Ayurveda', *Numen* 50, no. 4 (2003): 420; The dating of these texts is problematic as is their authorship. See for example G. Jan Meulenbeld, *A History of Indian Medical Literature*, Vol I. A (Groningen: Egbert Forsten, 1999): 105–15.

9 Engler, '"Science" vs. "Religion"', 417–18; for the integration of forest and tribal ritual and custom into Brahmanic high-culture Puranic Hinduism in ancient India, see Romila Thapar, 'Perceiving the Forest: Early India', *Studies in History* 17, no. 1. (2001): 14.

10 Norton, 'Useful Plants of Dermatology', 683; Angela Ki Che Leung, *Leprosy in China* (New York: Columbia University Press, 2009), 156.

11 Anna Winterbottom and Facil Tesfaye, eds, *Histories of Medicine and Healing in the Indian Ocean World, Volume One: The Medieval and Early Modern Period* (New York: Palgrave Macmillan, 2016); Anna Winterbottom and Facil Tesfaye, eds, *Histories of Medicine and Healing in the Indian Ocean World, Volume Two: The Modern Period* (New York: Palgrave Macmillan, 2016).

12 F. J. Mouat, 'Notes on Native Remedies: No. 1. The Chaulmoogra', *Indian Annals of Medical Science* 1 (1854): 646–52, reprinted in: *International Journal of Leprosy* 3, no. 2 (1935): 221–2.

13 Leonard Rogers, 'History of the Foundation and the First Decade's Work of the British Empire Leprosy Relief Association', *Leprosy Review* 5 (1933): 54–8.

14 J. Buckingham, 'The Inclusivity of Exclusion: Isolation and Community among Leprosy-Affected People in the South Pacific', *Health History* 13, no. 2 (2011): 65–8.

15 Buckingham, *Leprosy in Colonial South India: Medicine and Confinement* (Basingstoke: Palgrave Macmillan, 2002), 91–6.

16 Abraham Meima et al., 'Disappearance of Leprosy from Norway: An Exploration of Critical Factors Using an Epidemiological Modelling Approach', *International Journal of Epidemiology* 31, no. 5 (2002): 992–3.

17 Rod Edmond, 'Returning Fears: Tropical Medicine and the Metropolis', in *Tropical Visions in an Age of Empire,* ed. Felix Driver and Luciana Martins (Chicago: University of Chicago Press, 2005), 181–7.

18 Robert Charles Hope, *The Leper in England: With Some Account of English Lazar-Houses* (Scarborough, [1891]), 17–26; S. N. Brody, *Disease of the Soul: Leprosy in Medieval Literature* (Ithaca: Cornell University Press, 1974); Z. Gussow and G. S. Tracy, 'Stigma and the Leprosy Phenomenon: The Social History of a Disease in the Nineteenth and Twentieth Centuries', *Bulletin of the History of Medicine* 44, no. 5 (1970): 425–9.

19 Edmond, 'Returning Fears', 181–3.
20 Ibid., 175–7.
21 Arnold, *Colonizing the Body*, 18; Stephen Snelders, Leo van Bergen, and Frank Huisman, 'Leprosy and the Colonial Gaze: Comparing the Dutch West and East Indies, 1750–1950', *Social History of Medicine* 34, no. 2 (2021): 611–31.
22 Buckingham, *Leprosy in Colonial South India*, 76–96.
23 Ibid., 66–70.
24 Joseph F. Rock, 'Recent Information on the Chaulmoogra Tree and Some Related Species', in 'Chaulmoogra Tree and Some Related Species: A Survey Conducted in Siam, Burma, Assam, and Bengal', US Department of Agriculture, Bulletin No. 1057, Washington, DC, Professional Paper (24 April 1922), 24.
25 Joseph F. Rock, 'History of Chaulmoogra Oil', in 'Chaulmoogra Tree and Some Related Species: A Survey', 3–6.
26 Parascandola, 'Chaulmoogra Oil and the Treatment of Leprosy', 48.
27 Buckingham, *Leprosy in Colonial South India*, 140–4.
28 Parascandola, 'Chaulmoogra Oil and the Treatment of Leprosy', 49–50.
29 Leonard Rogers and Ernest Muir, *Leprosy*, 2nd ed. (London: Simkin Marshall, 1940), 232.
30 Shubhada S. Pandya, 'The First International Leprosy Conference, Berlin, 1897: The Politics of Segregation', *História, Ciências, Saúde-Manguinhos* 10, no. 1 (2003): 172–4.
31 Fernando Sergio Dumas dos Santos, Letícia Pumar Alves de Souza, and Antonio Carlos Siani, 'Chaulmoogra oil as Scientific Knowledge: The Construction of a Treatment for Leprosy', *História Ciências Saúde-Manguinhos* (2008): 37.
32 J. Buckingham, 'Indenture and the Indian Experience of Leprosy on Makogai Island, Fiji', *The Journal of Pacific History* 52, no. 3 (2017): 325–42.
33 J. Buckingham, 'Leprosy, Philanthropy and Social Capital in New Zealand/Pacific Relations 1950s–1960s', *Journal of New Zealand and Pacific Studies* 2, no. 1 (2014): 39–56.
34 Frank Oldrieve, Secretary, The British Empire Leprosy Relief Association, to Under Secretary of State, Colonial Office, London, 16 July 1925, H1 1299 131/12/15 9295 Archives New Zealand Te Rua Mahara o te Kāwanatanga, Wellington.
35 British Empire Leprosy Relief Association, 'Memorandum on the Prevalence of and Prophylaxis against Leprosy in the British Empire, Based on Replies to the Questionnaire of the British Empire Leprosy Relief Association; with Suggestions for Dealing with the Problem', 15, H1 1299 131/12/15 9295 Archives New Zealand Te Rua Mahara o te Kāwanatanga, Wellington. [Hereafter BELRA, Memorandum]; For 'Ball's method of making ethyl esters of the fatty acids of Chaulmoogra oil' see Harry T. Hollmann, The Fatty Acids of Chaulmoogra Oil in the Treatment of Leprosy and Other Diseases', *Archives of Dermatology* 5 (1922): 95.

36 BELRA, Memorandum, 18.
37 Ibid., 18.
38 Ibid.
39 'Chaulmugra Oil Produced at Makogai Leper Colony', *Manufacturing Chemist and Aerosol News* 17, no. 8 (1946): 345; Sr Mary Stella, *Makogai Image of Hope* (Christchurch: Lepers Trust Board, 1978), 149, note.
40 Norton, 'Useful Plants of Dermatology', 685.
41 Rock, 'History of Chaulmoogra Oil', in 'Chaulmoogra Tree and Some Related Species: A Survey', 6.
42 Philip E. Steinberg, 'Of Other Seas: Metaphors and Materialities in Maritime Regions', *Atlantic Studies* 10, no. 2 (2013): 165.
43 'Lyttelton News', *Press*, LXI, Issue 18446, 29 July (1925): 13 *Papers Past*. https://paperspast.natlib.govt.nz/newspapers/CHP19250729.2.94 (accessed 22 January 2022).
44 'Brave Nurses', *Evening Post*, CX, Issue 141, 11 December (1925): 9 *Papers Past* https://paperspast.natlib.govt.nz/newspapers/EP19251211.2.95 (accessed 22 January 2022).
45 C. J. Austin, 'A Study of Leprosy in Fiji', *International Journal of Leprosy* 4, no. 1 (1936): 55; Buckingham, 'Indenture', 329–32.
46 Buckingham, *Leprosy in Colonial South India*, 184–8.
47 *Jahaji bhandal* refers to the small bundle of belongings tied together in a piece of cloth and brought on board the ship by indentured labourers migrating to Fiji and other parts of the British empire. https://www.saada.org/thethingswecarried/part-ii (accessed 21 January 2022); Brij V. Lal, *Chalo Jahaji: On a Journey through Indenture in Fiji* (Canberra: Division of Pacific and Asian History, Australian National University and Fiji Museum, 2000).
48 Stella, *Makogai*, 149, note.
49 Benjamin Kingsbury, *The Dark Island: Leprosy in New Zealand and the Quail Island Colony* (Christchurch: Bridget Williams Books, 2019), 34–5; C. H. Upham, Lyttelton, to Dr Fletcher Telford, Ministry of Health, Christchurch, 12 April 1924, H1 1299 1311215 9295, Archives New Zealand Te Rua Mahara o te Kāwanatanga, Wellington.
50 Brave Nurses', *Evening Post*, CX, Issue 141, 11 December 1925, 9, *Papers Past*.
51 Department of Health Annual Report of Director-General of Health, 1922, *Appendix to the Journals of the House of Representatives*, H-31, 10.
52 C. H. Upham, Lyttelton, to Dr Fletcher Telford, Ministry of Health, Christchurch, 12 April, 1924, H1 1299 1311215 9295, Archives New Zealand Te Rua Mahara o te Kāwanatanga, Wellington.
53 Ibid.
54 Ibid.
55 Ibid.

56 Ibid.
57 T. Fletcher Telford, Medical Officer of Health to Director-General of Health, Wellington, 27 April 1925, H1 1956 131 12 16 3805, Archives New Zealand Te Rua Mahara o te Kāwanatanga, Wellington.
58 Ibid.
59 Advertisement, 'Chaulmoogra treatment of leprosy "Moogrol"', *Leprosy Review* XII, no. 3 (July 1941): ii.
60 'Brave Nurses', *Evening Post*, Volume CX, Issue 141, 11 December 1925, 9, *Papers Past*.
61 Managing Director, General Mercantile Corporation, LTD, Cochin, to Health Department, Wellington, 2 April 1936, H1 1694 131 12 26331, Archives New Zealand Te Rua Mahara o te Kāwanatanga, Wellington.
62 A. G. C. Deuber, Officer in Charge, Her Majesty's Trade Commissioner, Wellington, 17 May 1939 to Secretary, Health Department, Wellington, 17 May 1939, H1 1694 131 12 26331, Archives New Zealand Te Rua Mahara o te Kāwanatanga, Wellington.
63 T. R. Ritchie, Acting Director-General of Health, to His Majesty's Trade Commissioner, Wellington, 18 May 1939, H1 1694 131 12 26331, Archives New Zealand Te Rua Mahara o te Kāwanatanga, Wellington.
64 Advertisement, 'Chaulmoogra treatment of leprosy "Moogrol"', ii.
65 M. H. Watt, Director-General of Health, to Minister of Health, Wellington, 27 January 1944, H1 1574 131 12 44 23380, Archives New Zealand Te Rua Mahara o te Kāwanatanga, Wellington.
66 Telegram, Minister of External Affairs, Wellington, to Governor of Fiji, Suva, 27 January 1944, M. H. Watt, Director-General of Health, to Minister of Health, 27 January 1944, H1 1574 131 12 44 23380, Archives New Zealand Te Rua Mahara o te Kāwanatanga, Wellington.
67 BELRA, Memorandum, 18.

10

Bodies in circulation

Determining age and regulating health of transported convicts to the Andamans, c.1860s–1920s

Suparna Sengupta

Introduction

The Secretary of State of India, John Morley of Blackburn, writing from the India Office in London on 3 September 1909, brought to the attention of Gilbert Eliot, known as Lord Minto, Viceroy and Governor General of India (from 1905 to 1910), certain provisions of the 'Indian law' which he considered 'anomalous'.[1] He pointed out that the Executive Government in India was authorized to assign prisons in mainland India in which effect could be given to sentences of transportation passed by the courts. The consequences of such a legal provision implied that transportation in 'Indian legal parlance' did not imply punitive re-location 'beyond seas' to the Andamans and could effectively be a sentence for languishing in a mainland Indian jail! The issue threatened an imperial scandal and became a subject of bureaucratic deliberation, with 'seditionist' convicts being incarcerated in prisons in mainland India for a longer term than provided in the Indian Penal Code.[2]

This reveals the discretionary and arbitrary power of the Executive which was sanctioned as law in colonial India. The codification of laws and the commensurability of punishment to crime that were seen as typical and ideal characteristics of the Benthamite influence in the penal-judicial framework of colonial India were, thus, contradicted by such a legal provision that allowed for discretion in the execution of punishment. Punishment in the Empire did not, therefore, emerge as a semio-technique that represented careful calibration of offence to punishment as envisaged in an ideal penal code. The legal anomaly further reflected the 'hyperlegality' of the colonial state in which the judiciary had effectively become a department of the Executive.³ This Executive overreach, attested by several provisions of the Prisoners' Act, was partly a consequence of the classification of the able-bodied or healthy from the sick or unhealthy. Thus, the medical bipolarity of the healthy versus the sick intensely affected the penal-judicial administration in British India.

The policy of selective transportation to the Andamans was earlier subjected to critique by prison officials in mainland India for burdening them with the 'sick' and 'unhealthy' in their jails.⁴ It is important to note the dialectical tension of the administration of mainland Indian jails as well as the penal colony of Andamans in the distribution of the burden of the unhealthy criminal population. As observed by Padmini Swaminathan, the economy of running the jails through extraction of maximum profit from the prisoner's labour often conflicted with the objective of reform of the prisoner.⁵ Also, the punitive aspect of imprisonment, which was often exacting on the prisoners' health, contradicted the objective of reform and rehabilitation of the convict in the long-run – a feature which even plagued the administration of the penal colony.⁶ In the Andamans, the provision of select transportees was an outcome of the need for young labouring bodies in the penal settlement wherein convicts were also envisaged as colonists. Labour was intrinsic to the development of the island-colony in the Indian Ocean and the 'sick' had to be filtered out from being transported lest they became a financial and administrative liability to the Port Blair authority in the Andamans.

Morley's letter led to an enquiry within the colonial bureaucracy on the nature of legal 'anomalies' concerning penal transportation. The reply to the letter took over a year after various proposals were solicited by the local governments and after intense consultation with several officials of various departments.⁷ The arbitrariness in the penal policy of transportation to the Andamans was, however, strongly defended by the colonial state administration in British India as a humanitarian measure. It was argued that 'the old and decrepit criminals' who were to only consequently die in the Andamans for their 'lessened vitality' were barred from undergoing penal transportation and were, therefore, incarcerated in jails in mainland India. It was stated that 'the unsuitability of the climate of the Andamans to people of weak physique . . . make it inexpedient to send to those islands all persons sentenced to transportation.'⁸ Thus, only those who were assessed as physically and mentally fit were to be sent to the Andamans.⁹ Here, one witnesses the calibration of the humanitarian appeal of the imperialist civilizational discourse to the corporeality of punishment which, in its arbitrariness, reflected the political violence of the colonial state.¹⁰ Also, it is pertinent to note that it was not only the racialized constitution of the Europeans which were seen as vulnerable in the tropical climates of South Asia, as studied by Mark Harrison.[11] In fact, a portion of the native population, with age constituting an important differential, was identified as unsuitable for transportation to the monsoon-rich islands of the Andamans in the Indian Ocean – close to the pestilential mangrove forests and 'putrid shallows' of Sundarbans with 'poison' in the air of the Bay of Bengal.[12] Besides, the geographical diversity of the tropics was acknowledged and the specificity of the Andaman Islands was registered.[13] However, one notices here, with shifting valences in the administrative discourse, the transposition of an unhealthy climate to an unhealthy body, often identified as an ageing body – an extra-territorialization, somatization and objectification. Such bodies had to be classified, differentiated and excluded from transportation to the islands. It is worthwhile to note that the convict population in the Andamans also provided ready material for experimentations and advancement of medical research. For instance, by observing the prevalence of malaria in convict villages in the Andamans that were situated near the shores of the Bay of Bengal in the Indian Ocean, the idea was established that brackish water and salt swamps were responsible for the spread of malaria, via a particular species of Anopheles.[14] The Andamans was, therefore, not simply a peripheral region of the Empire for penal administration of British India but a crucial site for the advancement of medical knowledge that was akin to the experimentation on convict population in mainland Indian jails.[15]

This chapter investigates and highlights the policy of medical regulation of convicts who were judicially sentenced to penal transportation. In such a colonial policy, we observe that the definition of a 'healthy body' remained a source of contention within the colonial administration and there was no easy consensus on determining precisely how old was 'old'. Were the old to be determined chronologically or diagnosed biologically? What was the sign of age? Besides, one notices that sickness and age were inflected and refracted by racial prejudices in the medical discourse. I argue that 'old age' was perceived increasingly as a disability and a factor in the rate of mortality in Andamans which was itself an effect of the ethos of productivism in colonial capitalism that thrived on the statistical calculation of probability rates.[16] Although the extraction of convict labour in the penal colony, unlike a plantation colony or mainland jail manufactories, was not geared towards 'production of surplus value' in a Marxian sense, labour was important to sustain its economy, in which the 'self-supporting' system constituted its bulwark. In such a context, the pathological and the old became synonymous with incapacity to work. However, the visible sign of old age was difficult to translate to a fixed chronological marker that was required for classifying the old in official policy and the symptoms of ill-health as signs of unproductivity were often indeterminate and fraught within various spheres of colonial administration.[17]

Regulating transportation of convicts to Andamans: The 'selection of the fittest'

Morbidity and mortality of transported convicts to Andamans became an administrative concern from the early years of the penal settlement that was established for a second time post-Revolt of 1857. It may be noted that Andamans was briefly occupied by the English East India Company from 1789 to 1796 and the sickness and death among the transported convicts then led to its premature abandonment.[18] When the task of colonizing Andamans through convicts was contemplated for a second time, the insalubrity of the islands characterized as 'primeval jungle' became a matter of debate among the colonial officials.[19] It was argued with a hint of optimism that the effects of the topography of Andaman could be corrected like the coast of Arakan in colonized Burma even if it could not be imagined to be transformed into a Montpellier.[20] Also, the location of convict settlement had to be protected from the noxious and 'miasmatic' air brought by the south-west monsoon, characteristic of the Indian Ocean, through careful selection of site. It is important to note that Frederick J. Mouat, the Superintendent of Alipore Jail with a distinguished medical career, led an expedition as the president of the Committee to survey the Andaman Islands for the purpose of colonization in 1856–7. However, the very task of modification of ecological conditions through the clearing of jungles and swamps by convict labour, in a tautological manner and resulting irony, entailed the risk of suffering the loss of many transported convicts due to the double factors of death and diseases such as 'malarial fever' and gangrenous ulcers. As observed by Rohan Deb Roy, 'malaria' in the nineteenth-century medical correspondences was largely a 'multipotent, fluid, flexible, not-one diagnostic jargon' and many experimental measures were carried out to avoid what was vaguely perceived as 'malarial deaths'.[21] The rate of mortality among convicts which was concomitant with the very process of settlement was sought to be controlled by the colonial administration through a policy of selective transportation and the differentiation of 'healthy' and 'unhealthy' sites before the loss in the subject population threatened abandonment of the very imperial project of colonization.

In an initial medical report on the settlement of Port Blair in 1863, senior medical officer, Dr Gamack, observed that the dilapidated condition of accommodation of convicts and the nature of employment of convicts had resulted in increasing sickness and death among them. Labour in Andamans was principally extra-mural and 'heavy' which entailed 'cutting down jungle, quarrying stones, working in swamps, sawing timber, loading and unloading vessels with coal, building piers with huge stones, towing heavy barges, & c.'[22] Such a policy was rather a reversal of the emphasis on intramural labour in the penal administration of nineteenth-century mainland.[23] However, in further diagnosing the causes of mortality among the convict population, the factor of debilitating heavy labour to unacclimatized convicts was given short shrift in comparison to the very state of health and bodily condition of transported convicts. As early as 1859, within the first year of the penal settlement at Port Blair, Dr Gamack had recommended that aged men who were not fit to labour in the settlement should be sent back to India as they added to the mortality rate. The discursive ploy of internalizing the external causes of death as germane in the body of the convict further exonerated the colonial state administration from owning any responsibility in causing the deaths of the convict population by assignment of tasks such as jungle-clearing in heavy monsoons. Although the Government of India did not acquiesce with the recommendation of the senior medical officer for repatriation of old convicts as it could potentially deteriorate the deterrence of the punishment, the careful selection of convicts for transportation to Andamans on medical grounds was subject to serious deliberation by the colonial administration in the subsequent years.

In an inspection report on the settlement of Port Blair in 1867 by the medical officer, Major H. N. Davies, it was observed that 'importation of old, worn-out men' was one of the main causes of high mortality rate among the convicts in that year. Though other causes such as scarcity of animal and vegetable diet (mainly anti-scorbutic vegetables), inadequate clothing, congested barrack accommodation, clearing jungle for cultivation without being given adequate time for acclimatization to the newly arrived convicts were cited as various factors for the sickness and mortality among the convict population, age of the convicts, through an inductive reasoning, was attributed as the primary cause for the increasing mortality. It was observed that 'Out of 675 deaths which occurred in 1866, 473 were convicts who had been less than one year on the settlement, and 40 percent were men of 40 years old and upwards.'[24] It is significant that in the statement prepared by the officiating senior medical officer of Port Blair, Dr Gamack, 41.70 per cent of deaths occurred among convicts who were classified as being aged between twenty-five and thirty-five years. However, the colonial official concluded that the average age of forty was the limit above which convicts were susceptible to increasing mortality.

It was repeatedly reiterated by colonial officials that 'only healthy and vigorous prisoners' should be sent to Andamans. The mortality rate of convicts in Port Blair was put to cold calculation by the administration as it was complained by the officials that the deaths of the convicts resulted in a financial loss to an incipient colony in which the maintenance of a convict cost four to five times more than mainland Indian jails. Thus, public finances of the repressive colonial state were not geared towards healthcare but was rather sought to be managed through an exclusionary policy of selection of convicts.

The consequence of such economistic thinking was prohibition and proscribing of the seemingly old (classified as above forty-five), infirm and sick from being transported to the penal colony. A strict policy was initiated from the year 1867 and elaborate instructions were thereby issued to the local governments to bar the deportation of those who did not fit the criteria. In 1885, 55 per cent of convicts from Berar were barred from deportation to Andamans by the Alipore Medical Committee on account of 'bad physique'. However, it was complained by the Resident of Hyderabad that 'bad physique' was 'too difficult a term to define' and 'a physical standard should be fixed as to height, girth of chest, & c' as a verification procedure.[25] Subsequently, an extensive set of regulations were framed in a resolution passed in 1886. In accordance with the rules, the responsibility of selecting convicts for deportation to the Andamans vested with local governments and administrations, and the Alipore Medical Committee was empowered to detain any convict who suffered only from 'temporary indisposition'. In every Province, a local committee was constituted which, consisted of three members, one at least of whom was a medical officer, and inspected each batch of convicts before deportation with a view to eliminate 'all who were unfit for *ordinary labour*' (emphasis added).[26] A strict stipulation was laid down that all convicts who suffered from any of the following diseases, including blindness of both eyes to such an extent as to interfere with the performance of ordinary labour, insanity, idiocy, leprosy, pthisis pulmonalis and epilepsy, were to be barred from transportation.[27]

In this odd catalogue, each of the diseases that was listed formed a set which indexed functional decline and reduced capacity to labour adding to the administrative burden of hospitalizing the convalescent convict population and the 'Invalid Gang' in Andamans. Despite such stipulations, it was admitted that no 'hard-and-fast rule' could be laid down to regulate the transportation of convicts on medical grounds which became, thus, a ground for discretion that gambled on the physical potential for labour. This was testified earlier in an official correspondence in which the senior medical officer at Port Blair, Surgeon Major J. Dougall, was asked to indicate all the physical infirmities which incapacitated a convict from performing hard labour. The doctor stated in reply that 'to enumerate such infirmities it would be necessary to copy nearly the whole of the volume known as the "Nomenclature of Diseases"!' Despite such a reservation, he enumerated a list of thirty diseases or infirmities which could incapacitate a convict from performing *hard labour* ranging from heart disease to being 'debilitated, thin and weakly' (emphasis added).[28] The list indexes the possibility of restricting the wide array of diseases by estimating the capacity for hard labour in comparison to ordinary labour, which itself was not clearly defined. There were several other instances which the officials cited such as 'paralysis of one or both legs, elephantiasis of both feet, advanced disease of the heart & c', which incapacitated a convict from performing hard labour.[29] For detecting such ailments, it was, however, left to the experience and skilled knowledge of medical superintendents who were also doubling as jail officers. The simple test for the deportation of convicts, it was reiterated, was whether they could perform ordinary labour in an Indian jail. It was stated that 'convicts who, although of inferior physique, are not suffering from any organic disease, need not be rejected as being unfit for deportation, nor should such diseases as hydrocele, goitre and varicose veins, except in an aggravated form', unless it materially interfered with their capability of undergoing ordinary labour.[30] It was a difficult administrative task to draw the equivalence of the functioning capacity for ordinary labour in an Indian jail to the labouring tasks in the penal colony. This was largely because of the extra-mural nature of work in the penal settlement in which jungle reclamation was an important component. Labour in the penal colony was further differentiated into several grades in accordance to different classes of the penal regime for the ostensible objective of reform and rehabilitation as a convict graduated from the lowest in the hierarchy entailing the most laborious and punitive work to the top which comprised of lighter tasks and supervisory roles.[31] The assignment of newly arrived convicts to the lowest class entailing the hardest labour conflicted with the theory of gradual acclimatization. Also, a differentiation in the nosology is observed where organic diseases are attributed for reduced labouring capacity in comparison to functional disorder that had visible symptoms. It can be contended, in consonance with Foucault's argument on the politics of health in the eighteenth century, that although there was no medico-analytic precision to determine the 'healthy', the doctor as an administrator subjected the biological traits of the convict population to medical scrutiny for both economic management and utility.[32] It is the utilitarian calculation of the colonial state administration which sought to measure age and health and correspond it with vitality and mortality rates to assess which convicts could be transported, subjected to labour and utilized.

However, the Port Blair government often complained that unfit convicts or convicts of 'feeble constitutions', those suffering from 'enlarged spleen', anaemia and so on were being sent to Andamans.[33] This was primarily affected by administrative needs as the provincial governments in mainland India who sought to transport convicts to ease pressure of congested jails. It must be remembered that the colonial state was a carceral state which subjugated a substantial number of native populations under a variety of offences and in which, vagrancy was constructed as a crime and social disorder. The blind beggar, the insane criminal and the suffering leper implied important figures of 'dangerousness' who had to be put behind bars.[34]

However, quite paradoxically, the 'simple' deportation rule, that is, the transportation of convicts who passed the test of being able to perform ordinary labour in an Indian jail, did not improve the health statistics of the convict population in Port Blair. Although other causes such as water, diet, nature of work were counted as variables affecting the health of the convicts causing dysentery, diarrhoea and skin ulcers, they were given less significance in comparison to the very constitution of the transported convict. At times, an 'unhealthy season' was attributed as the primary cause affecting the health of the convicts in comparison to other factors which led to regulation of work regime as per seasonal cycles.[35] However, such restrictions were seen as obstructions to the pace of improvement of the settlement.

The sign of health: Debating symptoms of disease

Commenting on the medical gaze, Foucault had observed that it 'was not content to observe what was self-evident but also to make it possible to outline chances and risks, it was calculating'.[36] The Alipore Medical Committee which was vested with the responsibility of careful selection of convicts at the port of embarkation before they were deported to Andamans was at loggerheads with both the local committees of the provinces or the Port Blair administration over the interpretation as to who constituted 'healthy' and who were to be barred from penal transportation. Either the complaint was of leniency in transporting convicts (by the Port Blair administration) or for overt strictness (by the local committees).[37] Other than the ambiguities of medico-administrative knowledge, it is important to observe, as earlier hinted, of the contrary pressures of maintaining the overcrowded and congested jails in mainland India vis-à-vis the cost of maintaining convicts in the penal colony. Also, the contentious issue was compared to the emigration of Indian labourers to tea plantations in Assam in the official discourse.[38] The analogy of penal transportation to the emigration of indentured labour significantly shows how medical regulation of mobile bodies informed each other, in terms of policy. Also, the analogy of convicts to 'coolies' underscored the importance of convicts as workers.[39]

The following few cases illustrate the ambiguities of the medico-administrative knowledge. This was most pronounced in cases of detection of 'lunatic' convicts.[40] With regard to the examination of prisoners by the Alipore Committee, Dr C. J. J. Jackson, medical officer of the Alipore Jail and member of the Transportation Committee, presented two cases which became points of contention among the various medical committees. One was the case of Khorda Manjhee, who was returned by the Andaman Committee for being 'insane', and another convict named Budhu, who was returned from the Andamans for being a 'leper'.[41] According to C. J. J. Jackson, however, Khorda Manjhee was 'rational, coherent, and intelligent'. Earlier noted for not being as fluent in Bengali as he was a Santhali, Khorda Manjhee was observed to show no sign of insanity. As a testimony to his rational behaviour which was attested through the logic of work and utility, it was recorded that at the Alipore Jail, he worked at bag-sewing, did '22 bags a day', and fully comprehended the 'proportion this bears to his task'.[42] The other medical officer, G. D. Harris, concurred with C. J. J. Jackson and hypothesized,

> It is possible that the man being an uneducated, uncivilized Santhali, was somewhat dense and boorish, and not intellectually up to the standard required of convicts in the Andamans, and evinced a lot of unnatural dislike to penal labour whilst at the Settlement. That he is insane, I deny, but that he may be both clumsy, stupid and cunning I think quite possible.[43]

One may observe, here, the civilizational discourse of the colonial administration which inflected the perception of tribal communities as simultaneously 'uncivilized', 'stupid' and 'cunning'. Also, the utilitarian understanding of work and its symmetric correspondence with 'rationality' was embedded within the medical discourse. There was a slippery terrain where resistance to work and malingering could symbolize as 'irrational' and 'unnatural'. The ambiguities were confounding. It was often suspected by the colonial-medical officials that many convicts pretended to be insane to avoid penal labour in Andamans. In the 'peculiar case' of one Abdul Rahman, who was transferred from the Indore Jail to be only rejected by the Alipore Medical Committee as 'insane', there was a lot of back and forth in official correspondences in diagnosing the status of his mental health. He was noted as being capable of carrying 'rational conversation' and yet behaving in a 'very strange manner'. The Superintendent of the Presidency Jail surmised that his 'strange behaviour' could be a deliberate act of avoiding transportation to Andamans and yet, the absence of motive in committing murders as per his history sheet indexed his 'irrationality'. Abdul Rahman, was, therefore, not deported to Andamans and sent back to Indore Jail. It is important to note that such a policy was adopted because the transportation of criminal lunatics was strongly and frequently complained against by the Port Blair administration.[44] Special attention was demanded to be given to the mental condition of the convicts by taking recourse to the judgements which evidenced whether the convicted criminal was liable to fits of insanity or had such a tendency. Other than the implicit acknowledgement in several official correspondences that the settlement conditions itself could precipitate 'anxiety', 'sullenness' and consequent violence it was apprehended that 'convicts who are liable to paroxysms of mania' could get more violent due to the very laxity of adequate surveillance in the penal colony. The official discourse often emphasized upon the 'always-already' unhealthy convict who had to be barred from transportation and fused insanity with the notion of crime as being both sign of imminent danger. Such internal discussions on the settlement conditions as a possible trigger for insanity threatened into a public scandal via newspaper reports when seditionist convicts were transported in the early twentieth century leading to the deputation of medical administrator, C. P. Lukis. The torture in Andamans was described in the newspaper reports and autobiographical accounts mostly as the harshness of labour exacted from the 'gentlemanly terrorists' in the Cellular Jail and the settlement despite public official denial.[45]

It is important to note that it was not only the sign of insanity of convicted criminals, in the absence of manifest physiological evidence, that refuted medico-analytic precision. The visible symptoms of several diseases were as much disputed among doctors. The differences in diagnoses can be attributed to the distribution of medical examination of a convicted criminal among several committees for a duration until deportation. The reading of the signs over the course of a disease - the anamnestic sign (of what has happened), the diagnostic sign (of what is taking place) and the prognostic sign (what will happen) to the medical condition of the convicted criminal who was judicially sentenced to transportation was subjected to the medical gaze of several doctors at various stages and locations. For instance, in the case of Budhu, who was returned from Andamans for being a leper, it was observed by the medical officer of the Alipore Committee that during his examination, there was only slight puffiness of his face and there was no sign of leprosy as complained by the Andaman Committee such as skin thickening and loss of sensation on the cutaneous surface.[46] In another instance, two convicts, Badlu and Kammu, who were passed by the local committees, Bareilly and Jubbulpore respectively, were pronounced by the Medical Committee at Alipore as unfit for deportation to the Andamans. The Medical Officer at Alipore, W. D. Neal reported the condition of Badlu's heart as a reason for his unfitness for travel and Kammu was diagnosed as unfit for ordinary jail labour for his enlarged spleen.[47] In a representation by the Medical Committee of Bareilly Central Jail regarding its medical examination of life-convict Badlu, it was, however, contended by the medical officer, Colonel Woodwright, that the patient was not suffering from any organic heart disease when he was last examined and only suffered a temporary and functional condition of dilation of heart for having frequently suffered from malarial fever during the latter's residence in Badaun.[48] Similarly, Kammu's enlarged spleen was said to be only temporary in nature by the Jubbulpore Medical Committee.[49]

Besides, unlike the medical scrutiny of male convicts, there was an administrative reluctance and diffidence to subject female convicts to medical examination in Andamans. Anxious to maintain the code of heteronormativity in a convict population with a skewed sex-ratio as well as for the purpose of colonization by encouraging convicts to become settlers through the arrangement of marriages in the penal colony, female convicts were encouraged to be transported from the mainland Indian jails without many restrictions.[50] Any close medical examination of female convicts for venereal diseases on arrival in Port Blair was actively discouraged for causing 'undeserved mental pain and hardship' despite strongly expressed opinions of senior medical officers.[51] It was ordered that no female convict was to be medically examined 'previous to permission to marry from the Female Jail'.[52] It was observed that most convict women were already mothers before being transported to Port Blair and the status of health or to her antecedents before conviction must serve as points for reference to warrant a medical check-up.[53] This differential policy of treatment of male and female convicts demonstrates the gendered nature of colonial administration which determined medical regulations.

Debating the age clause: Defining the 'Norm'

In a letter to C. A. Elliott, secretary to the Government of North-Western Provinces, W. Walker, inspector general of prisons, North-Western Provinces, expressed his opinion with reference to two prisoners, Gyadeen and Kurreem, on whether they were to be deported or not, both being fifty years of age. He argued that every healthy man should have the sentence of transportation carried out on him irrespective of his age. According to Walker, age should not be the limit for the completion of a legal sentence. The correlation of the average age of forty-five and health, to him, was not so clear. He argued that young bodies, accustomed to the dry climate of North India could be more vulnerable to the corrosive damp climate of Andamans rather than physically mature, old men.[54] Apart from the legal anomaly of not executing the judicial sentence of penal transportation, we observe that old age was not perceived as functional decline with propensity for mortality and rather indicated maturity. This was an inversion of the perception of the metonymic association of age with vitality and acclimatization which belies the understanding that age was an empirical fact. Rather, age was assessed along several axes of ethical values, racial bias and gender.

This was especially evident in the medical and administrative concern of female convicts whose age was seen as determining their reproductive capacity. There was discussion among the administrative circles whether an age limit of thirty-five should be imposed on female convicts while deciding upon their marriages in the penal colony. In an article of the medical official, Major Woolley, it was observed that some of the women were allowed to marry rather old. He suggested that the disproportionate sex-ratio in the penal colony and 'consequent loose living' had further spread venereal diseases in convict villages which was partly responsible for 'unproductive marriages' besides age.[55] However, it was later decided by the Port Blair administration that it was not essential for women to be of child-bearing age and the main reason for encouraging convict marriages was to prevent the 'unnatural evil' of homosexuality than for motherhood.[56] Convict women in Andamans were employed in the weaving manufactories of the female jail and deployed for other gendered work such as wheat-cleaning, rice-husking, cooking food etc., but primarily, they were objectified for 'rationing sex' through the marriage-system in Andamans.[57] The sexual division of labour also implied that physical strength was equated with masculinity and household, sexual and other forms of work performed by women were represented as 'non-work' in the colonial discourse.

The imposition of the age limit for transportation of male convicts was a subject of fierce debate. In accordance with the inspection report of the penal settlement in 1867 by Major H. N. Davies, it was observed, as mentioned earlier, that no one above forty years of age was to be transported to Andamans. This age limit was, however, considered unnecessarily low by E. C. Bailey, another colonial administrator, when the policy of transportation of convicts under selective criteria was subjected to scrutiny. This debate was also spurred and inflected by the material needs of accommodation expressed by provincial jail administrators periodically for de-congesting the prisons which witnessed an increase in the number of inmates. According to Bailey, a man of fifty, *if in good health*, had probably a good chance of resisting the unfavourable climatic influences of Andamans as one of forty years of age and a compromise of age limit of forty-five years was reached to settle the dispute. This further illustrates that correspondence of biological ageing to chronological ageing was no easy task.

At this point, it might be engaging to ask, why was age considered as an objective indicator of labouring capacity and health rather than some other measure of capacity or index? Aditya Sarkar had observed that the criterion of age limit was the optimal benchmark for factory work and for regulation of child labour. The attestation of the age of the mill workers was conducted through medical tests such as the measure of height, girth and dental growth. He argues that the emergence of age as a suitable measure and as an objective standard was related to the nineteenth-century era of growing scientific expertise and codification when 'ad-hoc procedures of empirical investigation needed to be supplanted, or precisely given shape, by universal designators of truth, fact, and value'.[58] Age, in theory at least, as he argues, was a measure of capacity which could be applied across barriers of space and culture. However, I argue that in the context of convict transportation to Andamans, the veneer of 'objectivity' of old age to be determined physiologically or through empirical records was more difficult and was further refracted through the lens of race. The uncertainty in determining old age was due to the lack of precise symptoms and its symmetrical correspondence to vitality as well as the singularity of ageing despite being a common experience. In the instance of one prisoner Goomani, sent from Thannali jail, the Alipore Medical Committee rejected him as too old, but upon his return to Bombay, the Medical Committee there certified him to be below forty-five. The explanation offered by the Medical Officer at Alipore Jail, Dr C. J. J. Jackson, was that 'the man may have been tired with his long journey and have looked older here than after resting on his return!'[59]

Further, there were several queries. How was the chronological marker of age to be verified? Was age to be medically certified or the judicially recorded age at the trials of the convicts or in their descriptive rolls was to be accepted as 'facts'? Or, how was the age limit of forty or forty-five for classifying the old was to be arrived at?

That the age clause was subject to dispute can be demonstrated through several cases. In one of the several instances, life-convict Bhakta Patni was ordered to be re-transferred to Assam as he was declared to be permanently unfit for transportation to the Andamans by the Medical Committee at Alipore. According to the descriptive roll, Bhakta Patni was thirty-eight years of age, but the Alipore Committee certified him to be above forty which was accepted as final.[60] Convicts Pitambar Karwal and Baldeo Chaudhury were pronounced by the Alipore Medical Committee as unfit for deportation on account of overage. It was however acknowledged by the colonial administration that the 'determination of precise age by medical examination is apparently a controversial matter'.[61] It was speculated by a colonial official that due to the restriction of deportation for overage, the Bihar and the Orissa Committee could have diagnosed the age as less than the limit while the Alipore Committee 'followed the age recorded at the trial which of course would not be based on expert opinion'.[62] The administrative conundrum which hints a possible manipulation in certifying age by the provincial medical committees was driven by the same desire of increasing the upper limit of age for transportation, that is, de-congestion of local jails. Further, it was apprehended that if the Medical Committee at Alipore were to accept the age given at the convicts' trial in preference to the age given by the medical committees of up-country jails and this became generally known, a tendency would grow to overstate age at the time of conviction 'so long as the present anxiety to avoid deportation prevails in Upper India.'[63] The observation that the 'natives' in general in the Indian subcontinent - not necessarily limited to the lower classes or illiterate masses - could not be trusted or relied upon on stating their age accurately and might have ulterior motives to tamper with it was as much present in the discourse of census officials.[64]

In 1905, the superintendent of Port Blair brought to the notice of the Government of India the high proportion of deaths which occurred among the newly arrived convicts during the first year of residence in the settlement. He recommended the further reduction of age limit from forty-five to forty years as he assumed, in agreement with the senior medical officer, that 'advancing age seems to be a powerful factor in killing the new-arrival.'[65] According to him, 'in vitality and power of resistance the average native of India of 45 corresponds to the average European of 55'.[66] The analogy of the physical strength of a 'native' to that of a European and the former's decreased vitality and immunity on the scale of age shows the salience of racial discrimination and the bracketing of the peculiarity of 'Indianness' in colonial-medical discourse. It is significant that the senior medical officer had also ascribed the excessive mortality to the overcrowded and ill-ventilated state of the barracks, the quantity and quality of the diet, the employment of new arrivals on work unsuited to their physical condition and their exposure to malaria.[67] However, all these factors were dismissed by the superintendent of Port Blair, and the cause for excessive mortality was blamed upon the poor condition in which the men arrived at Port Blair.

The director-general of Indian Medical Service, G. Bomford, concurred in favour of reduction of age from forty-five to forty with the observation that '40 was a recognised turning point' and 'the signs which indicated that a man is on "the wrong side of 40" were better understood than otherwise'.[68] He reiterated that 'a native over 40 can generally be recognised to be so'.[69] Not many agreed with such an assessment. In accordance to H. Hendley, director-general of Indian Medical Service in the year 1916, G. Bomford's opinion of forty as a 'turning point' was not based on any 'physiological fact' but was merely a 'figure of speech'.[70] Asserting that he favoured dropping the age clause, he claimed, 'I have known young men of 50 and old men of 30' and reiterated that 'the exact determination of age of an Indian is frequently impossible'.[71] He suggested that rather than age being a determinant of deportation 'all deportees must be of sound health, capable of performing jail labour and free from communicable disease'. Such a stipulation, according to H. Hendley, would necessarily bar those who were 'aged' in 'medical sense'.[72] The emphasis upon age in 'medical sense' and its diagnosis through co-related factors such as health and labouring capacity was sought to be distinguished from age as a neutral vital statistical parameter. However, there was no consensus. The strong racialized perception of age was expressed again by C. P. Lukis, another director-general of India Medical Service, who had visited Andamans in 1912–13. He stated that 'we are dealing with Indians and not Europeans' and claimed that 'we all know how quickly Indians age after arriving at middle life'.[73] Agreeing that he had met old men at the age of thirty, he asserted that he had never met an Indian who was young at the age of fifty![74] He suggested that it was rather safe to continue forty-five as the maximum age for deportation than to extend it to fifty as was suggested by the Punjab Government. Despite such disputes of synchronizing chronological, physical time with biological ageing which was further complicated by racial somatization, the rules regulating transportation to Andamans remained in force till the Jail Committee Report of 1919 recommended the abolition of transportation to Andamans.

Conclusion

The colonial policy of medical regulation of convicts who were otherwise judicially sentenced to transportation demonstrates that health became a sign of the labouring capacity of the convicts. The colonial administration displaced the causes for sickness and mortality among the convict population in Andamans from 'external factors' such as the sanitary conditions of the penal settlement and labouring assignments to the very 'bodies' of the convicts themselves who had to be, thereby, placed under medical scrutiny. However, it has been shown that there was no medico-analytic precision for determining the health and inferring the age of transported convicts. Also, the differential treatment of male and female convicts demonstrates how administrative concern overdetermined medical regulation. It is argued that the correlation of age to physical qua labouring capacity was much disputed and debated within the colonial administration and this relation was perceived through the prism of race.

Notes

1 Home, Judicial, June 1910, no. 112–113, National Archives of India, New Delhi (hereafter, NAI), 17.
2 Home, Judicial., June 1910, no. 112–113, NAI.
3 Nasser Hussain, 'Hyperlegality', *New Criminal Review: An International and Interdisciplinary Journal* 10, no. 4 (2007): 514–31. Hussain describes administrative classification introduced by the state bureaucracy in the context of terror legislations in the UK. These classifications can be related to what Ian Hacking describes as 'Kinds of People' who are targeted in state policies. See Ian Hacking, 'Kinds of People: Moving Targets', *Journal of British Academy* 151 (2007): 285–318.
4 Report of the Indian Jail Conference, 1877 (Calcutta: Home Secretariat Press), 25.
5 Padmini Swaminathan, 'Prison as Factory: A Study of Jail Manufactures in the Madras Presidency', *Studies in History* 11, no. 1 (1995): 77–100.
6 See Satadru Sen, *Disciplining Punishment: Colonialism and Convict Society in the Andaman Islands* (Delhi: Oxford University Press, 2000), 131–65. Sen misreads Foucault's contribution by arguing that the latter emphasized on disciplinary mechanisms of the modern state which did not target the body. Also, Sen looks

principally at the conflict of medical administrators in Andamans with the settlement officials over the control of the transported convict. This chapter, in contrast, looks into the contradictions within the colonial administration at various levels in diagnosing the sign of age and health of a convicted criminal judicially sentenced to transportation.

7   Home, Judicial-A, August 1911, no. 69–79, NAI.
8   Home, Judicial-A, June, 1910, no. 112–113, NAI.
9   To summarize the statistics, in Madras nearly 100 per cent of those examined were rejected on medical grounds, and it was estimated that 25 per cent of those not examined would be rejected; in Bengal, 27.61 per cent, were rejected on medical grounds on an average of four years, in the North-Western Provinces, 6.2 per cent, in the Punjab, 63.7 per cent on medical grounds, and in Central Provinces, 19.7 per cent on medical grounds. Deportation of convicts to Port Blair, Home, Port Blair-A, May, 1885, no. 6–12, NAI.
10 See the tensions of Liberalism and Empire in Steven Pierce and Anupama Rao, eds, *Discipline and the Other Body: Correction, Corporeality Colonialism* (Durham: Duke University Press, 2006). The dialectics of the colonized subject's pathos and the subject's inadequacy for deploying corporeal form of punishment is elaborated in the set of essays in the edited volume.
11 Mark Harrison, *Climates and Constitutions: Health, Race, Environment and British Imperialism in India, 1600–1850* (Delhi: Oxford University Press, 1999).
12 From the Andaman Committee to C. Beadon. Secy. to Govt.of India, dated Port Andaman, 1 January, 1858. Selections from the Records of the Govt. of India (Home Dept.), Calcutta: Baptist Mission Press, 1859.
13 See David N. Livingstone, 'Tropical Climate and Moral Hygiene: The Anatomy of a Victorian Debate', *The British Journal for the History of Science* 32, no. 1 (1999): 93–110 on the dissection of 'not one, but infinite' tropical climates.
14 Anti-Mosquito Measures in India (1912), *British Medical Journal*, 1(2662): 23–5.
15 I owe this observation to the comment made by David Arnold on the paper presented at the workshop, Health and Materiality: Histories of Health, Medicine and Trade across cultures, 1600–2000, November, 2018. For jail population in colonial India as a site for experimentation to further medical knowledge, see David Arnold, *Colonizing the Body: State Medicine and Epidemic Disease in Nineteenth Century India* (Berkeley: University of California Press, 1993), 61–115.
16 See Ian Hacking, 'Nineteenth Century Cracks in the Concept of Determinism', *Journal of the History of Ideas* 44, no. 3 (1983): 455–75.
17 For elucidation on the valences of signs and symptoms to the medical gaze, see Michel Foucault, *The Birth of the Clinic: An Archaeology of Medical Perception*, trans. A. M. Sheridan (London: Routledge, 2003), 88–106, Taylor & Francis e-Library.

18 Satadru Sen, 'On the Beach in the Andaman Islands: Post Mortem of a Failed Colony', in *Disciplined Natives: Race, Freedom and Confinement in Colonial India*, ed. Satadru Sen (Delhi: Primus, 2012), 274–94.
19 Foreign, Political, 4 April, 1856, no. 13–14, NAI.
20 Ibid.
21 Rohan Deb Roy, 'Mal-Areas of Health: Dispersed Histories of a Diagnostic Category', *Economic and Political Weekly* 42, no. 2 (2007): 122–9.
22 Home, Port Blair-A, January 1873, no. 1–2, NAI, 12.
23 See Radhika Singha, *A Despotism of Law: Crime and Justice in Early Colonial India* (Delhi: Oxford University Press, 1998).
24 Home, Public-A, December, 1867, no. 89–97, NAI.
25 Home, Port Blair-A, July, 1885, no. 40–42, NAI.
26 Home, Port Blair-A, September, 1909, no. 65–69, NAI.
27 Ibid.
28 Home, Port Blair-A, June 1877, no. 6–8, NAI.
29 Home, Port Blair-A, March, 1886, no. 101–103, NAI.
30 Ibid.
31 For details on the six-tiered different classes of labour, see Sen, *Disciplining Punishment*, 86–130.
32 Michel Foucault, 'The Politics of Health in the Eighteenth Century', in *The Foucault Reader*, ed. Paul Rainbow (New York: Pantheon Books, 1984), 273–89.
33 Home, Port Blair-A, November, 1888, no. 15–17, NAI.
34 Radhika Singha, 'Punished by Surveillance: Policing Dangerousness in colonial India, 1872–1918', *Modern Asian Studies* 49, no. 2 (2015): 241–69.
35 Home, Port Blair-A, November, 1888, no. 15–17, NAI.
36 Foucault, *The Birth of the Clinic*, 89.
37 Home, Port Blair-A, May, 1885, no. 129–133, NAI.
38 Home, Judicial-A, August 1872, no. 228–232, NAI.
39 See Anand Yang, 'Indian Convict Workers in South-East Asia in Late Eighteenth and early Nineteenth Centuries', *Journal of World History* 14, no. 2 (2003): 179–208; Clare Anderson, 'Coolies and Convicts: Rethinking Indentured Labour in the Nineteenth Century', *Slavery and Abolition* 30, no. 1 (2009): 93–109.
40 Following the pioneering work of Michel Foucault, a large number of studies have been devoted to the study of insanity which would be difficult to list here for sheer lack of space. The peculiarity of 'madness' in its lack of manifest physiological symptoms has been argued to be the strong basis of psychiatric power despite its conjectural science and its difference from the empiricism of the medical gaze. See Michel Foucault, *History of Madness*, trans. Jonathan Murphy and Jean Khalfa (London: Routledge, [2006] 2009). In the context of colonial India, see Waltraud Ernst, *Mad Tales from the Raj: Colonial Psychiatry in South Asia, 1800–58*, rev. edn (London: Anthem Press, 2010) and James H. Mills, *Madness, Cannabis*

and Colonialism: The 'Native-Only' Lunatic Asylums in British India, 1857–1900 (London: Palgrave Macmillan, 2000).

41 Home, Port Blair-A., May 1885, no. 129–133, NAI.
42 Ibid.
43 Ibid.
44 Home, Port Blair-A December, 1907, no. 91, NAI. Noting the complaints, a colonial official remarked that he had discussed the matter with the director-general, Indian Medical Service, and if such stringency was stipulated, 'we shall eventually make jail superintendents afraid to pass *any* convicts as fit for transportation'.
45 Home, Political, August 1913, no. 67–68, NAI. On 'Gentlemanly Terrorists', see Durba Ghosh, *Gentlemanly Terrorists: Political Violence and the Colonial State in India, 1919–1947* (Cambridge: Cambridge University Press, 2017). Ullaskar Dutt recounts his delusional mental state which was triggered by the harsh conditions of labour and punishment in the penal settlement in his autobiography titled *Twelve Years of Prison Life* (Calcutta: Arya Publishing House, 1924).
46 Home, Port Blair-A., May 1885, no. 129–133, NAI.
47 Home, Port Blair-A. October, 1910, no. 79–81, NAI.
48 Home, Port Blair-B. February 1911, no. 22, Part-B, NAI.
49 Home, Port Blair-B, March, 1911, no. 7, NAI.
50 Satadru Sen, 'Rationing Sex: Female Convicts in Andaman Islands', in *Disciplined Natives, Race, Freedom and Confinement in Colonial India,* ed. Satadru Sen (Delhi: Primus, 2012), 243–73. Also, Aparna Vaidik, 'Settling the Convict: Matrimony and Domesticity in the Andaman Islands', *Studies in History* 22, no. 2 (2006): 221–51.
51 Home, Port Blair-A, August, 1902, no. 74–75, NAI.
52 Ibid.
53 Ibid.
54 Home, Judicial-A, January, 1873, no. 16–17, NAI.
55 J. M. Woolley, Convict Marriages in Andamans, Annual Administration Report of Port Blair Penal Settlement, March, 1912, 89–94.
56 Home, Port Blair-A, September, 1915, no. 37–40. NAI.
57 Sen, 'Rationing Sex'.
58 Aditya Sarkar, *Trouble at the Mill: Factory Law and the Emergence of the Labour Question in Nineteenth-Century Bombay* (Delhi: Oxford University Press, 2018), 191.
59 Home, Port Blair-A, May, 1885, no. 129–133, NAI.
60 Home, Port Blair-B, March, 1914, no. 25–26, NAI.
61 Home, Port Blair-B, November, 1912, no. 5–6, NAI.
62 Ibid.
63 Ibid.
64 Timothy Alborn, 'Age and Empire in the Indian Census: 1871–1931', *Journal of Interdisciplinary Studies* 30, no. 1 (1999): 61–89.

65 Home, Port Blair-A, May, 1906, no. 53–57, NAI.
66 Ibid., 20.
67 Ibid.
68 Ibid.
69 Ibid.
70 Home, Port Blair-A, September, 1916, no. 22–24, NAI.
71 Ibid.
72 Ibid.
73 Ibid.
74 Ibid.

11

From tribal knowledge to Ayurvedic medicine

Transition of *Arogyapacha*, the wonder herb of Kerala

Girija KP

Abbreviations

BSM	Benefit-Sharing Model
GI	Geographical Indications of Goods
IPR	Intellectual Property Rights
ITDP	Integrated Tribal Development Project
JNTBGRI	Jawaharlal Nehru Tropical Botanical Garden and Research Institute
KIRTADS	Kerala Institute for Research, Training and Development of Scheduled Castes and Tribes
RRL	Regional Research Laboratory
TKDL	Traditional Knowledge Digital Library
WIPO	World Intellectual Property Organisation

Introduction

The chapter focuses on the journey of *Arogyapacha* (green-health), a small plant with green leaves and brown seeds, identified as *Trichopus zeylanicus travancoricus* and found in the southern Western Ghats region in India.[1] It explores *Arogyapacha*'s transition from being a rejuvenating substance in indigenous knowledge to a key therapeutic polyherbal commodity named *Jeevani* in Ayurvedic medicine through 'retro-botanizing'.[2] The complex negotiations among multiple players with conflicting interests that emerged illustrate the ways in which the plant got shifted from a rejuvenating substance in nature to a commercially valuable medicine. During the span of ten years from 1987, the plant also came to be recognized as an endemic species that needs protection from massive commercial exploitation. The interpretations produced in every stage of the plant's journey through different regimes, including the transnational regime of intellectual property rights, the national biodiversity laws, the regional Panchayati Raj system and the knowledge of Kani tribes are examined. A plant referred to as *Chathankilangu* by the Kani tribes and locally known as *Arogyapacha* eventually came to be known as 'the wonder herb of Kerala' as well as 'the Ginseng of Kerala' in the course of this journey. This transition was not simple or linear; local, regional, national and international agencies and their networks contributed to this transformation. The subjective, oral knowledge (treated as experience) of a tribal community came to be seen as an objective knowledge with textual and scientific validation, for positioning it into a commercial and therapeutic product used for rejuvenation with anti-fatigue and immune-modulator properties.

The commercial utilization of the herb and the sharing of half of the profit accrued with the original owners of the knowledge made it an internationally acclaimed benefit-sharing model (hereinafter BSM). The model won the first Equator Initiative Price of 2002 for the sustainable utilization of local knowledge with a proper benefit-sharing with the indigenous people. The award was given in Johannesburg to a scientist of Jawaharlal Nehru Tropical Botanical Garden and Research Institute (JNTBGRI) and was received by him along with a member of the Kani community. This model which addressed the tense relationship between a community-owned sacred knowledge and its utilization by Ayurveda, biomedicine and the society hardly survived a decade. During this journey of *Arogyapacha*, several disputes erupted among different stakeholders with conflicting interests in supporting the knowledge and the knowledge bearers of the plant. *Arogyapacha* was like a genie let out of its bottle that opened up an array of discussions and dilemmas, many of them not yet sorted out. Most recently, the herb has fallen back to its original status of an endemic plant that grows in the hills of the Western Ghats. But this time, the status of the plant was elevated with a tremendous potential that could be exploited by any pharmaceuticals at any point of time with the support of a patent.

What came to be known as 'the *Jeevani* project' and its BSM is still seen as a global model for access and benefit-sharing among multiple stakeholders including indigenous community. However, it never led to the reshaping of international patent laws for preserving and protecting indigenous, oral knowledge of tribal communities.[3] In 2001, the Government of India decided to make a database called Traditional Knowledge Digital Library (TKDL) to prevent biopiracy of traditional knowledge, in accordance with the Convention of Biological Diversity, 1992. However, TKDL has so far documented knowledge only within Ayurveda, Unani, Siddha and Sowa Rigpa medical systems.[4] The myriad indigenous medicinal knowledge including *Adivasi vaidyam* (tribal medicine) are excluded from the purview of TKDL and hence from the protection under international patent laws. Some indigenous knowledge and herbs are included in the TKDL only through a reinterpretation as Ayurvedic herbs seen in the canonical texts.[5] Thus, they are refashioned from their original status of being an indigenous knowledge to a classical Ayurvedic knowledge. Inclusion of herbs and tribal knowledge into institutionalized Ayurveda leads to the exclusion of the original location of that knowledge and its ownership, rather than giving that knowledge an 'elevated' status. This exclusion is germane to the set norms of validation systems such as patent laws, TKDL and so on that prioritize textual evidence rather than empirical proof to establish the medicinal property of any herb. The rejuvenation property of *Arogyapacha* was equated with the aphrodisiac property of the herb *Varahi* mentioned in the canonical text. Tribal knowledge thus undergoes a translation and interpretation according to the conditions set by modern institutions in order to make it comprehensible to the world reshaped by the very same institutions. In the process, the meaning and the value of the herb for the community also get reinterpreted.

One of the outcomes of the process of the BSM was the formation of a Kerala Kani Samudaya Kshema Trust (Kerala Kani Community Welfare Trust), purported to represent the Kani community. Towards the end of the project, the Welfare Trust ended up destroying the mutual trust among the community and led to a rift among community groups living in different geographical locations. The nomadic imagination of the geographical territory of Kanis who lived on the fringes of two states was not accommodated in the BSM meant for the community. Because of this, the monetary benefits were shared to a limited section of the community living within the Kerala state and belonging to two panchayaths. The Kani people living in nearby panchayaths were not entitled to the monetary benefits of the BSM as they were not involved in the project.

Various regulatory authorities entered the scene and exerted their power and rules to regulate a community-owned knowledge related to the herb. With the cultivation and bulk production of *Arogyapacha* for the commercial market, the state Forest Department identified a hitherto nondescript plant in the forests as an endangered species. The department was initially unsure whether to include the plant in the list of Minor Forest Produce, a category of forest resource over which tribal communities had some granted access. An institute meant for the welfare of the tribal communities, the Kerala Institute for Research, Training and Development of Scheduled Castes and Tribes (KIRTADS) did not cooperate with a research institute and a pharmaceutical company in transforming a Kani knowledge into an immune-modulator polyherbal medicine. The institute assumed that the right to protect and support the tribal community was solely its prerogative under the conditions insisted by it and ended up in supporting some Kani members to file a case against the research institute that developed medicines out of *Arogyapacha*.

The effort to cultivate the plant outside its original ecosystem habitats in the forest turned out to be a failure as the properties of cultivated plants differed significantly. The plant needs shade, forest canopy and a natural habitat to infuse its herbal properties. The patent regime that was formulated elsewhere and was made applicable to India was not sufficient to protect a valuable community knowledge and the herb *Arogyapacha*. Instead of making the tribal community and their knowledge fit into the institutional imaginations of regulations, it would have been better to think the other way around and make necessary changes within the policies to accommodate the community ideas of geography and ownership on knowledge.

Kanikkar, the inhabitants of Agasthya hills

The physical properties of the herb *Arogyapacha* were only known to the members of the Kani tribe (*Kanikkar*) who live in the Agasthyamala (Agasthya hills).[6] The mountain (also known as Agasthyakoodam, Agasthyar hills) is unique for its rich flora which constitutes around 2,000 species of ferns, mosses, lichens and orchids apart from rare medicinal plants like *Arogyapacha*.[7] In 2016, Agasthya hills was classified under the World Network of Biosphere Reserves by UNESCO. The total area of the Biosphere reserve is 3,500.36 square kilometres, in which 1,828 square kilometres is in Kerala and 1,672.36 square kilometres is in Tamil Nadu. The name *Arogyapacha* – green-health – itself hints at the properties of the herb. The non-tribal people who live in the vicinity of Agasthya hills were also aware of *Arogyapacha*. Kanikkar, who reside in the Agasthya hills, are unofficially recognized as the knowledge bearers of the forests, its flora and fauna as well as the rare herbs and their medicinal values, as they serve as guides to tourists, environmentalists and scientists who trek in the Agasthya hills. Kanikkar do agricultural work, make handicrafts out of bamboo and reed, apart from gathering and selling Minor Forest Produce.[8] Kanis eat the fruit of the plant to survive for a day or two in the forest without fatigue when they go to collect Minor Forest Produce. They called the herb *Chathankilangu*, *Thenchikka*, *Chattukkodi* or *Arnanakkan* in their language apart from the regionally known name *Arogyapacha*.⁹

Trichopus zeylanicus – *Arogyapacha* – is a rhizomatous perennial small plant with green leaves and brown seeds, endemic to the Agasthya hills. It is also seen in Thailand, Malaysia and Sri Lanka, even though the energy-enhancing medicinal properties of the plant have not yet been tested and recorded.[10] The Kerala variety is named as *Trichopus zeylanicus travancoricus* as the plant is seen in the Ghats of the Travancore region (Thiruvananthapuram/Trivandrum), the southern part of Kerala.[11] The species had been identified from the Agasthya hills by the Botanical Survey of India, Southern Circle, Coimbatore, but the medicinal properties of the species were not known. In the 1861 botanical classification, the plant was named as *Trichopodium travancorium*, which was later renamed as *Trichopus zeylanicus*.[12] In 1997, *Arogyapacha* gained the status of 'wonder herb of Kerala', also claimed as the 'Ginseng of *Kanikkar*' because of its rejuvenating and anti-fatigue qualities which were hitherto unknown to the people outside of the Agasthya hills. When the plant was introduced by the *Kanikkar* reluctantly to a group of scientists who had gone to the forest for a scientific exploration with Kani men as their guides, the journey of the plant began from a local herbal plant to a pan-Indian Ayurvedic medicine and then to an internationally acclaimed BSM and a health product.

Discovering the wonder herb

In 1987, scientists from the JNTBGRI at Thiruvananthapuram and the Regional Research Laboratory (RRL) at Jammu went to the Agasthya hills for an ethnobotanical survey. They were guided by two local Kani men: Mallan and Kuttimathan.[13] The expedition included two senior scientists and two junior researchers. On the way, when the scientists felt tired and hungry, they rested and ate the food they carried. But the Kani people did not carry any food and they ate some small black-coloured berries that they had gathered from the forest. The Kani men were energetic and agile throughout the journey, but the scientists were not. The scientists were curious to know about the berries and the plant that bore the fruit. The Kani guides offered them the berries and the researchers felt 'a sudden flush of great energy and strength'.[14] Initially, the Kani men were reluctant to reveal their sacred ancestral knowledge because sanctity and secrecy constitute preservation techniques in traditional knowledge. Later on, with the persistent inquiry of the scientists, Mallan Kani and Kuttimathan Kani showed the plant, *Arogyapacha* to the scientists and informed them that the berries of the plant gave energy when they were hungry and tired.[15] The trust built up between the scientists and the Kani guides led to the sharing of the knowledge to an outside world which might otherwise have remained within the community.

The berries and leaves were tested for their anti-fatigue property in the RRL at Jammu. Such ethnopharmacological testing includes the parameters of modern science and traditional Ayurveda.[16] Throughout the course of the research, it was assumed that there would be no conflict of interest between the tribal understanding of a herb and the classical Ayurvedic understanding of it. Pharmacological investigations proved that the plant has anti-stress, anti-fatigue and immune-stimulating properties. After seven years of testing with various parts of the plant, in 1995, JNTBGRI developed a compound drug, known as *Jeevani* ('life-giver'). This compound consists of *Arogyapacha*, *Ashwagandha* (*Withanis somnifera*), *Pipali* (*Piper longuam* or long pepper) and *Vishnukranthi* (*Evolvalus alsinoides*).[17] An anti-diabetic drug and a sports medicine were also developed from this combination. The properties of *Piper longuam*, *Withanis somnifera* and *Evolvalus alsinoides* had long been known, as they were part and parcel of many Ayurvedic and Siddha medicines. It requires long years of research and laboratory testing to develop and prove the effectiveness of a drug from a single herb. This may explain why the scientists and Ayurveda experts developed a compound drug using many herbs within seven years. The scientists found that all parts of the plant have therapeutic benefits, although they used the leaves of the plant to make the medicine, because the berries used by the Kanis are very small and were available only seasonally.

Oral knowledge tradition at the mercy of textual validation

The medicine developed, *Jeevani*, came to be known for its immunity enhancing, anti-fatigue, anti-stress and liver-protective properties. The JNTBGRI obtained a process patent in 1996 for the drug formulation because until 2000, only process patents were permissible in India and many other 'developing countries'. In 2000, as per the requirement of the Trade-Related Aspects of Intellectual Property Rights law, the rules were amended to convert process patents into product patents. Process patents had facilitated many pharmaceuticals in India to produce low-cost generic medicines that were sold by colossal international pharmaceuticals. A slight tweak in any existing process of making medicines would allow for the pharmaceuticals to acquire a process patent for drugs with the same ingredients.[18] To obtain a process patent as well as the permission from the drug controller of India to manufacture a drug, it was essential to locate the herbs used in making a product within a codified text of Ayurveda/Siddha. So, JNTBGRI found an alternative to locate a plant with similar properties in the *Samhita* texts of Ayurveda. The foregrounding of texts as the prime validation of local knowledge had already happened in the late nineteenth century. The formation of 'classical Ayurveda' by consolidating and appropriating knowledge from diverse health traditions and legitimizing it by way of textual traditions has been well-documented by scholars.[19] The process of codification also occurred through interactions between health practitioners and those selling drugs, people like shepherds, tribes, mendicants and herb collectors from hills and forests.[20] However, from the early twentieth century onwards, these codified texts came to symbolize an everlasting truth-carrying capacity to demonstrate the evidence and the point of origin of a classical Ayurveda in India. By that time, finding a point of origin from a Sanskrit text to establish the divinity and age-old tradition for the practice of Ayurveda was imperative. So, a U-turn to a supposedly classical text to validate tribal knowledge happened in 1995 in the case of *Arogyapacha*.

The scientists found that in *Suśruta Samhitā*, a plant called *Varahi* (*Ioscorea bulbifera*) exhibits the characteristics of *Arogyapacha* in terms of its habitat. Currently, there is no information available on the Ayurvedic use or identity of this plant. From a critical survey of the various ancient Ayurvedic classics, the authors have come across some descriptions of a plant which matched strikingly with 'Arogyappacha'. Sushruta, while dealing with the various divine drugs along with 'Some' also described one 'Varahi' – which he described as 'Kandha sambhava' – rhizomatous, 'Ekapatra' single leaves arising from a stem and 'Anjana samaprabha' – shining like the grey-black stone. The leaves and flowers of this plant shine like grey-black stone. Sushruta also described the plant that with its railing stem with the raised leaves appears – 'Krishnasarpa swarupena' – like a black cobra with its raised hood. Sushruta ascribed great rejuvenating property to the divine 'Varahi' which is very true to 'Arogyappacha'. Sushruta has also described the habitat of this plant as a shade-loving herb found on the banks of rivers and natural ponds is also true to this plant. These descriptions given by Sushruta suggest that the divine 'Varahi' described by Sushruta may be about 'Arogyappacha', Sushruta has recorded the distribution of the divine 'Varahi' in the Kashmir region but has also mentioned that it may also be found in a similar habitat of other mountainous regions in the country.[21]

This ethnopharmacological research linked *Arogyapacha* with *Varahi,* a herb used mainly in aphrodisiac medicine. Thus, through an Ayurvedicalization process, the non-textual, subjective knowledge of *Kanikkar* was transformed into textual, Sanskritic, scholastic and objective knowledge tradition, through the validation of finding the herb (or a somewhat similar herb) in an approved text. Through this process of finding the herb in a text, an energy vitalizer and immuno-booster found within a tribal culture was linked to an aphrodisiac in Ayurveda. The validation of a local health tradition has happened by repositioning that knowledge, the very name of the herb and the qualities inherent in it into a different realm of textual knowledge. From the very beginning of the journey of *Chathankilangu,* the knowledge of the *Kanikkar* was comprehensible to the world only through the norms set within a language and structure of modern institutions. An oral knowledge can only survive by transforming itself into a textual knowledge through its assumed presence in a supposedly codified text. It is a process of validating a supposedly invalid knowledge of the tribal community through textual evidence. Pushpangadan further states that 'the anti-fatigue and spirit promoting properties of the fruits of Arogyapacha' was experienced by the scientists. This also means that the scientists subjectively experienced the properties after eating the fruits. But 'the rejuvenating, age stabilizing, disease resistance building etc.' properties claimed by the *Kanikkar* are deemed as lacking in evidence.[22] So, the immediate effect of the fruits is acceptable through the experience of scientists, which is considered to be more valid than that of *Kanikkar*. Though the remote effects need to be proven through ethnopharmacology and other methods, the plant was equated with *Varahi* which is mainly used in aphrodisiac medicine for rejuvenation and age stabilization to preserve sexual energy. The morphological property of *Arogyapacha* is equivalent to *Varahi* as per the description of the scientists, but there was no elaboration about the equivalence of the herbal properties of both plants except that of rejuvenation.

Wonder herb to Ginseng of Kanis/Kerala

In 1988, scientists wrote about *Arogyapacha* and its medicinal qualities in *Ancient Science of Life,* a journal published by the Ayurveda pharmaceutical company Arya Vaidya Pharmacy of Coimbatore. They equated the 'tonic effect of the plant' with the Korean health drug Ginseng.[23] The product brochure of Arya Vaidya Pharmacy, which produced and sold *Jeevani,* also claimed that *Arogyapacha* would compete with the 'billion-dollar international market of Ginseng'.[24] Later, *Arogyapacha* was also described by the journalists and scientists as the Ginseng of Kerala and even the Ginseng of India.[25] When the JNTBGRI scientists described the herb as the 'Ginseng of Kani tribes of Agasthyar hills (Kerala)', acknowledging the ample share of a specifically Kani community knowledge, the subsequent description by the journalists and other writers in naming the plant as the Ginseng of Kerala or India extended it to a whole region and a possession of that region which in turn reduced the specific contribution of the knowledge of the Kani tribes. However, in Kani description, the quality of the plant or its fruits they consume was never equated with that of an aphrodisiac.

On 10 November 1995, JNTBGRI transferred the technology to produce *Jeevani* to Arya Vaidya Pharmacy. Subsequently, *Jeevani* was sold through the outlets of the pharmacy from 1996 onwards at a rate of INR 160 per 75 grams. It was sold outside India to countries like Japan and United States. The licence was for seven years and according to the agreement, Arya Vaidya Pharmacy had to pay a licence fee of INR 10 lakhs and a royalty at the rate of 2 per cent of the profit from the annual turnover of the sale of the medicine to JNTBGRI. The name of the Kani tribe or individuals who shared the knowledge does not appear anywhere in acquiring the patent for *Jeevani*. However, JNTBGRI officials decided to share half of the licence fee and royalty with the Kani tribes. This was the first benefit-sharing model in India, which shared the profits of a product with the knowledge bearers, the Kani tribe. It was also a world-acclaimed model envisaged and implemented before the enactment of the Biological Diversity Act of 2002. However, the model was facilitated by the spirit of the first Convention on Biological Diversity signed at the Earth Summit at Rio de Janeiro in 1992. Article 8(j) of the Convention suggests for national legislation to protect and respect the 'innovations and practices of indigenous and local communities' as well as to 'encourage the equitable sharing of the benefits arising from the utilization of such knowledge innovations and practices'.[26] In 2005, the World Intellectual Property Organization (WIPO) also highlighted the BSM as a sui generis method to protect the traditional medicinal knowledge and the community ownership over it.[27] However, the internal incoherence of the intellectual property rights (IPR) and the patent laws in accommodating traditional knowledge as equivalent to any other knowledge has not been addressed and remedied yet.

From undistinguished plants to endangered species

Arya Vaidya Pharmacy needed the leaves of *Arogyapacha* in bulk for the production of *Jeevani*, which had a high demand in India and abroad. The Integrated Tribal Development Project (ITDP) and Arya Vaidya Pharmacy envisaged a plan in 1995, along with JNTBGRI to support the *Kanikkar* in cultivating the plant with a buy-back system. Fifty tribal families were selected and paid INR 1,000 each for the cultivation of the herb in their settlements in the forests.[28] Arya Vaidya Pharmacy bought the leaves by paying INR 500 per kilogram for the pilot programme of producing *Jeevani*.[29] According to this project, the leaves were to be given to JNTBGRI and they would transfer it to Arya Vaidya Pharmacy. *Kanikkar* managed to sell the leaves of the first harvest. However, during the second harvest, 10,500 plants were confiscated from a private nursery at Vithura, a village in Trivandrum.[30] When the cultivation and collection of the herb were commercialized for the first time, other agencies of the state intervened in policing and controlling the field of business. The Forest Department entered the scene by enforcing their official control and ownership in governing the forest. Since Kanis have no property rights or tenure rights on the forest land, they were at the mercy of the Forest Department to cultivate and collect the herb. The Forest law permits Kanis (and all tribes) to collect Minor Forest Produce, though not endangered species. Until that time *Arogyapacha* was neither included among Minor Forest Produce nor identified by the Forest Department as a valuable or endangered plant.

The consumption of *Arogyapacha* was not on a large scale and the knowledge was strictly restricted within the community as a local health tradition transferred from generation to generation. When the collection of the herb had started on a commercial basis with the increasing market demand, the Forest Department intervened. They filed cases against the unauthorized collection of the herbs by the tribes when they seized large quantities of leaves while Kanis took them out of the forest. From the knowledge bearers of *Arogyapacha*, Kanis became plunderers of this forest produce. Parallel to this, other non-tribal smugglers who unlike Kanis were well versed in the strategies of the market came into the scene to collect and sell the herb in bulk. Meanwhile, the Forest Department convened a meeting to decide whether *Arogyapacha* can be considered as Minor Forest Produce in order to make it available to the *Kanikkar*.[31] But no decision has been taken till date. This unnoticed plant became a puzzle for the Forest Department. The plant was stolen by many people and grown in their home gardens. JNTBGRI tried to culture the plant in their institute but found that the size of the leaves was smaller than those growing in the natural environment of the forest. The medicinal properties also differ when the plant is grown outside of its natural habitat without having the protection of the forest canopy. This could be the only reason that restricts the cultivation and sale of *Arogyapacha* in bulk within and outside of Kerala; perhaps a natural control to protect the herb from large-scale commercial exploitation. Eventually, Arya Vaidya Pharmacy withdrew from the contract in 2008 as there was a scarcity of supply and they were forced to buy the herb from Tamil Nadu.

In November 1997, a Kerala Kani Samudaya Kshema Trust was registered with nine members to ensure that the benefits of the commercial sale of the herbs would be available to the community rather than for a few individuals.[32] This was known as the first and best BSM in the world and won the 'UN-Equator initiative award' during the Earth Summit in 2002, held at Johannesburg.[33] Kuttimathan Kani, one of the guides who shared the knowledge about *Arogyapacha* also attended the summit along with Pushpangadan, the scientist of JNTBGRI, who received the award. The Agasthya hills spread across the states of Kerala and Tamil Nadu. But the financial benefits from *Jeevani* went to the Kanis of Kerala, that too limited to Kanikkar of just two panchayaths, because of the jurisdictional constraints of the government institutions in Kerala. Later, tension erupted within the Kani tribes living in other panchayaths in Kerala regarding the sharing and selling of their sacred knowledge of *Arogyapacha*'s properties to those outside of their community. A trust formed to protect the community's interest and welfare unfortunately became a reason for disrupting the trust within the members of *Kanikkar*.

Muddled territories

The hill tribe community of *Kanikkar*, with a population of 21,251, lives in and around the forests spread across the geographical boundaries of Kerala and Tamil Nadu. Around 16,000 members are from the hills of Kerala and the rest reside in the hills spread across the nearby state of Tamil Nadu.[34] In Kerala, they live within and adjacent to the forests of Trivandrum and Kollam districts, notably in places such as Vithura, Peringamala, Tholikkod, Pangode, Amboori and Kulathupuzha. In Tamil Nadu, they live in Kanyakumari and Tirunelveli districts.[35] Kanis speak a language based on both Malayalam and Tamil, which indicates that they live and move across the official territories of the two states.[36]

They move across the regions in the forest without bothering about the rigid political, geographical and linguistic divisions.

The inadequacy of addressing the issues of geographical and linguistic division was reflected in the BSM intended to advantage the Kani tribe. All the institutions involved in the transformation of Kani knowledge into a social knowledge worked under the state government of Kerala. It also signals the unsuccessful implementation of many of the welfare measures meant for the tribal communities who live on the fringes of the forest. The clan and the bonds of the *Kanikkar* are divided as Keralites and Tamils in all enumeration. Documents such as the Ration Card, meant for getting free provisions through the public distribution system of the state; the Aadhar Card, which serves as the unique identification number; and the Voter's Identification Card are given as per the state geographical boundary within which the *Kanikkar* live. There is no system to envisage a joint plan or programme of two or three states together to address the welfare of the communities who live on the fringes of those states. What could be the idea of citizenship for the Kani tribe (if at all there is any) is not yet addressed in the knowledge transfer and the subsequent resource-sharing model of *Arogyapacha*. The name of the Trust, Kerala Kani Samudaya Kshema Trust, itself hints that it is only meant for Kanis of Kerala state. The larger umbrella of the citizenship, statist ideologies and regionalism work to categorize people under rigid linguistic identities and geographical territories. *Kanikkar* fall beyond these categorizations of Tamil or Malayali linguistic and geographical identities. They occupy a liminal space and their idea of territory has never been addressed or accounted till date while involving them in any kind of knowledge-sharing process.

When the BSM was envisaged with *Arogyapacha*, the imagination of the officials about the Kani community was limited to the *Kanikkar* of Kerala, even though the Kanis did not have such a regional vision about their community. One of the disputes that erupted within *Kanikkar* was that the benefit-sharing model did not involve Kani tribes who live in panchayaths such as Vithura and Peringamala within Kerala state. But we do not know what the feeling could be of the Kanikkar who live adjacent to the Kerala border and move across the forest borders of Kerala and Tamil Nadu for their livelihood. Whether there was tension within the community in addressing their own people who live just outside the border, yet in the proximity of the Kerala state has not yet been addressed. On the other hand, the Kani tribe also has a sense of a state under which their jurisdiction has been regulated. This could be a reason for the Kani tribes who live in Tamil Nadu and in the threshold of the two states not raising any official complaints regarding the sharing of the benefits from the commercialization of *Arogyapacha*. When a BSM was proposed, the community's idea of their habitats, geographical boundary and linguistic ownership was not considered. In fact, this was the first BSM and the institutions involved in envisaging such a model also had been learning from the unaddressed issues arising from it.

Players with conflicting interests

To implement the BSM, the trust was registered with nine members of the Kanis in 1997 and the membership of the trust had increased to 500 from around forty settlements.[37] The executive committee of the trust decided to deposit INR 5 lakhs in the bank. They bought a vehicle to reduce the dearth of transportation from their region to the nearest market and to facilitate the transportation of locally harvested Minor Forest Produce to the market.[38] They paid INR 20,000 each to Kuttimathan Kani and Mallan Kani and INR 10,000 to Eachan Kani (the third person who shared the knowledge of *Arogyapacha*) for sharing the community knowledge with JNTBGRI. They also spent some money to construct a community hall-cum-office at Chonampara. The Kanis who lived at Amburi, Peringamala and Vithura were not happy with these activities as they could not enjoy the financial benefits because of their physical location being far from Chonampara. Meanwhile, another government agency, KIRTADS entered the scene to protect the rights of the tribes. Some of the Kani men, with the support of KIRTADS, wrote a letter to the government of Kerala, stating that JNTBGRI was stealing their secret and sacred tribal knowledge.

KIRTADS, located in the northern part of Kerala, carries out a series of activities to preserve and exhibit tribal knowledge. They conduct festivals of tribal food, art, medicine and undertake documentation of tribal culture. They also have an ethnological museum on tribes with artefacts, jewellery, musical instruments, agricultural tools and so on. KIRTADS rarely supports scientific research on the medicinal properties of herbs. In the case of *Arogyapacha*, they had sought the assistance of the RRL to produce an effective tribal medicine from the herb, but this did not materialize. Meanwhile, JNTBGRI contacted KIRTADS with a proposal to help the Kani tribes by providing land for cultivating *Arogyapacha*. KIRTADS refused this offer of support, stating that they did not want to enter a contract for profit-making with a private company like Arya Vaidya Pharmacy.[39] But the government institution succeeded in creating confusion and rivalry among the Kani tribes who stayed in different parts of the Agasthya hills. The

Kanis who stayed in Tamil Nadu had not turned up asking for benefit-sharing. Besides, the whole Kani community did not enjoy the benefit of their knowledge transfer. It was limited to a few members of the Kani Welfare Trust, especially those who were based in Chonampara and nearby areas. So, it was easy for an institution to create havoc among them in the name of preserving their knowledge instead of arriving at a creative and pragmatic solution. KIRTADS suggested to JNTBGRI to amend the benefit-sharing agreement with Kanis and to impart the know-how of medicine making to enable the community members in producing the medicine.[40]

In 2004, the JNTBGRI agreement with Arya Vaidya Pharmacy was extended for one year. Prior to that period, the production of *Jeevani* was not smooth with the scarcity of getting *Arogyapacha* leaves from the *Kanikkar*. In short, two government departments, including the one directly working for the welfare of the tribes did not creatively envisage a plan to overcome the lacuna in the existing rules and regulations to create an income-generating as well as a knowledge-sharing model for the Kanikkar. The tribal community needs creative support from the governing institutions to protect their knowledge, share it cautiously while ensuring the benefit from them and to prevent the misuse of the herbs only known to them. A community knowledge-transfer project for producing a commercial medicine ended up benefitting a few members of the community, inviting the intervention of the forest law to regulate the community members and bringing in new traders who were well versed in the intricacies of commercial marketing. Several players who had been 'positioned unequally, in their renegotiation of knowledge and power'[41] entered the scene for sharing different kinds of benefits and power among them, which lasted for a few years, but ended in generating tension. The questions of trust, access, power and knowledge are linked to a community's lack of ownership on resources like land and forest as well as the troubled relation of various institutions with the marginalized tribal community.

A community which did not get 'educated enough' to share their knowledge strategically with an institution; an institution with the good intention of innovating a polyherbal product from community knowledge; a pharmacy ready to manufacture and sell the medicine commercially, but could not procure enough herb; a department which wanted to enforce their regulating power by confiscating the plant cultivated in the forest; another department meant for the welfare of tribes intervene in producing tension among them – all these players entwined in such a way that the authority of certain players in terms of knowledge, power, resources and goodwill did not help in empowering others.

For the *Kanikkar*, mere knowledge of herbs-at-hand was not enough to assert the uniqueness of that knowledge and in gaining rights over that knowledge. The lack of right over land and forest resources increased their handicap in asserting their right and power over traditional knowledge. Assuring the ownership of rights, resources and knowledge of a community ended up in benefitting a few within the community and bringing in tension among the stakeholders and new commercial players outside of the community. The failure of the state agencies in assuring community rights for marginalized people by making national laws and policies flexible and in tune with the customary practices of the Kani tribes ended up in providing only monetary benefits to a few individuals. WIPO clearly states that 'the current international system for protecting intellectual property was fashioned during the age of industrialization in the West and developed subsequently in line with the perceived needs of technologically advanced societies'.[42] The TKDL, prepared by India as a remedial measure, also did not include medicinal knowledge other than Ayurveda, Unani, Siddha and Sowa Rigpa.

A supplier of nutritional supplements and sports medicine based in Connecticut, NutriScience Innovations, became the distributor of *Jeevani* in the United States, as Arya Vaidya Pharmacy could not directly sell the medicine there. In April 1999, NutriScience acquired the US trademark of *Jeevani*. However, under pressure from different agencies, they withdrew their trademark in 2001.[43] Great Earth Company Inc. New York also filed a trademark on *Jeevani Jolt* in March 2000. In 2015, a four-party agreement between Oushadhi – the Kerala government Ayurvedic medicine manufacturing company, JNTBGRI, Forest Development Agency and Kerala Kani Welfare Trust was conceived to produce and sell *Jeevani*.[44] The Kanis have been allowed to cultivate and harvest *Arogyapacha* in their settlements, but under the monitoring and control of Eco-development Committees started under the Participatory Forest Management programme. Oushadhi has not started making *Jeevani* yet. The current patent law in India and the Geographical Indications of Goods (Registration and Protection) Act 1999 are meant to protect tribal knowledge from misappropriation. But nothing has happened so far in terms of the protection and preservation of tribal knowledge and specifically the sustainability of *Arogyapacha*. The patent laws are formulated all over the world, envisaging liberal individuals. Community imagination of collective ownership and resource sharing has less space in such laws and is difficult to protect through such laws. However, medicinal plants belonging to particular regions which exhibit specific medicinal properties are eligible for protection under the Geographical Indications of Goods (Registration and Protection) Act, 1999. Medicinal plants or agricultural varieties registered under the GI of Goods (Registration and Protection) Act can obtain premium pricing in the market. This could also be a better protection measure for the wonder herb of the *Kanikkar*. Yet, the dilemmas in addressing the community imagination of *Kanikkar* as well as their geographical vision and community bonding may pause issues to the GI of Goods (Registration and Protection) Act too. If *Arogyapacha* is registered as a special medicinal herb of the Agasthya hills of Kerala isolating the nearby Tamil Nadu area, it could not accomplish the aspirations of a community who live on the fringes of two states.

Notes

1   Western Ghats is a chain of mountains situated in the western coast of India from the river Tapti in the north to the southern tip. They pass through the states of Gujarat, Maharashtra, Goa, Karnataka, Tamil Nadu and Kerala. The Ghats is a global biodiversity hotspot and covers an area of around 140,000 square kilometres in a 1,600-kilometre-long stretch with an interruption of 30 kilometres in the Palakkad district of Kerala.
2   Projit Bihari Mukharji, 'Vishalyakarani as Eupatorium Ayapana: Retro-Botanizing, Embedded Traditions, and Multiple Historicities of Plants in Colonial Bengal, 1890–1940', *The Journal of Asian Studies* 73, no. 1 (2014): 65–87. 'Retro-botanizing', according to Mukharji, is identifying botanical names for local species. He argues that botany, like any other scientific knowledge, is a historically contingent discipline and the meticulousness in naming plants are influenced by epistemic and political interests.
3   Harilala Madhavan and Jean-Paul Gaudillière, 'Reformulation and Appropriation of Traditional Knowledge in Industrial Ayurveda: The Trajectory of Jeevani', *East Asian Science, Technology and Society: An International Journal* 14, no. 4 (2020): 603–21, https://doi.org/10.1215/18752160-8771025.
4   See 'About TKDL', TKDL. http://www.tkdl.res.in/tkdl/langdefault/common/Abouttkdl.asp?GL=Eng (accessed 1 October 2021).
5   *Charaka Samhita*, *Suśruta Samhitā* and *Ashtanga Hridaya* constitute the canonical *Samhita* texts and known as the *Brhatrayis* or the great triad.
6   Agasthyakoodam hills (also known as Agasthyamala or Agasthyar hills) is the second highest peak in Kerala (1,868 metres) at the southern end of the Western Ghats. It is a trekking destination and a place of pilgrimage where sage Agasthya is believed to be the protector of the hills. Agasthya is believed to be a celibate sage, one among the eight *Siddhars*, the fathers of *Siddhavaidyam*, an indigenous health practice of Tamil Nadu and surrounding

areas. Trekking is seasonal and restricted for forty-one days from mid-January to March to a fixed number of 100 people per day. Kanis serve as guides for the tourists and pilgrims who visit the hills. The steep path through the forest takes one through deciduous forest, grass lands, semi-evergreen forests and evergreen forests.

7   Sathis Chandran Nair, *The Southern Western Ghats: A Biodiversity Conservation Plan* (Indian National Trust for Art and Cultural Heritage, 1991), 19–22.
8   The forest law gives right to the tribes who depend on the forest for survival to collect minor produce such as honey, Indian Olibanum (a fragrant gum used as an incense), bamboo, cane, tamarind, medicinal plants, herbs and tubers. Major Forest Produce includes timber, sandalwood and pulpwood. However, the Forest Department has the right to define contextually what constitutes Minor Forest Produce from time to time.
9   Kaumudy, 'What happened to Trichopus zeylanicus (Arogyapacha)? /Part1/ Kaumudy TV', YouTube Video, 9.14, 24 December 2017. https://www.youtube.com/watch?v=OKgiMRMHpn0. Unnikrishnan Payyappallimana, 'From Rio to Reality: A Case Study of Bio-Prospecting Local Health Knowledge in Kani Tribal Community of Kerala, India' (Masters's thesis, University of Amsterdam, 2000), 41.
10 In Sri Lanka, *Trichopus zeylanicus* is locally known as *Bimpol*, with the English name being snake guard. They use the plant to treat the poison of snakebite and for fractures. See 'Trichopus zeylanicus', Ayurvedic Medicinal Plants of Sri Lanka Compendium. http://www.instituteofayurveda.org/plants/plants_detail.php?i=1309&s=Local_name (accessed 25 October 2020); 'Bimpol/Trichopus zeylanicus', Herbal Plants Sri Lanka. https://herbalplantslanka.blogspot.com/2015/05/bimpoltrichopus-zeylanicus.html (accessed 25 October 2020).
11 The state of Kerala came into being on 1 November 1956 by integrating the regions held by the former princely states of Travancore and Cochin along with the Malabar province of the British Madras presidency.
12 Palpu Pushpangadan et al., '"Arogyappacha" (Trichopus Zeylanicus Gaerin), the "Ginseng" of Kani Tribes of Agasthyar Hills (Kerala) for Ever Green Health and Vitality', *Ancient Science of Life* 8, no. 1 (1988): 13–16.
13 Payyappallimana, 'From Rio to Reality'. The ethnobotanical survey was conducted jointly by the All India Coordinated Research Project on Ethnobiology (AICRPE) unit of the Postgraduate cum Research Centre in Ayurveda, Trivandrum, JNTBGRI and RRL. AICRPE was a programme coordinated by the Union Ministry of Environment and Forestry from 1982 to 1998, initially with headquarters at RRL, Jammu. Dr Pushpangadan, a senior scientist from RRL was the chief coordinator of the programme. It was a multidisciplinary, multi-institutional and action-oriented research programme. One of its major activities included inventorying tribal knowledge of local biological resources. Pushpangadan et al., '"Arogyappacha"

(Trichopus Zeylanicus Gaerin)'. Later, the institution was relocated to Trivandrum in 1990 at JNTBGRI when Pushpangadan become the director of JNTBGRI.

14 Pushpangadan was one of the senior scientists in the expedition to Agasthya hills in 1987. Pushpangadan et al., '"Arogyappacha" (Trichopus Zeylanicus Gaerin)'.

15 Payyappallimana, 'From Rio to Reality'; C. R. Bijoy, 'Access and Benefit Sharing from the Indigenous Peoples' Perspective: The TBGRI-Kani "model"', *Law, Environment and Development Journal* 3, no. 1 (2007): 1–23.

16 Ethnopharmacology research includes experts from Ayurveda and Siddha as well as from chemistry, pharmacognosy, pharmacology, molecular biology, biochemistry, etc. The objective of this collaboration is to understand the property of the herb from the perspective of the classical concepts of Ayurveda and to make it a scientifically proven one. Palpu Pushpangadan et al., 'All India Coordinated Research Project on Ethnobiology and Genesis of Ethnopharmacology Research in India Including Benefit Sharing', *Annals of Phytomedicine* 7, no. 1 (2018): 8.

17 Bijoy, 'Access and Benefit Sharing'; Payyappallimana, 'From Rio to Reality'. *Ashwagandha* is anti-inflammatory, reduces anxiety and pain. It is a well-known immunity booster. *Pipali* is used in Ayurveda for treating chronic bronchitis, asthma, constipation, gonorrhoea, paralysis of the tongue, diarrhoea, cholera, chronic malaria, viral hepatitis, respiratory infections, stomach ache, bronchitis, diseases of the spleen, cough and tumours. *Vishnukranthi* is good to reduce nerves debility, loss of memory, chronic bronchitis. It is also a blood purifier. Suresh Kumar et al., 'Overview for Various Aspects of the Health Benefits of Piper Longum Linn. Fruit', *Journal of Acupuncture and Meridian Studies* 4, no. 2 (2011): 134–40.

18 Sabil Francis, 'Who Speaks for the Tribe? The Arogyapacha Case in Kerala', in *Politics of Intellectual Property: Contestation over the Ownership, Use, and Control of Knowledge and Information*, ed. Sebastian Haunss and Kenneth C. Shadlen (Cheltenham: Edward Elgar Publishing, 2009), 80–106.

19 Kavita Sivaramakrishnan, *Old Potions, New Bottles: Recasting Indigenous Medicine in Colonial Punjab (1840–1945)* (Hyderabad: Orient Longman, 2006); K. P. Girija, 'Refiguring of Ayurveda as Classical Tradition', *Pragmata: Journal of Human Sciences* 3, no. 1 (2016): 43–62.

20 N. V. Krishnankutty Varier, *Ayurveda Charitram* (Kottakkal: Arya Vaidya Sala, 1980); Also see M. S. Valiathan, 'Traditional Medicine in Buddhist India', Module 1: Evolution of Ayurveda (video lecture, National Programme on Technology Enhanced Learning, IIT Madras). https://nptel.ac.in/courses/121/106/121106003/.

21 Pushpangadan et al., '"Arogyappacha" (Trichopus Zeylanicus Gaerin)', 13–16.

22 Ibid.

23 Pushpangadan et al., '"Arogyappacha" (Trichopus Zeylanicus Gaerin)', 14.

24 Payyappallimana, 'From Rio to Reality', 42.

25 'Kerala's Ginseng Project Grounded By Forest Officials', *Business Standard*, 26 February 2013. https://www.business-standard.com/article/specials/keralas-ginseng-project-grounded-by-forest-officials-198020301084_1.html (accessed 10 October 2020); K. S. Jayaraman, 'Indian Ginseng Brings Royalties for Tribe', *Nature* 381 (1996): 182.
26 'Introduction', Convention on Biological Diversity, last modified 19 October 2021, https://www.cbd.int/traditional/intro.shtml.
27 World Intellectual Property Organization (WIPO), 2005. Intellectual Property and Traditional Knowledge. Booklet No. 2. www.wipo.int/publications/en/details.jsp?id=123&plang=AR (accessed 2 October 2021).
28 R. V. Anuradha, 'Mainstreaming Indigenous Knowledge: Developing "Jeevani"', *Economic and Political Weekly* 33, no. 26 (1998): 1615–19.
29 Payyappallimana, 'From Rio to Reality'.
30 'The Red Tape vs Kanis', *Down to Earth*, 15 November 1998. https://www.downtoearth.org.in/coverage/the-red-tape-vs-kanis-22646.
31 Payyappallimana, 'From Rio to Reality', 11.
32 Anuradha, 'Mainstreaming Indigenous Knowledge'; Bijoy, 'Access and Benefit Sharing'.
33 'Achievements', KSCSTE – Jawaharlal Nehru Tropical Botanic Garden and Research Institute http://jntbgri.res.in/index.php/research/ethnomedicine-and-ethnopharmacology/achievements (accessed 2 October 2020).
34 The Census of India, 2011.
35 Kanyakumari was a part of Travancore before the linguistic state formation in 1956. Most people who live in this region are fluent in both Malayalam and Tamil.
36 All the tribes who live on the fringes of the states know and speak the language of both the states that they occupy as their habitats. In addition, sometimes they also speak a unique language of theirs. In the Karnataka–Kerala border, the tribal communities speak a mixed language of Kannada and Malayalam or Tulu and Malayalam. This does not imply that there is only one language in each state of India. Among the multiplicity of languages, each linguistic state represents an official language as that of the region.
37 Bijoy, 'Access and Benefit Sharing'.
38 Sachin Chaturvedi, 'Kani Case A Report for GenBenefit (2007)', *Research and Information System for Developing Countries* (New Delhi, India, 2007), 1–28, https://www.ris.org.in/images/RIS_images/pdf/Kani_Case.pdf.
39 Payyappallimana, 'From Rio to Reality'.
40 Chaturvedi, 'Kani Case'.
41 Gyan Prakash, *Another Reason: Science and the Imagination of Modern India* (Princeton: Princeton University Press, 1999).
42 See 'Traditional Knowledge and Intellectual Property – Background Brief', World Intellectual Property Organisation. https://www.wipo.int/pressroom/en/briefs/tk_ip.html (accessed 2 October 2021).

43 Chaturvedi, 'Kani Case'; Bijoy, 'Access and Benefit Sharing'; Anil Gupta, 'Value Addition to Local Kani Tribal Knowledge: Patenting, Licensing and Benefit-Sharing', *Research Gate*, 1 September2002. https://www.researchgate.net/publication/5113452_Value_Addition_to_Local_Kani_Tribal_Knowledge_Patenting_Licensing_and_Benefit-Sharing.
44 T. Nandakumar, 'Jeevani to Fetch Benefits for Kani Tribe', *The Hindu*, 3 October 2015. https://www.thehindu.com/news/national/kerala/jeevani-to-fetch-benefits-for-kani-tribe/article7718163.ece.

12

Of miracle drugs, Captain Hooks and Colonialism 2.0

Bioprospecting, biopiracy and the patenting of tribal bioresources and medicinal knowledge

Kaushiki Das

Bioprospecting projects in India

Across the world, there is a frantic, ongoing race between countries to gain exclusive control over plants of commercial value, be it for medicinal, agricultural or industrial purposes. The quest for 'green gold' has a long historical trajectory, dating back to the colonial era. The colonial expansion was built upon the expropriation of plants and knowledge from the colonies for serving European mercantilist interests and for self-sufficiency.[1] While turf wars and espionage missions were waged to extend control over commercially valuable plants and to sustain enslaved populations in the colonies, the drugs derived from native plants were imported into Europe, ensuring the flow of wealth into the government coffers.[2] Today the pursuit of biological resources has been bolstered by two landmark legal interventions. First, the bioprospecting race has been fuelled by Trade-Related Aspects of Intellectual Property Rights (TRIPS), established in 1995, which promises to grant monopoly and control over life forms as enshrined in Article 27.3(b). The ambiguities in TRIPS, including vague criteria for patentability and patentable subject matter, unclear distinctions between biological and non-biological, imprecise definitions of microorganisms and blurred lines between discovery and invention, offer loopholes to biotechnological firms for claiming exclusive rights over bioresources.[3] Second, the signing of the Convention on Biological Diversity (CBD) in 1992 at the UN Conference on Environment and Development in

Rio de Janeiro re-christened the utilization of biodiversity as 'bioprospecting': a formal, ethical and legal approach to discovering commercially valuable genetic and biochemical resources.[4] It is believed to mark a shift from indiscriminate exploitation of resources towards collaboration between bioprospectors and local communities. It dictated that the utilization of biodiversity be permitted as long as informed consent of the local communities is acquired, the benefits (monetary, technology transfer, sharing of intellectual property rights) are equally shared and biodiversity hotspots are preserved. The projects are expected to promote sustainable utilization of bioresources, to preserve indigenous knowledge and to enhance public health through the discovery of valuable drugs. Bioprospecting is viewed as favourable to the interests of all parties and hence, the projects are being undertaken with renewed vigour and anticipation.

In India, with their hopes pinned on discovering the new miracle drug, teams of ethnobotanists, taxonomists, microbiologists and chemists have been scouting areas occupied by tribal communities.[5] Since the 1980s till the present, biodiversity hotspots are being assiduously combed out and plants with any hint of pharmacological value are being collected, catalogued and screened.[6] Moreover, the knowledge of local communities is being meticulously documented to identify the plants. On 10 June 2008, Sangai Express reported that in Churchandpur district, Manipur, a plant called *Chawilien Damdei* had attracted considerable attention because of its miraculous therapeutic potential.[7] Used as veterinary medicine by the community, the plant was believed to hold potential cures for cancer, diabetes, malaria and indigestion. The Life Sciences Department of Manipur University researched its curative properties and reported to the Botanical Survey of India, Shillong. The Institute of Bioresource and Sustainable Development collected specimens for further analysis. In 2008, the Chawilien Cancer Medicine Research Agency was established.

Similarly, in 2016, under a collaborative project by the University of Madras, National Medicine Plants Board and IIT Madras, researchers were trying to derive a drug for curing various viruses, including those transmitted sexually, by investigating the native medicine of tribal communities living on a tiger reserve in Karnataka.[8] In Chhattisgarh, the government has extended its support to a self-help group of tribal women which procures raw materials and processes medicines for diabetes, cold, joint pain and indigestion.[9] The State Herbal Medicine Board and Forest Department provide the necessary equipment and infrastructure and sell the products to the Indo-Tibetan Border Police and in Raipur.

The impetus for bioprospecting can be traced to the implosion of herbal products in the domestic market since the 2000s.[10] As the demand for organic, chemical-free, no side effects and safe-to-consume products surged, pharmaceutical firms like Dr Vaidyas, Dabur, Patanjali and Himalaya launched a plethora of Ayurvedic products. While building a narrative of indigeneity, cultural specificity and tradition, they promise to revamp 'ancient knowledge' in a contemporary form. For instance, Dr Vaidyas (the 'New Age Ayurveda' as its tagline claims) sells LIVITUP, an Ayurvedic proprietary drug for curing hangovers. Its website advertises that the pills are an amalgamation of Ayurvedic ingredients like *Arogyavardhini ras* and *Kalmegh ghan* that break down the acetaldehyde produced by alcohol. Thus, the drugs are designed and packaged in ways to appease modern sensibilities. In light of the success of such ventures, the central government began focusing on tribal medicine. In 2015, the Ministry of Tribal Affairs issued a circular to all state tribal affairs departments, urging the documentation of medicinal plants and associated knowledge of these communities. Research teams had to record the names of the plants, description of the medical practice, the local name for the plant in Devanagiri script and the botanical name or English name.[11] The Ministry of Ayurveda, Yoga and Naturopathy, Unani, Siddha, Homeopathy and Sowa Rigpa (hereafter AYUSH Ministry)[12] was entrusted with the responsibility of validating the accumulated information.[13] In 2020, as the pandemic raged in the country, the government and domestic pharmaceutical firms accelerated their efforts to derive drugs from indigenous medical systems. For instance, in June 2020, Patanjali Ayurved Limited launched Coronil and Swasari medicine, claiming that tests conducted on 280 patients were found to cure Covid-19.[14] However, the Department of AYUSH in Uttarakhand barred Patanjali from advertising the drug because it had only granted approval for the production of immunity booster kits.[15] In September 2020, clinical trials of the Ayurvedic drug Immunofree and neutraceutical Reginmune were conducted in Gujarat, Maharashtra and Andhra Pradesh for assessing the impact on Covid-19 patients.[16] As the demand for drugs derived from indigenous medical systems surged, several bioprospecting projects mushroomed.

Such bioprospecting projects usually commence with the acquisition of the tribal community's consent and the signing of a contractual agreement which outlines the terms of resource and knowledge exchange between the two parties. Following this, databases are created to document the information about the plants (scientific names, local names, cultivation methods and sometimes cultural uses) and the medical knowledge of the healers. Second, the region where the plants grow is cordoned off for in-situ conservation and tribal self-help groups are recruited for the cultivation and accumulation of raw materials. The plants are cultivated under the supervision of ethnobotanists who spread awareness about the importance of conservation and instruct the community on the methods of sustainable utilization of plants. They monitor the extraction to ensure that no plant is uprooted and only the required amount is extracted. Third, after screening the plants to verify their healing properties, drugs are derived for specific disease categories such as cancer, diabetes, tuberculosis, liver damage and so on. The resultant drug is subjected to randomized clinical trials, quality control checks and product tests to ensure that it measures up to biomedical evaluation standards.[17] The profits earned from the drug sales are shared with the community and are used for developmental works in the region.

These bioprospecting projects are believed to herald a new age of formal, ethical and legal transactions between bioprospectors and tribal communities. There is a widespread notion that these projects mark a disjuncture from the colonial era of rampant biopiracy. However, this chapter argues that the existence of a formal, ethical and legal framework does not negate the violence perpetrated by bioprospecting projects. It seeks to push the conception of violence beyond the politico-legal framework in order to highlight the epistemic violence. The dominant debates in academic and activist circles have focused primarily on political-economic issues like violation of informed consent, inequitable benefit-sharing, threat to ecology and infringement of property rights.[18] Hence, they tend to obfuscate the epistemic violence inflicted on indigenous knowledge by the practices of cataloguing, environmental conservation, drug production and testing under bioprospecting projects. This is important because even if bioprospectors ensure that they acquire informed consent and share benefits equally, the cognitive regime that undergirds their project still inflicts violence.

At the same time, this chapter contends that bioprospecting projects today cannot simply be regarded as a continuation of the colonial patterns of exploitation. It contests the notion that expropriation of biological resources is largely undertaken by powerful Western pharmaceutical companies and governments from the Global South.[19] The chapter argues that domestic pharmaceutical firms, supported by governments in the Global South, are equally complicit in expropriation from tribal communities residing within its borders. The chapter also contends that the approach to expropriating plants and knowledge is being shaped in decisively novel ways due to the emergence of a new configuration of organizations, technologies and discourses. It draws attention to the specificities of bioprospecting in India where the projects are driven and legitimized by a unique set of political and economic agendas and discourses. It is important to move away from grand narratives and concepts of power towards a more fine-grained ethnographic engagement which takes into account the microprocesses that constitute the techno-politico assemblage of power.

The first section challenges the perception of bioprospecting projects as an ethical and legal approach to utilizing bioresources, by highlighting the epistemic violence perpetrated by them. It highlights the violence inflicted by cataloguing, environmental conservation, drug production and testing vis-à-vis the activities undertaken during the colonial era. The third section contests the notion that bioprospecting is a smokescreen for neocolonialism. It highlights the uniqueness of India's approach to bioprospecting. The final section stresses on the need to develop a nuanced critique of bioprospecting and to envisage new modes of resistance.

The violence of bioprospecting projects

There is a need to expand the scope of violence beyond the political economy framework which fixates on questions of benefit-sharing and consent. The extant literature on bioprospecting proposes that the problem of inequities in the exchanges of biomaterial and knowledge can be resolved through legal interventions such as acquisition of informed consent and equitable sharing of benefits.[20] However, the signing of prior informed consent forms and equitable sharing of benefits with communities alone do not guarantee transparency and fairness in the transactions. The knowledge exchanges under bioprospecting projects remain asymmetrical in nature due to the cognitive regime that undergirds these projects. Hence, there is a need to highlight the epistemic violence perpetrated by bioprospecting projects against indigenous knowledge, which includes delegitimization of native categories, imposition of alien theoretical and conceptual frameworks, and neglect of indigenous world view. Such epistemic violence is evident in the processes of cataloguing of plants and knowledge, cultivation practices, drug production and testing.

The violence of cataloguing

Under bioprospecting projects, cataloguing of plants is undergirded by a cognitive regime that favours scientific nomenclature over vernacular nomenclature, and renders distorted epistemological and ontological translations. Even though the vernacular names of the plant mentioned by the community are recorded and entered into the database after a series of stringent checks, eventually the botanical name (identified and categorized by the taxonomist according to the Linnaean taxonomic system) is prioritized. For instance, in the case of *Chawilien Damdei* plant, the Life Sciences Department of Manipur University replaced the local names *Kam-Sabut* and *Zanlung Damdei* by the botanical name *Croton Caudatus Gieseler*.[21] Databases also draw questionable equivalences between the aetiological and nosological categories of biomedicine and other medical systems.[22] Moreover, the knowledge is 'particularised (separated as types and fixed in time), validated (abstracted from context), and generalized (catalogued, archived and circulated)'.[23] The plant ingredients and formulations are pushed to the forefront while the multi-faceted therapeutic approach of tribal medicine is side-lined. Taxonomy is not a neutral plant reference system but perpetrates epistemic violence against tribal knowledge through the imposition of alien categories. Such 'linguistic imperialism' was also witnessed during the colonial era which aided in the promotion of European global expansion and colonization.[24] As the Linnaean classification system took over in eighteenth century, vernacular names of the plants (uprooted from their native environments) which revealed 'the medicinal value, biogeographical distribution and cultural valence' faded into oblivion; thereby reducing plant names to symbols.[25] European languages (except for Latin and Greek), non-European religious names, foreign names and names pertaining to uses of plants were obliterated.[26] The orientation towards homogenization and standardization created erroneous assumptions about the origin of some plants.[27] The Linnaean system celebrated the achievements of European male botanists and their 'noble sacrifices' for science while neglecting the contributions of other cultures to botany. In the exceptional case that the plant was named after a native informant for discovering its medicinal use, the wrong individual who had merely introduced it to Europe was acknowledged. Today, cataloguing under bioprospecting projects continues to delegitimize indigenous knowledge by failing to accommodate the native world view.

The violence of sustainable cultivation practices

Even as bioprospecting projects profess ethical intentions of environmental conservation, the language in which the concern for environmental sustainability is framed seems patronizing.[28] The emphasis on imparting 'environmental education' to the local community presumes that they have a short-sighted approach to utilizing the resources and do not appreciate the value of their resources.[29] The bioprospectors believe that the community can hamper conservation efforts because the healers tend to extract whole parts of the plant or even uproot the entire plant itself, rather than selectively culling few parts. Although the community has carefully nurtured the plant for years and their knowledge of its uses is deemed useful for scientific research, the community is engaged as mere plant collectors. For instance, in Kozhikode and Thiruvananthapuram, tribals have been recruited to collect medicinal plants in forest regions (including national parks and wildlife sanctuaries) identified by the Kerala Forest Department. These are then marketed by the Scheduled Caste Scheduled Tribes Development Cooperative Federation to pharmaceutical companies, wholesalers and retailers.[30] The tribals are not even allowed to grade or process the medicinal plants.[31] Similarly, in the Great Himalayan National Park, the local community had been hired to collect medicinal plants for pharmaceutical companies. Alternative employment opportunities were created for the locals to ensure that they do not engage in 'environmentally-destructive jobs'.[32] It is believed that only the bioprospectors' expert intervention can 'improve' upon the tribal approach to cultivation. The desire to 'improve' upon the indigenous cultivation method also provided the impetus for the attempts to rear native plants during the colonial era. For instance, Philip Miller at the Chelsea Physic Garden insisted that with 'proper cultivation techniques', the *Poinciana* would grow taller in England than in Barbados.[33] Today, bioprospecting firms delegitimize the contribution of tribal communities to environmental conservation by reducing them to parataxonomists.

The violence of drug production and testing

The current bioprospecting engagements with tribal medicine are undergirded by problematic translations between systems of medicine with disparate and often contradictory epistemologies and ontologies. The bioprospectors approach the tribal healer to enquire about specific biomedical disease categories whose cure they are seeking (diabetes, PCOD, urinary tract infection). They probe whether there are similar symptoms treated by the healer. They then interpret, co-relate and equate the symptoms mentioned by the healers with biomedical nosology. They also enquire about the ingredients of the formulations prescribed by the healer. For instance, in the case of the IIT project, the researchers believed that the tribal communities used the plants as 'immunomodulators' for treating various viruses, including those transmitted sexually.[34] Hence, they tried to isolate the biochemical molecules from the plant extracts to derive a drug for treating HIV/AIDS. The project had assumed an equivalence between biomedical nosology and tribal medicine's nosology.

Bioprospectors mistakenly assume that the translation between different systems of medicine would be a seamless process because biomedical disease categories will have equivalents in other medical systems, even if their labels vary. But equivalences cannot be simply drawn between indigenous medicine's nosology and biomedicine's nosology. For instance, the symptoms of the disease category of *mngal nad mkhris gryur* in Tibetan medicine do not correspond to symptoms of a single disease, but multiple diseases related to reproductive tract problems like STDs and dysmenorrhoea.[35] Moreover, Vincanne Adams argues that diseases are not considered to be consistent and they can morph depending on the duration of germination in the body and specificities of the patient. For instance, in Tibetan medicine, the *mngal nad mkhris gryur* may exhibit symptoms akin to reproductive tract infections in earlier stages, and in later stages, transmute into growths in the uterus.[36] Indigenous medicine does not believe that diseases are exclusively caused by physiological factors but also considers other causes such as deviant behaviour, spirit possession, social conflict or harbouring contempt towards elders.[37] Bioprospectors tend to ignore variations in epistemologies and ontologies and hence, their attempts to bridge the gap between the medical systems result in mistranslations. Harish Naraindas' ethnographic account of the production of Ayurvedic proprietary drugs demonstrates that attempts to draw equivalences between divergent registers introduce new complications in the drug formulation process. As pharmaceutical firms scan the Shastras[38] to identify potential symptoms that would align with a specific biomedical disease category and to determine corresponding formulations and their ingredients, biomedicine's nosology, pharmacological action or physiological description always gets prioritized over Ayurveda's holistic approach.[39] He argues that such kind of 'conceptual bilingualism condenses and morphs the entire panoply of Ayurveda's therapies and its endogenous logic into a "cookie jar", from which only the formulations get picked'.[40] The resultant creolized drugs of such precarious translational processes are what he terms 'halfway houses'.[41] Naraindas cautioned that the drugs born out of the problematic equivalences drawn between divergent epistemes pose a health risk.[42] Under bioprospecting projects, the evaluation protocols of indigenous medicine are ignored. There are no attempts to tweak the existing clinical trial procedures that prioritize biomedical nosological categories, aetiology, diagnostic tools and therapeutic approaches.[43] When it expectedly fails to measure up, it is dismissed at best, as inefficacious and at worst, as charlatanism.

Indigenous knowledge regarding plant uses was also delegitimized or supressed during the colonial period. Londa Schiebinger pointed out that the transfer of the knowledge from the colonies to the Empire was hindered due to cultural biases, circumstances and European medicine's theoretical and conceptual frameworks.[44] The native world views, schemas and spiritual elements were weeded out. Driven by the assumption that the natives had illogically mixed ingredients and produced ineffective drugs, the colonial botanists experimented on the drugs to 'improve' the potency and accuracy of dosage. Schiebinger argued that the drugs eventually included in the European Pharmacopoeia were sanitized versions, bereft of indigenous medicine's holistic therapeutic approach.

Current bioprospecting projects neglect indigenous medicine's conceptualization of anatomy, nosology, aetiology, prognosis, evaluation protocols, method of prepping and administering the medication and spiritual beliefs that are crucial for healing. Indigenous medical knowledge is merely used as a guide for identifying the plant ingredients while its social and cultural matrix is side-lined. Thus, bioprospecting projects inflict epistemic violence against indigenous knowledge, including its categories, ontologies, epistemologies and world view.

Colonialism 2.0

Given that the colonial plant trade and the activities undertaken under current bioprospecting projects appear similar, can the latter be regarded as colonialism 2.0?

Bioprospecting projects have been accused of re-packaging colonial interests and perpetuating biopiracy.[45] The Action Group on Erosion, Technology and Concentration (ETC Group)[46] has highlighted ethical violations of bioprospecting projects, branding them as Captain Hooks. They argue that like their colonial predecessors, bioprospecting projects undertaken by powerful corporations of the Global North encroach on the bioresources and knowledge of developing countries without compensation or acknowledgement of the source.

However, the label of neocolonialism presents a one-dimensional picture of both the past plant trade and the bioprospecting projects. Even as there were instances of espionage missions and violent clashes during the colonial era, the extraction was not as simple or intensely violent as the term biopiracy suggests. Schiebinger pointed out that it was a protracted struggle to extract the plants and knowledge, which was hindered by the clamour of languages, resistance and manipulation by non-Europeans and involved constant negotiation and coaxing.[47] The local population not only refrained from speaking the language of the Europeans whom they abhorred, but they also did not teach their language to protect their secrets.[48] Therefore, the colonial botanists had to resort to different tactics to gain the secrets of the indigenous people who refused to comply.

It will also be simplistic to conceive of current bioprospecting projects as a continuation of the colonial system of expropriation. There is a need to recognize that a new configuration of legitimizing discourses, technologies and organizations has emerged. In India, apart from the pecuniary motivation, bioprospecting is driven by the larger nationalism project which intends to highlight indigenous medical heritage of the country. The government's willingness to promote indigenous medical systems can be discerned from its latest policies. In 2018, the government issued a circular that state drug regulatory authorities can grant licences to patented or proprietary Ayurvedic, Siddha and Unani products without clinical trials or safety study reports.[49] The regulatory authorities have to rely on textual rationale or published literature as evidence of the drug's effectiveness and in case there is no such literature, then a pilot study has to be carried out. In 2019, the AYUSH Ministry issued an advisory that AYUSH experts would be enlisted during clinical trials undertaken by non-AYUSH institutions and the results would be screened to ensure that inaccurate conclusions are not drawn.[50] During the pandemic, a number of drugs derived from indigenous medical systems were promoted.

As such, the bioprospecting ventures being undertaken in the country aim to revive indigenous medicine. Medicinal plants are being demarcated as native to the country through cataloguing, cordoning biodiversity hotspots, drug production and marketing. The Traditional Knowledge Digital Library (TKDL)[51] is an outcome of the state's attempts to demarcate the boundaries of such knowledge. According to Sita Reddy, the state strives to create inventories, databases, texts and archives in order to codify, to make public and to stake ownership over such pharmacopoeia, formulations and healing practices.[52] This in turn enables domestic firms to stake claims to this knowledge for creating 'new' formulations, and to apply for trademarks and patents in the name of national appropriation.[53] Domestic firms claim that they are circumventing biopiracy perpetrated by foreign biotechnological firms. This is evident from the Divya Pharmacy case, wherein it was accused of not seeking the approval of the State Biodiversity Board prior to the extraction of biological resources, thereby violating the mandate of the Biological Diversity Act (2002). Moreover, it had not equally shared the benefits with the communities responsible for the conservation of the resources. The company argued that the charge of biopiracy could only be made against international companies and that it was entitled to appropriate the medicinal plants on the grounds of nationalism.[54] Thus, both the supposedly contradictory agendas – preservation of indigenous medical heritage and appropriation of indigenous medical knowledge – became inextricably linked.

The cultural boundaries of medical heritage tighten and mark the emergence of rigid cultural nationalism, heralding a new kind of enclosures movement.[55] This can be observed in the government's intention to open the TKDL to the domestic pharmaceutical industry under the Intellectual Property Rights policy in 2016.[56] It was proposed that the industry would be granted patent rights and in return, a share of the profits would be given to TKDL. According to Gaudillière, the nationalist dimension is further reinforced by the European patent offices that prioritize TKDL's claim that these ingredients were part of the indigenous medicine system of India. Patent applications which have incorporated ingredients that have for long been part of the European therapeutic inventory such as rose, mint and pepper tend to get rejected.[57] Interestingly, the defence put forth by activist Vandana Shiva in the Neem case was couched in the language of cultural nationalism, that the Neem tree is a sacred heritage of India and it was accepted by the patent office.[58] Also, domestic pharmaceutical firms draw upon a narrative of indigeneity, cultural specificity and tradition to market the drugs. For instance, Patanjali's marketing strategy of urging its consumers to buy its products as a nationalistic duty had helped garner 1.6 billion dollars in 2017.[59]

Moreover, the asymmetrical relationship between a codified system of medicine like Ayurveda and a non-codified system like tribal medicine introduces a new dimension to the drug formulation process in India. Tribal medicine's repository of medicinal plants is raided for merely procuring the drug ingredients. Due to state regulations that prioritize Ayurveda, the resultant drug is validated according to the Shastras and is ultimately categorized as an Ayurvedic proprietary drug. The drug ultimately lacks any recognizable trace of tribal medicine. Ayurveda is deemed to be primarily textual, grounded in philosophy and codified with complex theoretical and conceptual foundations as opposed to tribal medicine which is orally transmitted and practised in villages.[60] Tribal medicine has been treated as an unsafe, untested domain as compared to Ayurveda which is considered to be a relatively time-tested, legitimate tradition.

For instance, in Chhattisgarh, the formulations are monitored and validated by an Ayurvedic practitioner and a government lab.[61] Bioprospecting projects in India are thus driven and legitimized by a unique set of political and economic agendas and discourses. Therefore, labelling the current bioprospecting activities as neocolonialism would be a misnomer.

Conclusion

There is a need for increased critical scrutiny of bioprospecting projects in order to identify new patterns of violence and exploitation. A nuanced understanding is imperative because otherwise a stagnant critique of bioprospecting projects gets reiterated and new modes of resistance cannot be envisaged and forged. Both the prevailing notions of bioprospecting – as a potentially ethical and fair collaborative venture, and as neocolonialism – carry disconcerting implications. First, they do not recognize that in the Global South, domestic corporations, amply supported by the governments, engage in the expropriation of plants and knowledge from indigenous communities. The charge of biopiracy is always levied against foreign biotechnological firms while maintaining silence about the domestic firms' transgressions. Second, they obfuscate the epistemic violence inflicted on indigenous knowledge during the cataloguing, drug production and testing processes. Third, they do not recognize the complexities introduced by the intervention of a traditional medical system like Ayurveda. Fourth, the charge of neocolonialism does not recognize the intricacies of interactions between the tribal communities and bioprospectors. Tribal communities are willing participants in bioprospecting projects. They exercise their agency and strategically negotiate their contracts with the bioprospectors to derive benefits. For instance, the Kani tribals had made an informed decision to enter into an agreement with the institute, and they used the money for establishing hospitals, schools and for even buying TV sets.[62] At the same time, despite pressure from the community to share the knowledge, the healers may reveal only part of the knowledge to the bioprospectors and may share more information only after a lot of coaxing by the bioprospectors. Therefore, there is a need to re-imagine resistance. Resistance should not be conceptualized simply as an outright rejection of the project, but as a protracted give-and-take situation where the healer may use the information as leverage in further negotiations.

In conclusion, bioprospecting projects should be examined through a new lens which identifies and acknowledges the messy, prismatic picture created by the intersection of agendas of multiple actors (tribal communities, domestic pharmaceutical firms, government agencies like drug regulatory authorities), legitimizing discourses and the changing materiality of tribal therapeutic substances.

Notes

1. P. Fara, *Sex, Botany & Empire* (Cambridge: Icon Books, 2003); J. Merson, 'Bio-prospecting or Bio-piracy: Intellectual Property Rights and Biodiversity in a Colonial and Postcolonial Context', *Osiris* 15 (2000): 282–96; L. H. Brockway, 'Science and Colonial Expansion: The Role of the British Royal Botanic Gardens', *American Ethnologist* 6, no. 3 (1979): 449–65.
2. L. Schiebinger, *Plants and Empire: Colonial Bioprospecting in the Atlantic World*, 1st ed. (Cambridge, MA and London: Harvard University Press, 2007).
3. J. K. Plahe and C. Nyland, 'The WTO and Patenting of Life Forms: Policy Options for Developing Countries', *Third World Quarterly* 24, no. 1 (2003): 29–45; A. Coban, 'Caught Between State-sovereign Rights and Property Rights: Regulating Biodiversity', *Review of International Political Economy* 11, no. 4 (2004): 736–62.
4. N. Castree, 'Bioprospecting: From Theory to Practice (And Back Again)', *Transactions of the Institute of British Geographers* 28, no. 1 (2003): 35–55; C. Hamilton, 'Biodiversity, Biopiracy and Benefits: What Allegations of Biopiracy Tell Us About Intellectual Property', *Developing World Bioethics* 6, no. 3 (2006): 158–73.
5. The concept of tribe has been a bone of contention among anthropologists in India and, hence, it is not clearly defined. The earlier eighteenth-century colonial ethnographers used the term 'tribe' vaguely to denote common ancestry and interchangeably with castes. But from the 1901 census onwards, tribes were defined as those who practised animism, which was contested by scholars like G. S. Ghurye, who regarded them as backward Hindus. Tribal communities have been conventionally perceived as generally backward, having simple technology, illiterate, practising animism, living either in isolation from larger society (colonial ethnographies) or closer to larger civilization (native ethnographies), and as a society in transformation towards peasant society or caste society: V. Xaxa, 'Tribes as Indigenous People of India', *Economic and Political Weekly* 34, no. 51 (1999): 3589. Virginius Xaxa argues that tribes are not metamorphosing into caste society. Even as tribes have become peasants or socially differentiated entities, they have not lost their identities. Moreover, contrary to the notion that they are homogenous and are marked by the absence of exploitative classes, tribal societies are heterogeneous, with differences of religion, ideology, values, political orientation, way of life, resulting in conflicts between its members. Xaxa also differentiates between the

meanings attached to the term by administrators, academicians and tribals. While for the former, communities are tribes only if they are listed in the Constitution, the latter believes that the term gives a sense of belonging to the same community, irrespective of being listed in the Constitution. The term tribe has been embraced by the communities, not only to denote that they are the original inhabitants but also that they are marginalized as well (Xaxa, 'Tribes as Indigenous People of India', 3595). It has been the basis of several political movements for self-autonomy, such as in Chotanagpur in 1939. Although the term 'tribe' is largely a product of colonial construction, is riddled with contradictions and has been historically contested, I have referred to it for heuristic purposes.

6 The history of bioprospecting can be roughly traced to the All India Coordinated Research Project on Ethnobiology. It sought to conduct studies in tribal areas, regarding how bioresources can be preserved and utilized to ameliorate the state of the communities' lives as well as the country. It was launched in June 1982 by the Department of Science and Technology, but was later transferred to the Ministry of Environment and Forests: P. Pushpangadan, Varughese George, Thadiyan P. Ijinu, and Manikantan A. Chithra, 'Biodiversity, Bioprospecting, Traditional Knowledge, Sustainable Development and Value Added Products: A Review', *Journal of Traditional Medicine & Clinical Naturopathy* 7, no. 1 (2018): 256. In 1983, the Ministry established a coordination unit and Dr Pushpangadan was the chief coordinator of the project to monitor and execute the programmes under it. This later led to the first major bioprospecting agreement signed between the Jawaharlal Nehru Tropical Botanic Garden and Research Institute (JNTBGRI) and Kani tribals. In December 1987, a contract was signed stating the terms of benefit-sharing in exchange for deriving a drug from the Arogyapacha plant traditionally used by the community. The tribal guides who had accompanied the scientists on the ethnobotanical expedition were persuaded to reveal the source of their energy. The Jeevani drug was derived and patented by the institute and transferred to Arya Vaidya Pharmacy for manufacturing and sale. The Kani Samudaya Kshema Trust was established to ensure welfare of the community who were provided 50 per cent of the licence and 50 per cent of the royalty fees.

7 'Miracle Plant From Saikot: Curative Values Identified, Scientific Name Given', 10 June 2008. http://e-pao.net/GP.asp?src=1..110608.jun08 (accessed 10 August 2020).

8 S. V. K. Chaitanya, 'Is the Search Finally Over? Tribal Community May Hold the Answer to AIDS Cure', *New Indian Express*, 9 March 2016. https://www.newindianexpress.com/cities/chennai/2016/mar/09/Is-the-Search-Finally-Over-Tribal-Community-May-Hold-the-Answer-to-AIDS-Cure-901465.html (accessed 20 May 2016).

9 R. Mohanty, 'Tribal Women in Chattisgarh Beat the Poverty Trap with Fortunes from Indigenous Medicines', *Down to Earth*, 7 June 2008. https://www.downtoearth

.org.in/coverage/tribal-women-in-chattisgarh-beat-the-poverty-trap-with-fortunes-from-indigenous-medicines-4120 (accessed 15 April 2019).

10 One of the factors responsible for the popularizing of Ayurvedic products is Patanjali company's leveraging of the mass appeal of its founder, Baba Ramdev. Since 2001, his meteoric rise as a self-styled Godman and yoga guru attracted widespread attention to the Ayurvedic products manufactured by the company. His constant calls for the need to use only Swadeshi products and to refrain from using products of foreign multinational corporations helped the company rake in tremendous profits, around $1.6 billion in 2017 alone: R. Bhatia and T. Lasseter, 'As Modi and his Hindu Base Rise, so too does Yoga Tycoon Baba Ramdev', *Reuters*, 23 May 2017. https://in.reuters.com/article/india-modi-ramdev/special-report-as-modi-and-his-hindu-base-rise-so-too-does-yoga-tycoon-baba-ramdev-idINKBN18J1HJ (accessed 4 April 2019). The company's branding had leveraged a potent combination of Hindu nationalism and revival of the 'ancient tradition' of Ayurveda. For instance, its promotion of the cow-urine floor cleaner emphasized the need 'to rescue the country from the economic exploitation of foreign companies and to save the cow, the holy mother': B. Crair, 'This Multibillion-Dollar Corporation Is Controlled by a Penniless Yoga Superstar', *Bloomberg Businessweek*, 15 March 2018. https://www.bloomberg.com/news/features/2018-03-15/this-multibillion-dollar-corporation-is-controlled-by-a-penniless-yoga-superstar (accessed 4 June 2021). Its mass success reinvigorated public interest in Ayurvedic products which pushed other companies to launch products derived from local medical systems.

11 'Govt to Document Tribal Medicinal Practices', *Economic Times*, 5 July 2015. https://economictimes.indiatimes.com/news/politics-and-nation/govt-to-document-tribal-medicinal-practices/articleshow/47944528.cms (accessed 10 January 2019).

12 Ayurveda, Siddha, Unani and Sowa Rigpa are codified and organized systems of medicine that are grounded in philosophy and have complex theoretical and conceptual principles: Maria-Costanza Torri, 'Bioprospecting and Commercialisation of Biological Resources by Indigenous Communities in India: Moving Towards a New Paradigm?', *Science, Technology and Society* 16, no. 2 (2011): 123–46. They are deemed to be primarily textual, rooted in texts like Charaka Samhita, Sushruta Samhita, Bhela Samhita, etc. Such 'classical/scientific stream' of medicine is distinguished from the 'folk stream' which includes local health traditions that are orally transmitted and practised in villages by birth attendants, herbal healers, tribal physicians, bone setters and housewives: Planning Commission, 'Report of the Task Force on Conservation & Sustainable use of Medicinal Plants', 2002. https://niti.gov.in/planningcommission.gov.in/docs/aboutus/taskforce/tsk_medi.pdf (accessed 29 October 2021), 25.

13 The AYUSH Ministry was established in 2014 to revive and promote traditional systems of medicine; Ayurveda, Yoga and Naturopathy, Unani, Siddha, Homeopathy

and Sowa Rigpa. For this purpose, AYUSH pursues a fourfold strategy: to develop pharmacopeial standards of Indian systems of medicine and homeopathy drugs, to urge timely research on specific diseases addressed by these systems, to implement schemes for rearing medicinal plants and to bolster educational standards in the traditional medical system colleges: AYUSH Ministry, 'Background of Ayush Ministry', 6 May 2021, https://main.ayush.gov.in/background/ (accessed 1 July 2021).

14 Patanjali Ayurved Limited is a private Indian pharmaceutical company, incorporated in 2006, which manufactures Ayurvedic formulations, food supplements and herbal cosmetics. Its rising profits helped it challenge major industry stakeholders like Hindustan Unilever Limited and Nestle. The company's marketing strategy emphasizes the purity, non-toxicity and more importantly, swadeshi (national) origin of its products, unlike its competitors' products. Its products were mainly distributed through chikitsalayas (dispensaries), arogya kendras (health centres) and defence canteens. Moreover, Patanjali has received support from the central government and several state governments. For instance, while Maharashtra government granted 600 acres of land to Patanjali Yogpeeth for establishing ayurvedic products processing plant, Haryana government allotted twenty acres of land for establishing a university and school: K. Deka, 'Power Yogi: How Baba Ramdev Became India's Swadeshi FMCG Baron', *India Today*, 25 July 2016. https://www.indiatoday.in/magazine/cover-story/story/20160725-baba-ramdev-patanjali-yoga-829230-2016-07-13 (accessed 20 May 2021). It was also granted $46 million in discounts for land acquisitions in states controlled by the ruling party: R. Bhatia and T. Lasseter, 'As Modi and his Hindu Base Rise, so too does Yoga Tycoon Baba Ramdev', *Reuters*, 23 May 2017. https://in.reuters.com/article/india-modi-ramdev/special-report-as-modi-and-his-hindu-base-rise-so-too-does-yoga-tycoon-baba-ramdev-idINKBN18J1HJ (accessed 4 April 2019). R. Shukla, 'Coronil: All You Need To Know About Controversy Around Baba Ramdev's Ayurvedic Medicine For COVID-19', *Healthwire*, 25 June 2020. https://www.healthwire.co/coronil-all-you-need-to-know-about-controversy-around-baba-ramdevs-ayurvedic-medicine-for-covid-19/ (accessed 10 August 2020).

15 The Department of AYUSH was set up in 2010 by the Government of Uttarakhand primarily to promote the state as a premier Ayurveda treatment and wellness destination. It strives to mainstream AYUSH systems of medicine by developing AYUSH health and wellness centres and educational institutes, enhancing quality control of AYUSH drugs and launching community based AYUSH interventions: Uttarakhand AYUSH Department, 'Uttarakhand Ayush Policy 2018', 2018. https://investuttarakhand.com/themes/backend/acts/act_english1554790886.pdf (accessed 15 July 2021).

16 'Coronavirus Treatment: Ayurveda More Powerful than Indigenous Medicines, Finds a Study', *Times of India*, 29 September 2020. https://timesofindia.indiatimes

.com/life-style/health-fitness/health-news/coronavirus-treatment-ayurveda-more
-powerful-than-indigenous-medicines-finds-a-study/photostory/78384407.cms
(accessed 29 September 2020).

17 L. Pordié, 'The Politics of Therapeutic Evaluation in Asian Medicine', *Economic and Political Weekly* 45, no. 18 (2010): 57–64; S. R. Craig, '"Good" Manufacturing by Whose Standards? Remaking Concepts of Quality, Safety, and Value in the Production of Tibetan Medicines', *Anthropological Quarterly* 84, no. 2 (2011): 331–78.

18 To understand how databases have enabled pharmaceutical firms to access indigenous knowledge, see Devinder Sharma, 'Digital Library: Another Tool for Biopiracy', *The Business Line*, 12 June 2002. https://indiatogether.org/agriculture/opinions/ds_tkdl.htm (accessed 29 October 2021), Sita Reddy, 'Making Heritage Legible: Who Owns Indigenous Medical Knowledge?', *International Journal of Cultural Property* 13, no. 2 (2006): 161–88, and Jaideep Singh, 'Preempting Piracy, Foreign Policy', *Foreign Policy*, no. 144 (2004): 93. To understand how bioprospecting activities harm ecology, see Karim-Aly Kassam, Munira Karamkhudoeva, M. Ruelle, and M. Baumflek, 'Medicinal Plant Use and Health Sovereignty: Findings from the Tajik and Afghan Pamirs', *Human Ecology* 38, no. 6 (2010): 817–29, and Amita Baviskar, 'Claims to Knowledge, Claims to Control Environmental Conflict in the Great Himalayan National Park India', in *Indigenous Environmental Knowledge and Its Transformations*, ed. R. F. Ellen, P. Parkes and A. Bicker (Amsterdam: Harwood Academic Publishers, 2005), 101–19. To understand the asymmetries in benefit-sharing arrangements, see Chikako Takeshita, 'Bioprospecting and its Discontents: Indigenous Resistances as Legitimate Politics', *Alternatives: Global, Local, Political* 26, no. 3 (2001): 259–82, Cori Hayden, 'Taking as Giving: Bioscience, Exchange, and the Politics of Benefit-Sharing', *Social Studies of Science* 37, no. 5 (2007): 729–58, and S. Francis, 'Who Speaks for the Tribe? The Arogyapacha Case in Kerala', in *Politics of Intellectual Property: Contestation over the Ownership, Use and Control of Knowledge and Information*, ed. K. C. Shadlen and S. Haunss (Cheltenham: Edward Elgar Publishing Ltd., 2009), 80–106.

19 ETC Group, 'Biopiracy Update: A Global Pandemic', September/October 1995. https://www.etcgroup.org/sites/www.etcgroup.org/files/publication/473/01/raf icom45biopupdate95.pdf (accessed 9 May 2016); V. Shiva, 'Bioprospecting as Sophisticated Biopiracy', *Signs* 32, no. 2 (2007): 307–13; M. E. DeGeer, *Biopiracy: The Appropriation of Indigenous Peoples' Cultural Knowledge*, 2003. https://ipmall.info/sites/default/files/hosted_resources/PLANT_PATENT_ARTICLES/biopiracy_and_indigenous_knowledges.pdf (accessed 29 October 2021); A. Isla, 'An Ecofeminist Perspective on Biopiracy in Latin America', *Signs* 32, no. 2 (2007): 323–32; G. C. Delgado, 'Biopiracy and Intellectual Property as the Basis for Biotechnological Development: The Case of Mexico', *International Journal of Politics, Culture, and Society* 16, no. 2 (2002): 297–318; S. Mulligan and P. Stoett,

'A Global Bioprospecting Regime: Partnership or Piracy?', *International Journal* 55, no. 2 (2000): 224–46.
20 Leif P. Christoffersen and Eric J. Mathur, 'Bioprospecting Ethics & Benefits; A Model for Effective Benefit-Sharing', *Industrial Biotechnology* 1, no. 4 (2005): 255–9; C. Zerner and Kelly Kennedy, 'Equity Issues in Bioprospecting', in *The Life Industry: Biodiversity, People and Profits*, ed. M. Baumann, J. Bell, M. Pimbert, and Florianne Koechlin (London: Intermediate Technology Publications, 1996), 96–109; J. Millum, 'How Should the Benefits of Bio-Prospecting Be Shared?', *Hastings Center Report* 40, no. 1 (2010): 24–33.
21 The chapter deliberately includes both the vernacular names to contest the Linnaean taxonomic mandate of relying on a single botanical nomenclature to identify plants.
22 J. P. Gaudilliére, 'An Indian Path to Biocapital? The Indigenous Knowledge Digital Library, Drug Patents and the Reformulation Regime of Contemporary Ayurveda', *East Asian Science, Technology and Society: An International Journal* 8, no. 4 (2014): 399.
23 Reddy, 'Making Heritage Legible', 175.
24 Schiebinger, *Plants and Empire*; Fara, *Sex, Botany & Empire*.
25 Schiebinger, *Plants and Empire*, 197–8.
26 Ibid., 200.
27 Ibid., 205.
28 C. Hayden, *When Nature Goes Public: The Making and Unmaking of Bioprospecting in Mexico* (Princeton: Princeton University Press, 2003); ETC Group, 'Biopiracy Update'.
29 However, the tribals follow a regimented approach to nurturing the natural resources. For instance, Bhil and Bhilala tribal communities in Alirajpur tehsil, Madhya Pradesh, refrained from cutting green fodder and teak leaves during monsoon: Baviskar, 'Claims to Knowledge', 101–19. Even measures like slash and burn cultivation were driven by the rationale of leaving the land fallow for restoring its productivity: Christoph von Fürer-Haimendorf, *Tribes of India: The Struggle for Survival* (Berkeley: University of California Press, 1982).
30 T. P. Bharath Kumar, M. T. Lakshminarayan, and A. T. Krishnamurthy, 'Extraction of Medicinal Plants by Tribals in Kerala', *Journal of Pharmacognosy and Phytochemistry* 7, SP 3 (2018): 242.
31 Ibid., 243.
32 Baviskar, 'Claims to Knowledge', 101–19.
33 Schiebinger, *Plants and Empire*, 152.
34 S. V. K. Chaitanya, 'Is the Search Finally Over? Tribal Community May Hold the Answer to AIDS Cure', *New Indian Express*, 9 March 2016. https://www.newindianexpress.com/cities/chennai/2016/mar/09/Is-the-Search-Finally-Over-Tribal-Community-May-Hold-the-Answer-to-AIDS-Cure-901465.html (accessed 20 May 2016).

35 V. Adams, 'Randomized Controlled Crime: Postcolonial Sciences in Alternative Medicine Research', *Social Studies of Science* 32, no. 5/6 (2002): 670.
36 Ibid., 671.
37 R. Nigh, 'Maya Medicine in the Biological Gaze: Bioprospecting Research as Herbal Fetishism', *Current Anthropology* 43, no. 3 (2002): 451–77. The concepts of health, disease, cure and illness may not even be part of the vocabulary of indigenous medicine. For instance, among the Cree of James Bay, there is no linguistic equivalent to the English word 'health' and they instead use the word miyupimaatisiiun which can be roughly translated as 'being alive well': J. B. Waldram, 'The Efficacy of Indigenous Medicine: Current Theoretical and Methodological Issues', *Medical Anthropology Quarterly* 14, no. 4 (2000): 608.
38 According to Naraindas, shastras can be roughly defined as the science of formulating drugs. He adds that shastras can be regarded as part of a triptych – tatva (the axioms such as 'the five elements'/panca mahābhūta, the three 'humours'/dosa and seven 'tissues'/dhātu); śāstra (the science of joining them in a union/yogam) and vyavhar (applications): Harish Naraindas, 'Of Shastric "Yogams" and Polyherbals: Exogenous Logics and the Creolisation of the Contemporary Ayurvedic Formulary', *Asian Medicine* 9, no. 1–2 (2014): 14.
39 To understand the complications and asymmetries in epistemic translations between biomedicine and Ayurveda, see Harish Naraindas, Johannes Quack and William Sax, eds, *Asymmetrical Conversations: Contestations, Circumventions, and the Blurring of Therapeutic Boundaries*, 1st ed. (New York: Berghahn Books, 2014); Harish Naraindas, 'Nosopolitics, Epistemic Mangling and the Creolization of Contemporary Ayurveda', in *Medical Pluralism and Homeopathy in India and Germany (1810–2010)*, ed. M. Dinges (Stuggart: Franz Steiner Verlag, 2014), 105–36; and Naraindas, 'Of Shastric "Yogams" and Polyherbals'.
40 Naraindas, 'Of Shastric "Yogams" and Polyherbals', 34.
41 Ibid., 21. The resultant drugs neither lead to a full biomedicalization of Ayurveda nor to a herbalization in the western sense of 'the herbal', but to its creolization.
42 For instance, Piper longum was used as a bio-enhancer in anti-tuberculosis and anti-leprosy drugs to facilitate increased absorption of the 'active drug', thereby reducing the required drug quantity: Naraindas, 'Of Shastric "Yogams" and Polyherbals', 38. But, the Ayurvedic Shastra prohibits its long-term use because it may cause other ailments.
43 Adams, 'Randomized Controlled Crime', 669.
44 Schiebinger, *Plants and Empire*, 3–87.
45 Shiva, 'Bioprospecting as Sophisticated Biopiracy'; DeGeer, *Biopiracy*; Isla, 'An Ecofeminist Perspective on Biopiracy in Latin America'; Delgado, 'Biopiracy and Intellectual Property'; Mulligan and Stoett, 'A Global Bioprospecting Regime'.
46 The ETC Group is a non-profit research organization in Canada and Netherlands committed to issues of biopiracy, human genomics, intellectual property and

community knowledge systems. Since the late 1970s, the ETC Group has been contesting patents on plant genetic material and human tissue material, and has spread awareness about the ramifications of seed sterilization technology.
47 Schiebinger, *Plants and Empire*, 84.
48 Ibid., 87
49 A. Sreenivasan, 'Clinical trials not Mandatory for Licensing ASU drugs, says Govt; Researchers Warn of Fraud, Textual Data Manipulation', *Pharmabiz*, 9 July 2018. http://www.pharmabiz.com/NewsDetails.aspx?aid=109873&sid=1 (accessed 19 July 2019).
50 R. Prasad, 'Study of AYUSH Drugs must Involve Domain Expert, says AYUSH Advisory', *The Hindu*, 7 April 2019. https://www.thehindu.com/sci-tech/science/study-of-ayush-drugs-must-involve-domain-expert-says-ayush-advisory/article26763958.ece (accessed 10 October 2019).
51 In 2000, the Traditional Knowledge Digital Library (TKDL) was set up to digitalize traditional knowledge pertaining to Ayurveda, Unani, Siddha and Yoga. It was to be jointly managed by the Council of Scientific and Industrial Research and the Department of AYUSH under the Ministry of Health. The database was meant to curate details about the formulations, the plant ingredients, their botanical identities, use, preparation method and sources that documented the formulation: Gaudilliére, 'An Indian Path to Biocapital?', 400. By 2010, the TKDL had digitized two lakh medical formulations and the data was intended to verify the novelty claim of patent applications.
52 Reddy, 'Making Heritage Legible', 162.
53 L. Pordié and J. P. Gaudillière, 'The Reformulation Regime in Drug Discovery: Revisiting Polyherbals and Property Rights in the Ayurvedic Industry', *East Asian Science, Technology and Society: An International Journal* 8, no. 1 (2014): 68.
54 R. Dutta, 'The Divya Pharmacy Case: An Important Precedent on Biological Resource Use', *The Telegraph India*, 6 February 2019. https://www.telegraphindia.com/opinion/the-divya-pharmacy-case-uttarakhand-court-sets-an-important-legal-precedent-on-benefit-sharing-from-biological-resources/cid/1683795 (accessed 6 August 2020).
55 Reddy, 'Making Heritage Legible', 166–7.
56 D. Abrol, 'Who Gains from the Modi Government's Intellectual Property Rights Policy?', *The Wire*, 22 May 2016. https://thewire.in/economy/who-gains-from-the-modi-governments-intellectual-property-rights-policy (accessed 29 October 2021).
57 Gaudillière, 'An Indian Path to Biocapital?', 406.
58 Reddy, 'Making Heritage Legible', 173.
59 R. Bhatia and T. Lasseter, 'As Modi and his Hindu Base Rise, So Too Does Yoga Tycoon Baba Ramdev', *Reuters*, 23 May 2017. https://in.reuters.com/article/india

-modi-ramdev/special-report-as-modi-and-his-hindu-base-rise-so-too-does-yoga-tycoon-baba-ramdev-idINKBN18J1HJ (accessed 4 April 2019).
60 Torri, 'Bioprospecting and Commercialisation'; Planning Commission, 'Report of the Task Force'.
61 Mohanty, 'Tribal Women in Chattisgarh Beat the Poverty Trap With Fortunes From Indigenous Medicines'.
62 Francis, 'Who Speaks for the Tribe?'.

13

Privileging the body

The bio-materialization of medicine and the asymmetrical production of pluralism

Harish Naraindas

Ethnographic vignette

Ram was a 37-year-old chemical engineer. He suffered from renal failure. He was on a tri-weekly dialysis at a hospital in Madras (Chennai). He decided to skip his dialysis for a week: the week his nephrologist went out of town. Teresa, his Ayurvedic doctor, treated him for the week his nephrologist was away. A friend of his and I accompanied him on his first visit to the nephrologist after his 'hooky' week. He was petrified about confronting his nephrologist. He was sure the nephrologist would be deeply upset because he had skipped his dialysis, and worse for having subjected himself to an Ayurvedic therapy. His worst fears came true as the nephrologist, as predicted, was furious on both counts. The consultation turned into an extraordinary harangue. The nephrologist berated him for his appalling judgement. He wanted to know whether the patient had pawned his brains at the local pawn shop and taken leave of his senses; and whether he had written his last will and testament as he evidently wanted to die. He said he was surprised that he was still alive, and asked how an educated man like him, and a father of two young children, could be so utterly irresponsible and subject himself to such unbridled quackery. He wanted to sue the Ayurvedic doctor for offering to treat him and ended by issuing an ultimatum: that if he ever missed his dialysis again and stepped into her clinic, he need never come back, as he did not want to waste his time treating an imbecile and did not want the ignominy of being held responsible for his death that would certainly ensue if he followed the Ayurvedic treatment. In fact, he was convinced that his renal failure had been brought on by his previous encounters with Ayurveda and its herbal concoctions, with their dubious mineral and metal ingredients. The harangue was so devastating that it made me wonder if his renal failure had indeed been brought on by his previous history of engagement with Ayurveda. It gave me pause and made me quietly bury a medical concoction specially prepared for my eyes by Teresa.

Ram was back the next evening to report the encounter to Teresa. She had successfully treated him and his family, including his children and parents, for all their ailments over several years. But he and his wife were now fearful and confused after the meeting with the nephrologist. Ram, with some help from me, managed to convey the tone, tenor and texture of the entire encounter to Teresa. An extremely annoyed, worried and beleaguered Teresa began to consult her text to see what therapy could be given for his condition while he continued with his dialysis. She opened the text and began to read the relevant 'stanza' and, to my surprise, I found that the verse, in the same breath, recommended *oushadi* (medicine), *homa* (fire offering), *bali* (sacrifice), *dana* (giving of alms) and *puja* (prayer/worship). I asked her quietly (by then I had followed her practice continuously for about six months and knew her well) as to whether she was going to recommend all that was prescribed in the text apart from the *oushadi* (medicine). This agitated and annoyed her further, and she looked as if she wanted me out of there. One of Ram's children began to cry at that moment and his wife decided to take the child out of the consulting room and into the veranda. I followed suit. Between us we distracted the child and I struck up one of my several conversations with her on her husband's condition and their predicament. It transpired that Teresa had only prescribed medicine along with an extremely strict regimen of diet and other 'therapeutic' protocols. But the wife, on behalf of her spouse, unbeknownst of the textual 'prescriptions', had carried out all that was suggested in the text: the *puja*, the *dana*, the *homa* and the *bali*. She was very pleased and enormously reassured when I told her that all the things she was doing were part of the 'prescribed' therapy, at least according to the text. When I subsequently raised this with Teresa, who prided herself on treating her patients only according to the genius of her Ayurvedic system, she was furious. She said that all that was not part of her provenance and she was only concerned with the *oushadi*. But I persisted in the form of a gentle banter and asked whether any of this was part of her curriculum and was addressed in the pedagogy when she was training to be an Ayurvedic physician. She said no and threatened to throw me out if I insisted on pursuing this ridiculous line of inquiry. I then told her of my conversation with the wife, and how Mrs Ram had seemingly followed all that was prescribed in the text. The mood changed.

Teresa beamed and said it was evident that patients knew what they needed to do apart from taking her medicines and following the regimen. That they were obviously plugged into a 'cultural grid' and did not need her to prescribe all that was not part of her provenance.

I raised this episode later with Maavi, one of Teresa's young interns. Unlike Teresa, who was a sociologist before she 'defected' during her doctoral fieldwork on Ayurveda to become a fully qualified Ayurvedic doctor, her young intern was a third-generation Ayurvedic physician in the making. Unlike his father and him, both of whom were trained in a 'modern' Ayurvedic college like Teresa, his grandfather had presumably not been so trained. The grandfather had practised, according to the young physician, what he roughly called 'tantra, mantra and oushadi', and was hence in a position to address some if not all of what was prescribed in the text, particularly the stanza in question; and his grand uncle was an astrologer, and the brothers would often refer patients to each other.[1] He said his grandfather was particularly gifted and straddled several realms that may have been the provenance of different specialists. But during his grandfather's era, the patients – depending on the diagnosis and the condition – would often be pointed, if not referred, to these other specialists and other realms, if the physician was either not so trained, or chose not to practice things other than *oushadi*. He said that the current college pedagogy muted, if not annulled, these other facets of the treatment as both teachers and students were often embarrassed by the presence of these clearly 'non-medical' and 'superstitious' prescriptions in a 'medical text', and hence they were quietly – but often explicitly – subject to gloss and excision. He said that like Teresa, he too was unlikely to broach any of this with the patients, unless they explicitly raised it.

Bio-materialization: Pedagogy, practice and the formulary

It is evident from the vignette that the locus is the present. The vignette – from 2001 – is set in the principal metropolis of Southern India, whose Anglophone history nominally starts in 1639 with the founding of Fort St George. And we are concerned with Teresa and Maavi, who are what I have elsewhere christened as MDTMs: modern doctors of traditional medicine.[2] These MDTMs like Maavi, or his father and Teresa, both of whom were contemporaries, were formally trained in an Ayurveda college for roughly the same duration as their biomedical counterparts, granted a university degree and licensed to practice by the Indian state. It is also evident from the vignette that the curriculum and the pedagogy have a cardinal bearing on the clinical practice of these MDTMs, unlike Maavi's grandfather, who was not trained in such an institution.

There are several moments of inflection in the vignette. But there was certainly a moment of bewilderment when I, so to speak, 'looked over' Teresa's shoulder and, to my surprise, I found that the verse, in the same breath, recommended *oushadi* (medicine), *homa* (fire offering), *bali* (sacrifice), *dana* (giving of alms) and *puja* (prayer/worship). Why was I surprised? I was surprised because the text, and a canonical one by contemporary scholarly consensus, brought together the realms of 'medicine' and 'religion' within the ambit of a 'medical' text and offered them as a prescriptive panoply to address Ram's 'renal failure' – although it is wholly moot as to whether anything like 'renal failure', or even the very organ called a 'kidney', was part of its conceptual corpus. In other words, my surprise came from the fact that I was not prepared to see what I had been led to believe was a set of religious/magical practices, studied by most disciplines, but especially sociologists/anthropologists, under the broad rubric of 'culture', to find mention in an avowedly medical treatise.

I then made – because I was startled – an ethnographic faux pas: my impromptu query, right in the middle of a highly charged and fraught moment, of this 'mixing' of religion and medicine. But the faux pas fortuitously paid off because of the child's crying, the revelations of Mrs Ram, and my subsequent conversations with Teresa and Maavi. But faux pas have a context: and the context was my broad enquiry into the contemporary practice of Ayurveda as practised by those formally trained in a modern college of traditional medicine, and what bearing, if any, their curriculum and pedagogy had on a) their clinical practice, and b) on the making, or formulating to be more precise, of contemporary Ayurvedic medicines.

This enquiry was in part prompted by the extant literature, which outlined the pitched battle over the curriculum for the better part of the twentieth century, but especially after Indian independence.[3] And the battle lines were nominally drawn between two principal camps, leaving in its wake several possible shades and amalgams between these camps and perhaps outside of them.[4] These two camps, indexed under the epithets of 'purists' (*shudda*) and 'integrationists', have argued and continue to argue for either reviving a 'pure' form of Ayurveda ostensibly 'sullied' by the modern institutions, or of 'integrating' Ayurveda (or Unani and Siddha) and biomedicine under the very aegis of these institutions, with what exactly is meant by 'integration' being the subject of emic contestation and etic scholarly interpretation.[5] There is a substantial body of literature – if not almost all the anthropological literature on Asian Medicine – that addresses, in some form, this epistemic, professional and ontological politics, both in South Asia and in China (and elsewhere too), where something similar is played out vis-à-vis Traditional Chinese Medicine (TCM).[6]

But irrespective of who the victors were or are – as it is nominally an ongoing agon, although increasingly less so as the 'integrationists' seem to have largely won the day – and the styles of practice it has spawned, it may be safely argued that the pedagogy, practice and the formulary of the contemporary MDTM are premised on an avowed bio-materialism, resulting in the privileging of certain corpuses and substances, downplaying and muting others and excluding if not annulling yet others. This was partly evident from Teresa's irritation with my queries, exacerbated no doubt by the fraught moment. Despite her attempted repudiation of her formal 'integrated' training, and her desire to practice Ayurveda in a 'pure' form, she too was unable to countenance all the seemingly 'religious' elements in the stanza on the grounds that it was not part of her provenance. And when her mood changed with the revelation about Mrs Ram, rather than countenancing it as a legitimate part of her medical cannon, despite the fact that it was there in black and white in her medical text, she 'reduced it' to culture, which often functions as a euphemism for religion/magic.

But it was apparent, as both she and Maavi had pointed out, that these elements were glossed or excised in their pedagogy because they were seen to be religious/superstitious. Hence, it is moot as to what extent such gloss and excision had a bearing on her reaction, despite her often-stated desire to remain 'true' to the corpus. This was buttressed by the fact that Maavi too never raised these facets with his patients, let alone prescribe it, despite his nodding acquaintance with them, thus indexing the general run of clinical practice in 2001. This was further borne out by the fact that I had already interviewed scores of students about their syllabus, classroom teaching, exam questions and expected ways of answering these questions[7], all of which pointed up what Teresa and Maavi had vocalized about the pedagogy and its bearing, willy-nilly, on their practice.

We could thus advance the argument that these exclusions (and inclusions), premised on a tacit materialism, are cardinal in producing the contemporary therapeutic topoi where certain texts, substances and modalities constitute the major keys, while others are the minor keys. These therapeutic topoi will allow us to index, if not place, the entire gamut of not only South Asian therapeutic practices but also all alternative therapeutic practices worldwide, in their relation to biomedicine. In other words, the South Asian therapeutic topoi that we hope to presently elucidate will function as a prism if not a fractal of the way contemporary therapeutic practice is organized globally. We hope to thus

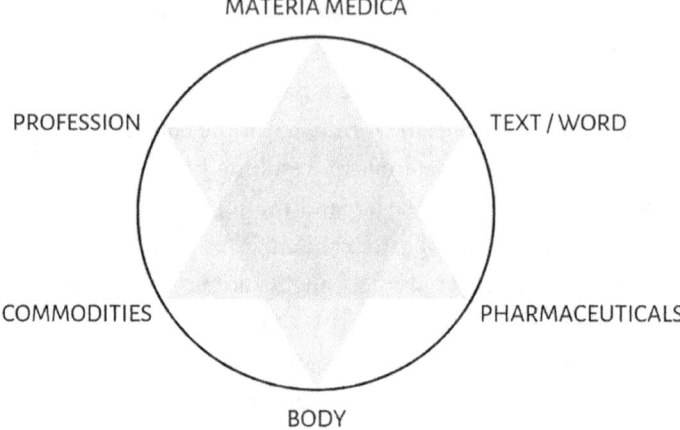

Figure 13.1 The bio-materialized world of medicine. ©Harish Naraindas.

advance a general theory of the co-emergence of (bio)medicine and alternative medicine, and the relationship that obtains between them, with the claim that materialism is a fundamental wedge: one that sets up an asymmetrical distinction between biomedicine and the rest. Hence the claim that the bio-materialization of medicine leads to an asymmetrical production of pluralism. The figure that I have drawn (Figure 13.1) is emblematic of our argument and will be used as a point of departure to explicate the topoi of the general theory I am attempting to advance.

Privileged bodies

Body, text and profession

Contemporary medicine is characterized by three privileged corpuses: the material body of the patient; the professional body of doctors and all the associated professions; and a body of written texts, whose codified acme is the International Classification of Diseases (ICD), which is at once a medical, legal and 'financial' codex in so far as it is a diagnostic manual that has a legal status and, in several parts of the world (Germany being exemplary), the fulcrum for the billing and reimbursement of medical expenses.

None of the above may have obtained in the past either to the same degree or, more importantly, in kind. Circumscribing the ambit of the disease by the ambit of material bodies and making the body of the patient as the local and causal space for the origin of diseases may be nominally said to begin in 1800 with the founding of histology. And coeval with this epistemic shift indexed by histology is the steady solidification of the profession through a particular form of institutionalized pedagogy called the 'teaching hospital', which re-draws the relationship between knowledge and its object, between teacher and student, between doctor and patient, and between philanthropy, public assistance and the state, to the institution of medicine.[8]

Materia medica, pharmaceuticals and commodities

While the privileging of these three bodies is marked by the triangle of the body, the profession and the text/word, the other triangle – *materia medica*, pharmaceuticals and commodities – marks the privileging and the materialization of another corpus: namely, the possible reduction of the *materia medica* to a mere materiality, which is the fulcrum around which this volume is built. While *materia medicas* have been around for millennia, and the substances therein have been traded and spawned empires, its form as a codex of exclusively material substances with therapeutic value, or as the principal if not the exclusive therapeutic codex, may not have obtained in the past. As we can see from the vignette earlier, for Maavi's grandfather, neither of the them may have been true: the *materia medica* may have included incantations (mantra); or if it did not, things outside the *materia medica*, such as prayer, talismans, the movement of planets, sacrifice, alms giving or the transmutation of *pret* (ghosts) into *pitr* (ancestors), may have been efficacious and legitimate therapeutic forms. In the present, however, many of these may be legally problematic in India under the Drugs and Magic Remedies Act of 1954,[9] or Maharashtra's Black Magic Act of 2013.[10] In any case, as is clear from the vignette, all these are mentioned in the same breath in what are now seen as 'ancient and canonical texts' but are either quietly buried or explicitly excluded from the current pedagogy; and if perchance publicly practised, they could be legally challenged and be criminally liable, although this is unlikely.

Finally, the privileging of the *materia medica* in the contemporary world also means it spawns fascinating histories, as is the case in this volume. But equally, if not more importantly, is the advent of something that was perhaps unknown within the *materia medica* as a therapeutic commodity in the past:

namely, its pharmaceuticalization. By that one does not only mean 'the process by which social, behavioural, or bodily conditions are treated, or deemed to be in need of treatment/intervention, with pharmaceuticals by doctors, patients or both'.[11] This process is merely part of the larger process of what is now called medicalization.[12] But these processes are fundamentally predicated on the industrial manufacture of drugs, which is now carried out through the isolation and chemical synthetization of their active ingredients, along with all the paraphernalia such as randomized clinical trials, the placebo test and so on, all of which in turn is predicated upon an epistemic shift marked by the notion of 'causal specificity', where ideally diseases are seen to have a single cause and a single cure.[13] The current pandemic, for example, is 'caused' by SARS-Cov-2 and is to be ideally 'nullified' by a vaccine or an anti-viral. In the interim, on the presumption that a vaccine or anti-viral is on the anvil (as is now the case), or if one comes down with the infection due to the unavailability of the vaccine, or despite being vaccinated, one then addresses the symptomatology of the 'infection', and the patho-physiological processes it leaves in its wake, with greater or lesser success.

Other medical systems may not work with such a notion of 'causal specificity'; and their 'drugs' may be a theoretically suave concoction of several drugs – for example, 16 or 108 drugs – put together according to a therapeutic logic, which in turn is invariably part of a larger therapeutic regimen, where the drug may not be the prima donna that we presume it to be in the present.[14] Hence, the *materia medica* triangle, through its pharmaceuticalization and commoditization, together make it something more and other than what it was earlier, leading to privileging it to the exclusion (or muting) of other therapeutic strategies and also excising possible immaterialities – such as incantations/mantra – from its body or corpus in the bargain.

Animism and esoteric exclusions

These two interlaced triangles (body triangle and *materia medica* triangle) are thus not only emblematic of the current state of medicine but, as is evident, they are also in an implicit relationship both to their own past and to all the alternative systems of medicine in the present. And this relationship is based on the fact that 'biomedicine' focuses exclusively on the 'bio' and is based on an avowed 'materialism'. This double reduction – to biology and a 'materialistic monism' – is understandably the wellspring of Hans Jonas' philosophical excursus in his *The*

Phenomenon of Life, which is aptly subtitled *Toward a Philosophical Biology*.[15] But Jonas' 'philosophical excursus' on life, unsurprisingly doubles up as a historical narrative and an anthropological stock-in-trade – the movement from simple to complex organisms, with metabolism as the principle that drives it, mirrors the evolutionary movement from simple to complex societies – of modern Western civilization, and tacitly functions as the apogee to an imputed perigee that is both the Past and the East. And the caesura that divides the Past/East from the present in Jonas' work is panpsychism, hylozoism and, fundamentally, animism. This leads to the claim that non-Western cultures posit sentience and agency to inanimate objects in quite the same way that Western 'civilization' presumably did in the past – thus making them 'the past in the present'. This bequeaths to the Western scholarly canon, and especially anthropology, the notion of the fetish, which, incidentally, is central to Marx in his explication of historical materialism.[16]

Hence, it is none too surprising that for Isabelle Stengers, as it is for Hans Jonas, 'reclaiming animism'[17] is an avowed preoccupation; while for Elizabeth Povinelli, her entire oeuvre is built on animism as the distinction: a distinction and a mode of governance that leads to the us-them binary on which anthropology as a colonial artefact is premised, leading her to say that 'the attribution of an inability of various colonized people to identify the kind of things that have agency, subjectivity, and intentionality of the sort that emerges with life has been the grounds of casting them into a premodern mentality and post-recognition difference'.[18] This is a difference the so-called ontological and animistic turns grapple with, and are a symptom of, with the works of Viveiros de Castro and Descola being the most popular anthropological instances, while Goff's plea for a 'return to panpsychism', and Stengers' attempt at 'reclaiming animism' are their philosophical counterparts.[19]

Given this nested historical, philosophical and anthropological trajectory, it is none too surprising that the so-called alternative therapeutic 'canons' also become bio-materialized. Having been unenviably cast into a 'premodern mentality and postrecognition difference' because of the spectre of 'animism' that haunts their corpus, they are reduced to a 'primitivism': a past in the present, and the ignominy of a living relic. These allochronic canons,[20] labouring under the yoke of primitivism, then clamour to step up and demonstrate that they too have the ability to distinguish life from non-life; and that they are both willing and able not to attribute 'agency, subjectivity and intentionality' to non-life. In other words, they are willing, often with alacrity, to jettison animism as the sine qua non for a passport to the present, in a vain attempt to establish parity with the colonizer's spectre – science – that haunts them and relegates them, despite their coevalness, to an antiquated and subordinate status. Our ethnographic vignette bears ample testimony to this jettisoning of the ineffable and the immaterial, resulting in reconfigured therapeutic systems that are now tacitly, if not explicitly, also predicated on a materialistic monism. In this new dispensation, as we will presently see, the text and the written word become the privileged centre, and the classroom the privileged pedagogic site, where prose rather than prosody is the new form, and materialism the metaphysical premise.

The proof of this pudding, as far as Ayurveda is concerned, is the gloss and excision of one of the eight branches of Ayurveda called *bhut vidya*, or the science/knowledge of *bhut*: which could simply mean past tense in Sanskrit grammar, or all those who have 'passed' and become ghosts (*pret*) instead of turning into ancestors (*pitr*); and these unincorporated ghosts (*bhut*), unlike the incorporated ancestors, could, as liminal Beings, then come back to afflict the living. One exemplary instance of such a gloss in the *Ayurvedic Pharmacopeia of India*, published in 1990 by the Government of India, is the translation of *graha dosha* (planet affliction) as psychosis; while the gloss in the 1930s for *graha dosha* was infection.[21] The 1930s gloss of infection still maintains the causal arrow of an affliction that comes from the outside to the inside; and in so far as it does, it is still true to the spirit of a causal scheme called *agunta* – that which comes from outside – under which such afflictions were listed in the Ayurvedic corpus. This gloss from the 1930s is not wholly surprising as the microbe that causes infection, as Ludwik Fleck pointed out a long time ago, is nothing but the Devil reincarnate, affording us, as Canguilhem says, an ontological point of view and the soothing certitude of a Being against which one can do battle.[22] But the latter-day gloss of *graha dosha* as psychosis banishes ontology by circumscribing the ambit of the disease entirely by the ambit of the body and thereby annuls the ghost of an aetiological resemblance between the two causal schemes, marked by planets/demons/ghosts on the one hand, and the microbe on the other.[23] But both of them – infection and psychosis – signal a passport to the present by jettisoning planets, along with deities, ghosts or one's shadow, as disease-causing agents/beings, and hence as real and substantive aetiologies. For planets – apart from shadows, ghosts, demons and deities – in the new dispensation are embarrassing. They are part of what is called astrology, whose rightful place is the leisure columns of Sunday morning newspapers rather than medical textbooks, diagnostic manuals or the pharmacopeia. And they are, to boot, legally problematic in so far as such claims may be culpable under the Magic Remedies Act, especially if one were to perform a caesarean under astrological dictum (presumably quite common in India),[24] and the mother or child were to die. Hence their practice may not be formally recorded, although they may be empirically widespread.

This formal jettisoning of animism, or the 'mistaken' attribution of causal agency to planets, idols, rocks and clouds as disease aetiologies – the clouds change shape and move because they can smell us (and not metaphorically) say the Australian aboriginals to Povinelli[25] – is an exclusionary mode through which the two corpuses, earlier marked by the 'body' and 'materia' triangles, are privileged. These esoteric exclusions, which mark the so-called demise of animism, may be schematically captured by the two interlaced triangles – the mantra-tantra-yantra triangle and the spirit-adept-possession triangle – in the diagram that follows (Figure 13.2).

Maavi's grandfather, if we recall, could inhabit some if not all the positions on this excluded esoteric circle. He was evidently adept at practising not just medicine (*oushadi*) but also *tantra*, which could have two cognate meanings in contemporary English: a Hindu or Buddhist mystical or magical text, dating from the seventh century or earlier; and, as a mass noun, it could mean adherence to tantric doctrines that involve *mantras* (incantations) and *yantras* (designs, diagrams, objects used as aids in tantric practices).[26] Evidently, not all physicians may have been as 'gifted' as Maavi's grandfather, as these practices may presuppose that one is an adept (Guni and Fakir are among the words in eighteenth and nineteenth-century British sources to describe the adept, with

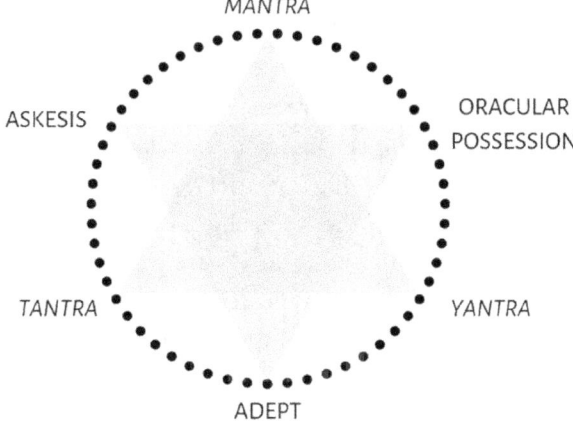

Figure 13.2 Excluded esoteric circle. ©Harish Naraindas.

the 'naked fakir' being the well-known pejorative epithet that has been handed down to us), through an act of initiation and training, at these esoteric practices. And such practices evidently involved forms of *askesis* and spiritual training and could also involve forms of 'oracular possession' and divination.[27] But we may not presume that all practitioners, in the past or the present, necessarily had the training and the wherewithal to practice these esoteric forms along with the *oushadi*.

Hence, Teresa was perhaps more than right when she claimed that these are not part of her provenance, which in turn was buttressed by Maavi alluding to the fact that not all physicians in the past may have necessarily been either privy to such esoteric knowledge or had the skill and the desire to practice them. But the fact remains that the non-material world of ghosts, spirits and ancestors, or the effects of the very material planets, were indeed part of her textual corpus and often functioned as aetiological agents, and/or set up nosological and diagnostic distinctions, or, as was the case in our opening vignette, present as therapeutic strategies, all of which, as we saw, had to be either excised or glossed as infection in the 1930s and psychosis in the 1970s.

Such forms of translation and gloss are legion in all forms of non-Western alternative systems, with the word *xie* in TCM suffering a similar fate.[28] They are an ongoing and continuous phenomenon, best imagined as updating to new versions of a software, or the periodic transition to a new operating system, necessitated by both the spectre of animism, and the continuous recasting of scientific theories, leading forever to allochrony between biomedicine and its others.

Zwingli and the demise of magic

The etymology of fever, from *februare*, means to ritually expel from a house the shades of the dead.[29] The image in Figure 13.3 dates from 1788 and depicts the personification of fever and Ague (malarial fever), indexing the fact that the 'rationality of life is identical to the rationality of that which threatens it',[30] as both life and death, and health and disease were grounded in an 'ontology of life',[31] where both death and disease appeared as a form of life. The transition from such an 'ontology of life', where the 'divine constancy of being was marked by the constancy of life',[32] which in defiance of death and its apparent verdict transmuted the dead into the living as ancestors or ghosts with a capacity to intercede in the world of the living, to an 'ontology of death', results in a lifeless

Privileging the Body 265

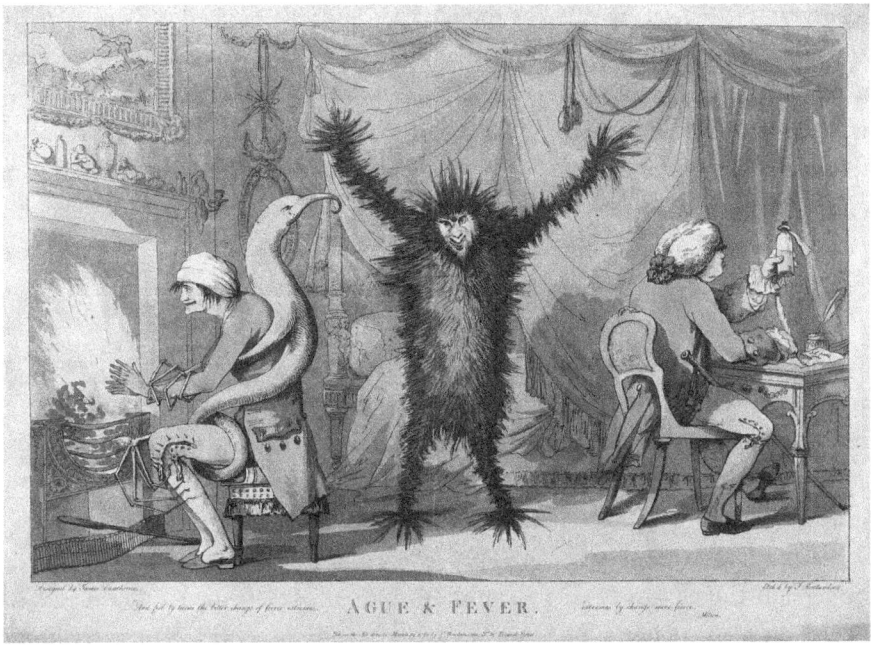

Figure 13.3 Fever, represented as a frenzied beast, stands racked in the centre of a room, while a monster, representing Ague, ensnares his victim by the fireside; a doctor writes prescriptions to the right. Coloured etching, 1788 by James Dunthorne, after Thomas Rowlandson and John Milton. Wellcome Library Catalogue.

nature save for the bios. This led, ironically, to a science of life grounded in an ontology of death. This understandably leads Stengers, in her 'reclaiming animism', to bemoan the extruded residue as that 'sad nature devoid of life'.[33]

A 'sad nature' that she – like scores before and after her – desires to 'reclaim': a reclamation set in motion by the Reformation which, in the singular figure of Zwingli, reduces the sacrament to mere bread rather than the transubstantiated Body of Christ, and makes of the communion a social and commemorative act instead of a magical one.[34] This banishing of the material presence of the divine indexes the permanent tearing apart of Western ontology into the real (bread) and the symbolic (Body of Christ); into the material (bread) and the metaphorical (Body of Christ); or the historical Body of Christ that was crucified on the cross (the past) and the commemorative bread on Sunday morning (the present). Zwingli thus abolishes the Mass to demonstrate that the Eucharistic communion is not a re-enactment of the sacrifice of Christ on the cross, for the risen Christ sits, he said, on the right hand of God in heaven and hence cannot also be literally and materially present on Sunday mornings in church. Hereafter,

Jesus, rather than being eaten as the ultimate and salvific medicament, is to be apprehended only through the inner eye of faith, and the sacrament is to be seen as an 'outward sign of an inner state'. This banishing of the divine as an everyday material presence is perhaps finally indexed by the demise of the tabernacle in the Reformed churches, which once marked the literal presence of the Body of Christ. In fact, it was His presence, marked by the ever-burning candle at the tabernacle (except on Holy Saturday when Christ is dead), which housed the reserved Eucharist for the sick and the dying, that ostensibly made the church a church rather than a mere prayer hall.

Hence, in the anthropological canon when the word religion is used, it is, willy-nilly, and in fundamentally important ways, Zwingli's new religion – premised on the doctrine of non-substantiation, rather than Luther's 'sacramental union' or Calvin's 'pneumatic union' – that is being secretly indexed. And it is Zwingli's version of Protestantism in particular, and Protestantism more broadly in all its avatars, and not science as it is usually understood, that slowly sets in motion the demise of magic, or the steady extrusion of the material presence of divinity from the world. Hence, it is none too surprising that Keith Thomas' book is called *Religion and the Decline of Magic in Eighteenth-century England* and not 'science and the decline of magic in eighteenth-century England'.

Two telling examples from Thomas' book make this amply clear. He tells us that 'the conventional distinction between a prayer and a spell', for example, 'seems to have been first hammered out, not by the nineteenth-century anthropologists, with whom it is usually associated, but by sixteenth-century Protestant theologians';[35] or, 'many post-Reformation writers busied themselves establishing the criteria by which one might distinguish a divine intimation from a diabolical imposture or the effects of indigestion'.[36] It is thus evident that by religion Thomas meant Protestantism, which is tacitly what is meant by religion in the anthropological triad of magic, religion and science (bequeathed to us by Tylor, Frazer and Malinowski) – though this is almost never explicitly admitted to in Anglo-European scholarly writing. For it is Protestantism that is the other to magic (false science) and science (true magic), as opposed to Catholicism and its magic of the sacrament, which was, with the passage of time, explicitly attacked by various Protestant denominations, including the Methodists in England. In opposition to Protestantism, and especially the one bequeathed by Zwingli, all other religions are at best magico-religious, and at worst shade into animism. And the origin of this slow demise of magic and the ineffable lies in the recasting of the sacrament.

It is therefore extremely unlikely that Stengers' exertions (or Harraway's, Latour's or Povinelli's – all, incidentally, Catholics) are likely to bear fruit, as it is on the sacrament – or solely on the question of the material presence of divinity in the world – that Luther and Zwingli fell out at the Marburg Colloquy of 1529.[37] The colloquy presumably began with Luther throwing down the gauntlet and asking Zwingli to prove that the sacrament was symbolic rather than assuming it was so. Finally, his angry retort to Zwingli's disassociation of the material and physical from the spiritual – through John 6:63 – was to disparage him by saying:

> [O]ur fanatics, however, are full of fraud and humbug. They think nothing spiritual can be present where there is anything material and physical, and assert that flesh is of no avail. Actually, the opposite is true. The spirit cannot be with us except in material and physical things such as the Word, water, and Christ's body and his saints on earth. . . . The mouth eats physically for the heart and the heart eats spiritually for the mouth, and thus both are satisfied and saved by one and the same food.[38]

But Zwingli was steadfast in his point of view and ultimately martyred himself to his cause when he refused the last rites as he lay wounded and dying in the Battle of Kappel against the Catholics in 1531.[39] He was then presumably slayed by his Catholic adversary, who had his head cut off, and his body hacked, burnt and mixed with pig entrails so that his bones could not be used as relics, which, ironically, was perhaps most befitting as that was the last thing Zwingli may have wanted. And Luther, who evidently disliked him, said that his denial of the last rites – which would have meant confessing and having the sacrament as the salvific Body of Christ – meant that he was hell-bound, as the denial was the denial of Christ and his offer of salvation.

This radical falling out on the sacrament between Luther and Zwingli, far more significant than the one between Luther and the Pope, turned on the question of the real, literal and material presence of the divine and the ineffable in the world.[40] It has reverberated for the last 500 years and has led to the principal and insurmountable fault lines in the Western philosophical tradition, including all the familiar dualisms that every discipline has flogged to death for half a millennium. It also continues to reverberate theologically and politically, ranging from 'the troubles' in Ireland, to the refusal of communion to Joe Biden and Nancy Pelosi over their abortion endorsement, to the current imbroglio over the communion in the case of mixed marriages (of Catholics and Protestants) in Germany, which is likely to founder as it did in 1529, on the understanding and meaning of the sacrament.

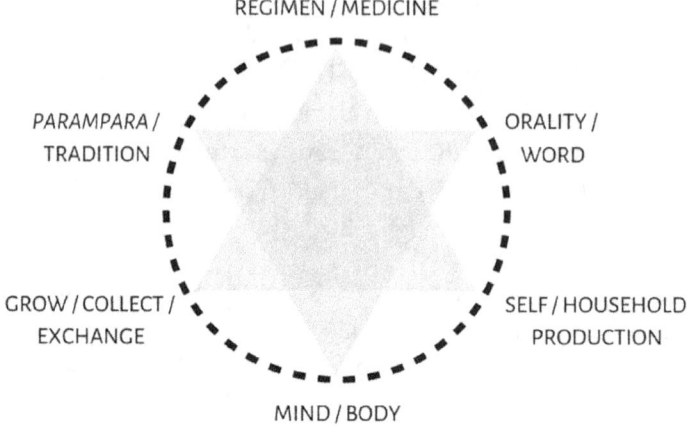

Figure 13.4 Excluded exoteric circle. ©Harish Naraindas.

Apart from the esoteric exclusions thus set in motion by the metamorphosis of the sacrament, which in turn led to the slow demise of magic/animism, and the continuing litany of lament it has evoked ever since the Enlightenment, there are also the exoteric and quite 'material' exclusions that equally mark the passage to the present – or produce the present and the past, coeval in time, as allochronic. We will now, through two ethnographic vignettes, attempt to elucidate the 'excluded exoteric circle' above (Figure 13.4).

Regimen and exoteric exclusions

Gayathri, Curd and pain

Gayathri was sixty-seven. She was arthritic. She was in pain. Constant pain that had grown worse with every passing year. She had run the entire gamut of systems and therapies. She turned up one morning at Teresa's clinic and said that Teresa had been highly recommended by the secretary of a drug-manufacturing cooperative in Madras, which also ran a full-fledged clinic on its premises. She told Teresa that she was her last hope. And how her pain was driving her up the wall and making her suicidal. Teresa did an anamnesis and discovered that her principal diet was 'curd rice' (yoghurt mixed with rice and often seasoned with spices). This was wholly unsurprising for Teresa, as Gayathri, an elderly Tamil Brahmin woman and a vegetarian, was consuming what was a staple for her caste, age and community at that particular historical juncture and region of South India. At sixty-seven, she had evidently been consuming this for decades, which according to Teresa was among the principal causes for her chronic condition. The clinical consultation ended badly. In fact, it exploded when Teresa told her, at length and quite categorically, that she should give up on curd if she wanted to be cured of her pain. Gayathri was outraged. She asked Teresa, and quite sharply, what was she supposed to eat if curd was disallowed to her hereafter. It was a rhetorical statement. She didn't wait for Teresa to reply. She got up, her eyes blazing, as quickly as she could on her arthritic and wobbly feet. She looked at all the young interns in the consulting room and asked them to ask Teresa what she was expected to eat if she couldn't eat curd rice. Without waiting for a reply, she stormed out of the room. For Gayathri – the playful epithet for her sect was curd rice (*thayir-sadam*), and perhaps her existential ground – curd trumped her suicidal pain.

The drug as the prima donna

Fiona was fourteen. She was asthmatic. She had found succour with Teresa after being buffeted by doctors, systems and therapies. She arrived one morning with her mother who was Teresa's long-standing patient. She had come down with a skin condition which was, much to her dismay, marring her face. After an anamnesis, Teresa wrote out a prescription and held it out for Fiona's mother. But Fiona quickly reached out, took the prescription from Teresa, immediately stood up, and said to her mother: 'mum, let's beat it, before she tells me not to eat this or that, sleep early, and what not'. Teresa began to laugh and the mother, deeply embarrassed by the unruly behaviour, asked her daughter to sit down. But Fiona ignored her, waved breezily at Teresa and her mum and left the room with a parting shot: 'I've got what I wanted, mum. I'll take the medicines and you can follow the *pathyam* (regimen)!'

Proscriptions and prescriptions

It is evident from these two vignettes – also from 2001 – that regimen (*pathyam* in Tamil), including dietetics, is central to Ayurveda, as it was to Galenic medicine, whose testimony comes from the *Regimen Sanitatis Salernitanum*, which was written sometime between the eleventh and thirteenth centuries. Its purportedly original 364 lines, expanded to 3,536 hexameter verses, were translated from Latin into almost all European languages over the course of a millennium; and it ran into more than 300 editions, with perhaps the final English translation by Ordonoaux coming as late as 1871.[41] Based on the Galenic distinction between the four humours and the six non-naturals of 'airs, diet, sleep, exercise, evacuation, and the perturbations of the soul', the regimen's focus was on the six non-naturals, based on the theoretical premise (which has unsurprisingly reappeared as the premise of contemporary epigenetics and, through it, Ayurgenomics, personalised medicine and pre-conception clinics) that not being mindful of the non-naturals led to the vitiation of the humours and thence to disease.

We can see from the already discussed vignettes the fundamental and continuing importance of regimen for Teresa's practice, as it was seen by her as the lynchpin that vitiated the humours (three in Ayurveda) and caused the disease; hence, it needed to be squarely addressed if a cure was to be effected. But irrespective of generation – Gayathri, b.1934; Fiona, b.1987 – persons often found it difficult, and sometimes well-nigh impossible, to follow the regimen, especially if it meant sacrificing, like Gayathri, a staple that was experienced as the defining food of one's community; while for the fourteen-year-old, the regimen was anathema, as it evidently straight-jacketed her and gave her little or no wiggle-room.

But for the majority of MDTMs such clinical encounters were unlikely, as the drug was the mainstay of their prescription. In fact, many if not most MDTMs ran their modest private practices with the five biomedical A's: anti-pyretics, antibiotics, anti-histamines, anti-inflammatories and analgesics.[42] These biomedical drugs, along with sundry Ayurvedic 'tonics', were their prescriptive mainstays, which also meant that their diagnosis largely followed (mimesis) a biomedical rather than an Ayurvedic aetiology and nosology.[43] And for those who used the Ayurvedic pharmacopeia more extensively, or exclusively, the Ayurvedic drug was the prima donna, and the *pathyam* (regimen) was played, if at all, in a minor key.

One of the arguments put forward by the MDTMs for downplaying the *pathyam* was that their patients would flee if the *pathyam* – often translated by Tamilians into English as 'restrictions' – was imposed on them. Gayathri's stormy exit, and Fiona's breezy one, with her attempt to outsource the *pathyam* to her mother, who was probably keeping her in line for her asthmatic condition, bears testimony. But they are merely exemplary and dramatic instances of the daily and plaintive tussle over the regimen, especially dietetics, between Teresa and her patients that one has repeatedly witnessed with hundreds of her patients. And for Teresa, unlike many if not most of her contemporaries, the 'drugs and the regimen', where both 'body and mind', best captured by being mindful of the six Galenic non-naturals, were fundamental to her practice.

But apart from the challenges posed by a refusal to jettison her proscriptions under the rubric of regimen, Teresa suffered from yet another infirmity with her prescriptions, despite her exclusive use of the Ayurvedic pharmacopeia, and despite her concomitant attempt to diagnose or re-diagnose her patients in Ayurvedic terms, as they invariably came to her pre-diagnosed with a biomedical disease category.[44] She was saddled, unlike Maavi's grandfather and the generations before him, with a full-fledged Ayurvedic drug-manufacturing industry that presented her with two different kinds of drugs: *shastric* and proprietary.

Shastric medicines were made according to the recipes in the traditional pharmacopeias or formularies; while proprietary medicines were new formulations where each individual drug was from the traditional pharmacopeias but put together in a new composition. But that was the least of it. While *shastric* medicines addressed an Ayurvedic nosology (or disease classification), the proprietary medicines invariably addressed a biomedical disease entity. They were thus primarily meant (a) for the MDTMs who used the five A's mentioned earlier; (b) to be sold as 'over the counter' (OTC) drugs directly to the 'modern' patient, who was invariably conversant with biomedical diseases, which they tacitly presumed to be universal disease entities'; and finally, (c) for biomedical doctors who used them as 'supplements', or when they were at sea with their disease conditions for which they had nothing to offer from their biomedical armoury.[45]

While Teresa exclusively used *shastric* medicines, she was still confronted by the industrial manufacture of these medicines and the challenges, albeit seemingly lesser ones, that they posed. Ayurvedic medicines are, unlike biomedicines, predominantly multi-drug compounds (there are 8,000 currently in vogue) formulated according to an Ayurvedic logic. For example, a *shastric* formulation called Daśamūla Kaṭutraya Kaṣāyam (DKK) is a decoction made up of fourteen ingredients and contains two *pancamūla* (two sets of *panca* (five) *mūla* (drugs) each, which makes up *Daśa* (ten) *mūla* (drugs)), and four more individual drugs. These compound formulations are called *yogam* – as in yoga, meaning union, which here would be the union (*yogam*) of these fourteen drugs. These fourteen drugs, however, are not simply additive, where each drug is addressing a discrete symptom (as they presumably are in Western polyherbals) but are assembled according to a therapeutic logic premised on Ayurvedic theory. Hence, the word synergy, which is usually defined as 'the interaction or cooperation of two or more substances to produce a combined effect greater than the sum of their separate effects', may not quite capture what is meant by a *yogam*.⁴⁶ These *shastric yogams*, in this case the DKK, may be given for a variety of conditions, such as a bad and persistent cold. When so prescribed, the DKK will ideally be given with a *vadagam* (another kind of drug) that will localize its action in the 'upper clavicle' region and amplify its effect. Otherwise, the DKK may act on the entire body, making it less effective, or, if not so localized, lead to other problems, which will vary depending on the patient, his constitution and his diseases.⁴⁷

But these shastric *yogams*, when they are industrially mass-produced, are, among other things, compounded according to a fixed ratio and proportion. But as Maavi pointed out to me, this was not always the case in his grandfather's time. His grandfather, said Maavi, would write out the ingredients of the DKK, and may, depending on the patient, his presenting symptoms, his constitution, the season, the stage of the disease, or his comorbidities, vary the ratio and proportion of some of the ingredients, or the *vadagam*, to tailor it to the individual patient. The patients would, in turn, collect some of the ingredients from their surroundings where they grew, or source it from neighbours, and buy the rest from a traditional druggist. They would then prepare the decoction at home, thus ensuring that the freshly made decoction was indeed made up of the fourteen ingredients with no adulterations or excipients, nor preservatives to enhance shelf life, and in the sure knowledge that it was tailored for them.

Exclusions and transmutations

We have, from what we have said so far, traversed most of the points in the excluded exoteric circle earlier. It is evident that neither was the material body of the patient the exclusive locus of either the cause of disease or its recovery, nor was the material drug the exclusive substance that was called upon to address the disease. The intangible facets (*mantra-tantra-yantra*) of the esoteric circle, along with the more tangible 'non-naturals' of the exoteric circle (which became central to 'life-style diseases' and are now the epicentre of epigenetics and personalized medicine) were fundamental earlier. It is through their muting, exclusion and often transmutation by creolization⁴⁸ that the bio-materialized world of medicine, outlined in Figure 13.1, makes its appearance. Maavi's grandfather, as a titular figure, is emblematic of a practitioner who was traditionally (*parampara*) trained, where the written text, often set to verse (e.g. the *Ashtanga Hyrdyam* in Kerala, quite like the *Regimen Sanitatis Salernitanum* set to hexameter verse) is memorized from a very young age, followed by a long apprenticeship in the pharmacy and the forest, and finally in the clinic. And for whom mind-body, drug-regimen and *mantra-tantra-yantra* were an intrinsic part of both aetiology and therapeutics. He was perhaps at the fag end of an era where drugs were not yet mass-produced in fixed ratio and proportion, or industrially manufactured according to an exogenous protocol derived from the biomedical pharmacopeia, and approved by a bio-medically trained drug controller, for whom the *yogam* was beyond his ken.[49] This made for flexible and tailored prescriptive practices and allowed both him and his patients to source them in some measure (though many of these drugs for millennia have been traded and come from faraway places) locally, and make them personally or as a cottage industry.

The asymmetrical production of pluralism

What then are the consequences of this therapeutic topoi? It leads to a form of asymmetry that flows from the privileging in biomedicine of the material over the immaterial, which in turn leads to privileging the somatic over the psychological, or the body over the mind. The mind in turn is subject to the same dualism where the brain as a material entity with its neurons and synapses is privileged over the mind. The cognate homologues are the textual over the oral, the literate over the non-literate and the institutionalized as against the non-institutionalized. This in turn leads to legitimate as opposed to illegitimate medical practices, with the best example being the relegation of other Beings (planets, deities, demons, spirits etc.) as possible aetiologies to the realm of religion, faith or culture, under the various possible rubrics of possession, trance and so on, and their relegation in contemporary Ayurveda, for example, to the realm of 'folk practices', or the more dignified term of 'local health traditions'. These local traditions are then muted, or altogether excised from the formal curriculum of institutionalized Ayurveda.

These local health traditions are, in turn, subject to the same law of fractals and divide once again into those that deal with plants and herbs (material substances), or bone-setting or nerve practices (the body), as opposed to those that deal with *tantra-mantra-yantra* (TMY), with the former being supported by both the state and non-governmental organizations as part of either a global bioprospecting value chain, or its obverse in the form of 'sustainable herbalism', respectively.

Interestingly, both the esoteric and exoteric circles, excluded or muted in the East, reappear in the West. The latter, under the rubrics of Ayurvedic Massage, Deitetics and *Panchakarma*, have become the mainstay of Western Ayurvedic practice, as they are non-drug based 'external' therapies which, among other things, do not require the import or ingestion of compound drugs, many of which have ingredients that are banned in the Western pharmacopeias, including their herbal pharmacopeias. And the esoteric circle, often stigmatized in the East, is routinely purveyed by entrepreneurs from the West, who then expropriate and transmute these practices, either as stand-alone practices under the epithet of 'spiritual healing', or by marrying them to Western psychoanalytical theory and offering them under rubrics such as past-life regression, or therapeutic trance.[50] In other words, if the drug is increasingly played as the major key in the South, the regimen and spiritualised magic are often played as the major keys in the North.

The exemplum of this argument is best captured by the terms 'Culture, Medicine and Psychiatry', which unsurprisingly is the title of a prestigious American journal, where medicine and psychiatry stand in for the body and the mind: divided again into the brain and the mind, with the brain and pharmaceuticals being the fulcrum and the therapeutic mainstay for psychiatry, while the mind and the talking cure is the mainstay for psychoanalysis; while culture, as the third term, not only becomes a euphemism for faith, religion and ritual but, under the rubric of anthropology (and Indology, Sinology and history), also renders invisible other systems of medicine through one of the principal binaries that has bedevilled medical anthropology: disease and illness. A binary that hands over 'disease' to the doctor and biomedicine, while anthropology occupies itself with what is called 'illness behaviour', which is seen to be the patient's subjective experience and the product of his *culture*. This preoccupation, especially when such an ethnography is set in the Global South, rather than seeing such 'illness behaviour' as being conditioned by, or exhibiting, an alternative nosology or aetiology (e.g. possession) based on an alternative epistemology, reduces it to the patient's culture of superstition, faith or belief (increasing ways of being 'progressive'); while psychiatry, as the biomedical arm (with its privileged access to the truth of the disease) often pathologizes such 'illness behaviour', especially 'possession', which it sees as a misapprehension of what, according to psychiatry, is truly a 'dissociative identity disorder'.[51]

This epistemic division of labour, as is by now evident, sets up a hierarchy between 'medicine, psychiatry and culture', which is ostensibly marked by decreasing levels of certainty and increasing levels of mutability, arising from the materialization of medicine by somaticizing (the body, the brain) disease and pathogenesis, and by privileging the *materia medica* (the drug) as the principal form of therapy. And cognate to this privileging, if not leading from it, is the industrial production of the *materia medica* in the form of pharmaceuticals, which are prescribed by a professionalized and licensed body of practitioners and sold as commodities.

This bio-materialization of medicine, where the ambit of the disease is circumscribed by the ambit of the body, with the drug as the new sacrament, inaugurates and produces a global division of labour within biomedicine and between biomedicine and alternative medicine, West and East, present and past. Asian and European alternative medical practices become, in this disciplinary and therapeutic landscape, the other of biomedicine in the West, while in the East the Asian medical practices fall prey to three possible and blurred trajectories of mimesis, bilingualism and creolization that I have delineated briefly above and at length elsewhere.[52]

Notes

1. M. Nichter, 'Negotiation of the Illness Experience: Ayurvedic Therapy and the Psychosocial Dimension of Illness', *Culture, Medicine, Psychiatry* 5, no. 1 (1981): 5–24; C. Leslie, *Asian Medical Systems: A Comparative Study* (Berkeley: University of California Press, 1976); C. Leslie, 'Interpretations of Illness: Syncretism in Modern Ayurveda', in *Paths to Asian Medical Knowledge*, ed. L. Charles and A. Young (London: University of California Press, 1992), 177–209; F. Smith, *The Self Possessed: Deity and Spirit Possession in South Asian Literature and Civilization* (Columbia: Columbia University Press, 2006).

2. H. Naraindas, 'Of Spineless Babies and Folic Acid: Evidence and Efficacy in Biomedicine and Ayurvedic Medicine', *Social Science and Medicine* 62, no. 11 (2006): 2658–69; H. Naraindas, 'Nosopolitics: Epistemic Mangling and the Creolisation of Contemporary Ayurveda', in *Medical Pluralism and Homeopathy in India and Germany (1810–2010): Practices in a Comparative Perspective*, ed. M. Dinges (Stuttgart: Steiner Verlag, 2014), 105–36; H. Naraindas, 'Of Shastric "Yogams" and Polyherbals: The Creolisation of the Contemporary Ayurvedic Formulary', *Asian Medicine* 9 (2014): 12–48; H. Naraindas, 'My Vaidya and my Gynaecologist: Narrative of a Post-modern Birth', in *Asymmetrical Conversations: Contestations, Circumventions and the Blurring of Therapeutic Boundaries*, ed. H. Naraindas, J. Quack, and W. Sax (Oxford: Berghahn, 2014), 150–209.

3. P. Brass, 'The Politics of Ayurvedic Education: A Case Study of Revivalism and Modernization in India', in *Education and Politics in India: Studies in Organization, Society and Policy*, ed. S. H. Rudolph and L. I. Rudolph (Cambridge: Cambridge University Press, 1972), 342–71.

4. Leslie, *Asian Medical Systems*; Leslie, 'Interpretations of Illness'.

5 Brass, 'The Politics of Ayurvedic Education'.
6 For Ayurveda see Brass, 'The Politics of Ayurvedic Education'; D. Tabor, 'Ripe and Unripe: Concepts of Health and Sickness', *Social Science and Medicine* 15 (1981): 439–55; Leslie, *Asian Medical Systems*; Leslie, 'Interpretation of Illness'; T. Nisula, 'In the Presence of Biomedicine: Ayurveda, Medical Integration and Health Seeking in Mysore, South India' *Anthropology and Medicine* 13 (2006): 207–24; M. Banerjee, *Power, Knowledge, Medicine: Ayurvedic Pharmaceuticals at Home and in the World* (Hyderabad: Orient Blackswan, 2009); M. Bode, *Taking Traditional Knowledge to the Market: The Modern Image of the Ayurvedic and Unani Industry, 1980–2000* (Hyderabad: Orient Blackswan, 2008); M. S. Harilal, 'Commercialising Traditional Medicine: Ayurvedic Manufacturing in Kerala', *Economic and Political Weekly* XLIV, no. 16 (2009): 44–51; V. Sujatha, 'What Could "Integrative" Medicine Mean? Social Science Perspectives on Contemporary Ayurveda', *Journal of Ayurveda and Integrative Medicine* 2 (2011): 115–23. For other Asian systems of medicine, see Cai Jingfeng, 'Integration of Traditional Chinese Medicine with Western Medicine – Right or Wrong?', *Social Science and Medicine* 27, no. 5 (1988): 521–9; V. Scheid, 'Shaping Chinese Medicine: Two Case Studies from Contemporary China', *Innovation in Chinese Medicine*, ed. E. Hsu (Cambridge: Cambridge University Press, 2001), 370–404; V. Adams, 'Randomised Controlled Crime: Postcolonial Sciences in Alternative Medicine Research', *Social Studies of Science* 32 (2002): 659–90; R. Fan and I. Holliday, 'Which Medicine? Whose Standard? Critical Reflections on Medical Integration in China', *Journal of Medical Ethics* 33 (2007): 454–61; J. Kim, 'Alternative Medicine's Encounter with Laboratory Science: The Scientific Construction of Korean Medicine in a Global Age', *Social Studies of Science* 37 (2007): 855–80; V. Adams and Fei-Fei Li, 'Integration or Erasure? Modernising Medicine at Lhasa's Mentsikhang', in *Tibetan Medicine in the Contemporary World: Global Politics of Medical Knowledge and Practice*, ed. L. Pordié (London: Routledge, 2008), 105–31; L. Pordié, 'Tibetan Medicine Today: Neo-traditionalism as an Analytical Lens and a Political Tool', in *Tibetan Medicine in the Contemporary World: Global Politics of Medical Knowledge and Practice*, ed. L. Pordié (London: Routledge, 2008), 3–32; J. Farquhar, *A Way of Life: Things, Thought, and Action in Chinese Medicine* (New Haven and London: Yale University Press, 2020). South Asian historians, by and large, rather than addressing the epistemic conflict and its fallout, often use Asian Medicine as a prism to address other (equally important) themes such as Nationalism or linguistic nationalism. For example, see J. Alter, *Gandhi's Body: Sex, Diet, and the Politics of Nationalism* (Philadelphia: University of Pennsylvania Press, 2000); P. Mukharji, *Nationalizing the Body: The Medical Market, Print and Daktari Medicine* (London, New York and Delhi: Anthem Press, 2009); K. Sivaramakrishnan, *Old Potions, New Bottles: Recasting Indigenous Medicine in Colonial Punjab 1850–1940* (New Delhi: Orient Longman, 2006); R. Berger, *Ayurveda Made Modern: Political Histories of*

Indigenous Medicine in North India 1900–1955 (Basingstoke: Palgrave Macmillan Press, 2013).
7   Naraindas, 'Of Spineless Babies and Folic Acid'.
8   M. Foucault, *The Birth of the Clinic. An Archaeology of Medical Perception* (London: Tavistock, 1973); N. D. Jewson, 'The Disappearance of Sick Man from Medical Cosmology, 1770–1870', *Sociology* 10 (1976): 225–44; M. E. Fissell, 'The Disappearance of the Patient's Narrative and the Invention of Hospital Medicine', in *British Medicine in an Age of Reform*, ed. R. French, and A. Wear (London and New York: Routledge), 92–109; Paul Atkinson's book *Medical Talk and Medical Work: The Liturgy of the Clinic* (London: Sage, 1995) is the contemporary demonstration of how the pathologist continues to be the lynchpin of modern clinical medicine. This in turn is problematized by Annemarie Mol, *The Body Multiple: Ontology in Medical Practice* (Durham: Duke University Press, 2003), which works in part because of her choice of disease (atherosclerosis), through which she wants to re-inscribe the clinician as an equally important part of the orchestra. But there is no wishing away of the histologist/pathologist/haematologist from the ensemble – at least for now.
9   http://www.accmumbai.gov.in/aircargo/pdf/drug_objectional_advertisement_act.pdf. The act defines 'magic remedy' as any talisman, mantra, amulet or any other object which is claimed to have miraculous powers to cure, diagnose, prevent or mitigate a disease in humans or animals. It also includes such devices that are claimed to have power to influence structure or function of an organ in humans or animals.
10 http://www.bombayhighcourt.nic.in/libweb/acts/Mah.Ord.2013.14.PDF. This Act was opposed by both Hindu and Muslim religious functionaries as an attack on their religious beliefs. And the Rationalist, Dabolkar, had to pay with his life by being assassinated on 20 August 2013. On 21 August, in the wake of his assassination, the Maharashtra Legislative Assembly adopted it as an ordinance, and it finally became law in December 2013. For a perceptive study on Dabholkar and Rationalism, and the possible implications for our argument, see J. Quack, *Disenchanting India: Organized Rationalism and Criticism of Religion in India* (Oxford: Oxford University Press, 2011).
11 J. Abraham, 'The Sociological Concomitants of the Pharmaceutical Industry and Medications', in *Handbook of Medical Sociology*, ed. C. Bird, P. Conrad, A. Fremont, and S. Timmermans (Nashville: Vanderbilt, 2010), 290–308.
12 A. Maturo, 'Medicalization: Current Concept and Future Directions in a Bionic Society', *Mens Sana Monographs* 10, no. 1 (2012): 122–33. As Maturo points out: 'even the treatment of heart-disease risk factors with cholesterol-lowering drugs, such as statins, may be considered an example of pharmaceuticalization. 'It should be noted', says Maturo, 'that all the conditions mentioned above could also be treated in non-pharmaceutical ways – **as they were in the past** (emphasis added).

The treatments could be medical, such as a psychotherapy, or non-medical, such as a change in lifestyle.' But this is as far as Maturo will, understandably, go. But it could also be, as we have pointed out earlier, by invoking spirits or ghosts, or in other words, through *immaterialities*, or forms of *animism*, on which more below. In other words, Maturo's tacit *materialism* will not permit him to countenance animism.

13 C. K. Carter, *The Rise of Causal Concepts of Disease* (Farnham: Ashgate Publishing, 2003).
14 Naraindas, 'Of Shastric "Yogams" and Polyherbals'.
15 H. Jonas, *The Phenomenon of Life: Toward a Philosophical Biology* (Chicago: University of Chicago Press, 1982).
16 Karl Marx, *Capital: A Critique of Political Economy. Vol. I.*, trans. Ben Fowkes (Middlesex: Penguin Books, 1976).
17 I. Stengers, 'Reclaiming Animism', *e-flux* 36 (2012). http://www.e-flux.com/journal/reclaiming-animism/ (accessed 6 October 2019).
18 E. Povinelli, *Geontologies: A Requiem to Late Liberalism* (London: Duke University Press, 2016). See also 'Life/Nonlife: A Response', http://somatosphere.net/forumpost/life-nonlife-a-response/ (accessed 10 August 2019).
19 V. De Castro, 'Cosmological Deixis and Amerindian Perspectivism', *The Journal of the Royal Anthropological Institute* 4, no. 3 (1998): 469–88; *Cannibal Metaphysics* (Minneapolis: Univocal Publishing, 2014; P. Descola, *Beyond Nature and Culture* (Chicago: University of Chicago Press, 2014); P. Goff, *Galileo's Error: Foundations for a New Science of Consciousness* (London: Rider, 2019); Stengers, 'Reclaiming Animism'.
20 J. Fabian, *Time and the Other: How Anthropology Makes its Object* (New York: Columbia University Press, 2014).
21 *The Ayurvedic Pharmacopeia of India*. Government of India, Ministry of Health and Family Welfare, Department of Indian Systems of Medicine and Homeopathy, Part One Volume 1, first edition (1990); and second edition (2003).
22 L. Fleck, *Genesis and Development of a Scientific Fact* (Chicago: University of Chicago Press, 1979); G. Canguilhem, *On the Normal and the Pathological* (Dordrecht: Reidel, 1978).
23 The gloss and its consequences index the fact that the word 'pharmacopeia' may itself be a gloss in the 'Ayurvedic Pharmacopeia of India', as modern pharmacopeias are unlikely to have 'planet affliction' as an aetiology. Hence, whether the *Bhavaprakasha*, *Sahasra Yogam*, etc., from where these 'pharmacopeias' are complied, can in turn be called/translated as 'materia medica' is moot; and if they are so translated, they may not conform to our purely 'material' conception of a materia medica.
24 S. G. Kabra, R. Narayanan, M. Chaturvedi, and P. Anand, 'What Is Happening to Caesarean Section Rates?', *The Lancet* 343, no. 8890 (1994): 179–80.

25 Povinelli, *Geontologies*.
26 In fact, the three diagrams – of a circle and two interlaced triangles – that I have created in this chapter to elucidate my arguments coincidentally mimic stock *yantras*!
27 Smith, *The Self Possessed*; for a recently published account of 'Eight Generations of Tantrics', see the small but important write up on the tantric Govinda Achari (c.1850s-1944), by his great-grandnephew Sharat Sundar Rajeev in the Indian Memory Project. https://www.indianmemoryproject.com/120/ (accessed 24 January 2022).
28 V. Lo and S. Schroer, 'Deviant Airs in "Traditional" Chinese Medicine', in *Asian Medicine and Globalization*, ed. J. Alter (Philadelphia: University of Philadelphia Press, 2005), 45–67.
29 Foucault, *The Birth of the Clinic*.
30 Ibid.
31 Jonas, *The Phenomenon of Life*.
32 Ibid.
33 Stengers, 'Reclaiming Animism'.
34 J. P. S. Uberoi, *Science and Culture* (Delhi: Oxford University Press, 1978).
35 K. Thomas, *Religion and the Decline of Magic: Studies in Popular Beliefs in Sixteenth and Seventeenth Century England* (London: Weidenfeld and Nicolson, 1971), 69.
36 Ibid., 151. But the standard narrative is to offer the ready and stock opposition of science and religion, or science and magic: a form of well-entrenched schoolboy reasoning. It is often difficult to disabuse contemporary scholarship, let alone 'lay' people, of this dictum. I have argued elsewhere that 'modern subjects' are, irrespective of their creed, willy-nilly Zwinglians when it comes to their 'official' explanations of the world, in so far as they are not able to countenance theurgic explanations. See H. Naraindas, 'Of Sacraments, Sacramentals and Anthropology: Is Anthropological Explanation Sacramental?' *Anthropology & Medicine* 24, no. 3 (2017): 276–300.
37 Uberoi, *Science and Culture*; B. Latour, *We Have Never Been Modern*, trans. Catherine Porter (Cambridge, MA: Harvard University Press, 1993).
38 John B. Payne, 'Luther and Zwingli: The Giant vs. Hercules', in *Christianity Today*, 1984. https://www.christianitytoday.com/history/issues/issue-4/zwingli-and-luther-giant-vs-hercules.html (accessed 20 October 2021).
39 Akin to Christopher Hitchens – the atheist – and his refusal to have a deathbed conversion as he lay dying of esophageal cancer. Zwingli could well be the Protestant prototype martyr of the atheistic Hitchens.
40 Uberoi, *Science and Culture*.
41 J. Ordronaux, *Translation into English Verse of the Regimen Sanitatis Salernitanum*. (Philadelphia: Lippincott, 1871).
42 Naraindas, 'Nosopolitics'.

43 Ibid.
44 Naraindas, 'Of Spineless Babies and Folic Acid'.
45 Naraindas, 'Nosopolitics'.
46 Naraindas, 'Of Shastric "Yogams" and Polyherbals'.
47 Ibid.
48 Naraindas, 'Nosopolitics'; Naraindas, 'Of Shastric "Yogams" and Polyherbals'.
49 Ibid.
50 H. Naraindas, 'Psychedelic Therapy: Diplomatic Re-compositions of Life/Non-life, the Living and the Dead', in *The Movement for Global Mental Health: Critical Views from South and Southeast Asia*, ed. William Sax and Claudia Lang (Amsterdam: Amsterdam University Press, 2021), 165–209.
51 D. Padmnabhan, 'From Distress to Disease: A Critique of the Medicalisation of Possession in DSM-5', *Anthropology and Medicine* 24, no. 3 (2017): 261–75.
52 Naraindas, 'Of Sacraments, Sacramentals and Anthropology'; Naraindas, 'Of Spineless Babies and Folic Acid'; Naraindas, 'Nosopolitics'; Naraindas, 'Of Shastric "Yogams" and Polyherbals'; Naraindas, 'My Vaidya and my Gynaecologist'; H. Naraindas et al., 'Introduction: Entangled Epistemes', in *Asymmetrical Conversations: Contestations, Circumventions and the Blurring of Therapeutic Boundaries*, ed. H. Naraindas, J. Quack, and W. Sax (Oxford: Berghahn, 2014).

Select Bibliography

Abraham, John. 'The Sociological Concomitants of the Pharmaceutical Industry and Medications'. In *Handbook of Medical Sociology*, edited by C. Bird, P. Conrad, A. Fremont, and S. Timmermans, 290–308. Nashville: Vanderbilt, 2010.

Abu-Lughod, Janet Lippman. *Before European Hegemony: The World System A.D. 1250–1350*. New York: Oxford University Press, 1989.

Adams, Vincanne. 'Randomized Controlled Crime: Postcolonial Sciences in Alternative Medicine Research'. *Social Studies of Science* 32, no. 5–6 (2002): 659–90.

Alam, Muzaffar. *The Languages of Political Islam, India 1200–1800*. London: Hurst and Company, 2004.

Alborn, Timothy. 'Age and Empire in the Indian Census: 1871–1931'. *Journal of Interdisciplinary Studies* 30, no. 1 (1999): 61–89.

Aloysius, G. *Interpreting Kerala's Social Development*. New Delhi: Critical Quest, 2005.

Amrith, Sunil S. *Crossing the Bay of Bengal: The Furies of Nature and the Fortunes of Migrants*. Cambridge, MA: Harvard University Press, 2013.

Anderson, Clare. 'Coolies and Convicts: Rethinking Indentured Labour in the Nineteenth Century'. *Slavery and Abolition* 30, no. 1 (2009): 93–109.

Anderson, Clare. *Subaltern Lives: Biographies of Colonialism in the Indian Ocean World, 1790–1920*. Cambridge: Cambridge University Press, 2012.

Anuradha, R. V. 'Mainstreaming Indigenous Knowledge: Developing "Jeevani"'. *Economic and Political Weekly* 33, no. 26 (1998): 1615–19.

Appadurai, Arjun, ed. *The Social Life of Things: Commodities in Cultural Perspective*. Cambridge: Cambridge University Press, 1986.

Arasaratnam, Sinnappah. 'India and the Indian Ocean in the Seventeenth Century'. In *India and the Indian Ocean, 1500–1800*, edited by Ashin Das Gupta and M. N. Pearson, 94–130. Calcutta: Oxford University Press, 1987.

Arnold, David. 'The Indian Ocean as a Disease Zone, 1500–1950'. *South Asia* 14, no. 2 (1991): 1–21.

Arnold, David. *Colonizing the Body: State Medicine and Epidemic Disease in Nineteenth-Century India*. Berkeley: University of California Press, 1993.

Arnold, David. *Science, Technology and Medicine in Colonial India*. Cambridge: Cambridge University Press, 2000.

Arnold, David. *Everyday Technology: Machines and the Making of India's Modernity*. Chicago: University of Chicago Press, 2013.

Arnold, David. *Toxic Histories: Poison and Pollution in Modern India*. Cambridge: Cambridge University Press, 2016.

Arunima, G. 'Imagining Communities–Differently: Print, Language and the (Public Sphere) in Colonial Kerala'. *The Indian Economic and Social History Review* 43, no. 1 (2006): 63–76.

Attewell, Guy. *Refiguring Unani Tibb: Plural Healing in Late Colonial India*. Hyderabad: Orient Blackswan, 2007.

Austin, C. J. 'A Study of Leprosy in Fiji'. *International Journal of Leprosy* 4, no. 1 (1936): 55–70.

Azhar, Misbahuddin and Nighat Anjum. 'Revand Chini (Chinese Rhubarb): A Review on Historical and Unani Classical Prospect'. *International Journal of Unani and Integrative Medicine* 3, no. 1 (2019): 11–18.

Barnes, Ruth, ed. *Textiles in Indian Ocean Studies*. London and New York: Routledge, 2005.

Bayly, Christopher. '"Archaic" and "Modern" Globalization in the Eurasian and African Arena, ca. 1750-1850'. In *Globalization in World History*, edited by Anthony Hopkins, 47–73. New York: W.W. Norton, 2002.

Behal, Rana P. 'Power Structure, Discipline, and Labour in Assam Tea Plantations under Colonial Rule'. *International Review of Social History* 51 (S14), (2006): 143–72.

Bellorini, Cristina. *The World of Plants in Renaissance Tuscany; Medicine and Botany*. New York: Ashgate, 2016.

Berg, Maxine. 'In Pursuit of Luxury: Global History and British Consumer Goods in the Eighteenth Century'. *Past & Present* 182, no. 1 (2004): 85–142.

Berg, Maxine, ed. *Goods from the East, 1600–1800: Trading Eurasia*. Basingstoke: Palgrave Macmillan, 2015.

Bian, He. 'Assembling the Cure: Materia Medica and the Culture of Healing in Late Imperial China'. PhD, Harvard, 2014.

Bian, He. *Know Your Remedies: Pharmacy and Culture in Early Modern China*. Princeton: Princeton University Press, 2020.

Bijoy, C. R. 'Access and Benefit Sharing from the Indigenous Peoples' Perspective: The TBGRI-Kani "model"'. *Law, Environment and Development Journal* 3, no. 1 (2007): 1–23.

Binsbergen, Wim M. J. van. 'Commodification: Things, Agency, and Identities: Introduction'. In *Commodification: Things, Agency, and Identities (The Social Life of Things Revisited)*, edited by Wim M. J. van Binsbergen and Peter Geschiere, 9–51. Münster: Lit Verlag, 2005.

Birdwood, George C. M. *Catalogue of the Economic Products of the Presidency of Bombay*. Bombay: Education Society's Press, 1862.

Blake, Stephen. 'The Urban Economy in Premodern Muslim India: Shahjahanabad 639–1739'. *Modern Asian Studies* 21, no. 3 (1987): 447–71.

Blake, Stephen. *Shahjahanabad, The Sovereign City in Mughal India 1639–1739*. Cambridge: Cambridge University Press, 1991.

Boivin, Nicole, Alison Crowther, Richard Helm, and Dorian Q. Fuller. 'East Africa and Madagascar in the Indian Ocean World'. *Journal of World Prehistory* 26, no. 3 (2013): 213–81.

Boivin, Nicole, Dorian Fuller, and Alison Crowther. 'Old World Globalization and the Columbian Exchange: Comparison and Contrast'. *World Archaeology* 44, no. 3 (2012): 452–69.

Bouchon, Genevieve and Denys Lombard. 'The Indian Ocean in The Fifteenth Century'. In *India and the Indian Ocean 1500–1800*, edited by Ashin Das Gupta and M. N. Pearson, 46–70. Calcutta: Oxford University Press, 1987.

Boxer, C. R. 'A Note on Portuguese Reactions to the Revival of the Red Sea Spice Trade and the Rise of Atjeh, 1540–1600'. *Journal of Southeast Asian History* 10, no. 3 (1969): 415–28.

Brass, Paul. 'The Politics of Ayurvedic Education: A Case Study of Revivalism and Modernization in India'. In *Education and Politics in India: Studies in Organization, Society and Policy*, edited by S. H. Rudolph and L. I. Rudolph, 342–71. Cambridge: Cambridge University Press, 1972.

Buckingham, J. *Leprosy in Colonial South India: Medicine and Confinement*. Basingstoke: Palgrave Macmillan, 2002.

Buckingham, J. 'Indenture and the Indian Experience of Leprosy on Makogai Island, Fiji'. *The Journal of Pacific History* 52, no. 3 (2017): 325–42.

Butterfield, Herbert. *The Origins of Modern Science*. London: G. Bell & Sons, 1949.

Campbell, Gwyn. 'The Indian Ocean World Global Economy in the Context of Human-Environment Interaction, 300 BCE –1750'. *Global Environment* 13, no. 1 (2020): 30–66.

Campbell, Gwyn and Eva-Maria Knoll, eds. *Disease Dispersion and Impact in the Indian Ocean World*. Basingstoke: Palgrave Macmillan, 2020.

Carter, C. K. *The Rise of Causal Concepts of Disease*. Farnham: Ashgate Publishing, 2003.

Chakrabarti, Pratik. *Materials and Medicine: Trade, Conquest and Therapeutics in the Eighteenth Century*. Manchester: Manchester University Press, 2010.

Chakravarti, Ranabir. *The Pull Towards the Coast and Other Essays: The Indian Ocean History and the Subcontinent Before 1500 CE*. Delhi: Primus Books, 2020.

Chandra, Bipan. *India's Struggle for Independence*. New Delhi: Penguin Books, 1989.

Chang, Che-Chia. 'Origins of a Misunderstanding: The Qianlong Emperor's Embargo on Rhubarb Exports to Russia, the Scenario and Its Consequences'. *Asian Medicine* 1, no. 2 (2005): 335–54.

Chatterjee, Kumkum. *Merchants, Politics and Society in Early Modern India, Bihar: 1733–1820*. Leiden: Brill, 1996.

Chatterjee, Partha. *The Nation and Its Fragments: Colonial and Postcolonial Histories*. Princeton: Princeton University Press, 1994.

Chaudhuri, K. N. *Trade and Civilisation in the Indian Ocean: An Economic History from the Rise of Islam to 1750*. Cambridge: Cambridge University Press, 1985.

Chavan, V. P. *Vaishnavism of the Gowd Saraswat Brahmins: And a Few Konkani Folklore Tales*. New Delhi: Asian Educational Services, 1991.

Christison, Robert. *A Treatise on Poisons*. Philadelphia: Edward Barrington and George D. Haswell, 1845.

Christoffersen, Leif P. and Eric J. Mathur. 'Bioprospecting Ethics & Benefits; A Model for Effective Benefit-Sharing'. *Industrial Biotechnology* 1, no. 4 (2005): 255–9.

Cleetus, Burton. 'Subaltern Medicine and Social Mobility: The Experience of the Ezhava in Kerala'. *Indian Anthropologist* 37, no. 1 (2007): 147–72.

Cobb, Matthew. 'Malpighi, Swammerdam and the Colourful Silkworm: Replication and Visual Representation in Early Modern Science'. *Annals of Science* 59, no. 2 (2002): 111–47.

Cobb, Matthew, ed. *The Indian Ocean Trade in Antiquity Political, Cultural and Economic Impacts*. London: Taylor and Francis, 2018.

Cohn, Bernard S. *Colonialism and its Forms of Knowledge: The British in India*. Princeton: Princeton University Press, 1996.

Cook, Harold and Timothy D. Walker. 'Circulation of Medicine in the Early Modern Atlantic World'. *Social History of Medicine* 26, no. 3 (2013): 337–351.

Cook, Harold John. *Matters of Exchange: Commerce, Medicine, and Science in the Dutch Golden Age*. New Haven and London: Yale University Press, 2007.

Corbin, Alain. *The Foul and The Fragrant: Odor and the French Social Imagination*. Cambridge, MA: Harvard University Press, 1986.

Craig, S. R. '"Good" Manufacturing by Whose Standards? Remaking Concepts of Quality, Safety, and Value in the Production of Tibetan Medicines'. *Anthropological Quarterly* 84, no. 2 (2011): 331–78.

Da Costa, Palmira Fontes, ed. *Medicine Trade and Empire: Garcia de Orta's Colloquies on the Simples and Drugs of India (1563) in Context*. London: Routledge, 2016.

Da Costa, Palmira Fontes and Teresa Nobre De Carvalho. 'Between East And West: Garcia de Orta's Colloquies and the Circulation of Medical Knowledge in the Sixteenth Century'. *Asclepio* 65, no. 1 (2013): 1–13.

Das Gupta, Ashin. 'Introduction II: The Story'. In *India and the Indian Ocean, 1500–1800*, edited by Ashin Das Gupta and M. N. Pearson, 25–45. Calcutta: Oxford University Press, 1987.

Das Gupta, Ashin. *Malabar in Asian Trade; 1740–1800*. Cambridge: Cambridge University Press, 1967.

Dash, Bhagwan and Acharya Manfred M. Jounious. *Handbook of Ayurveda*. New Delhi: Concept Publishing, 1983.

Daston, Lorraine. *Things That Talk: Object Lessons from Art and Science*. New York: Zone Books, 2004.

Datta, Rajat. *Society, Economy and the Market. Commercialization in Rural Bengal c. 1760–1800*. Delhi: Manohar Publishers, 2000.

De Castro, Eduardo V. 'Cosmological Deixis and Amerindian Perspectivism'. *The Journal of the Royal Anthropological Institute* 4, no. 3 (1998): 469–88.

De Orta, Garcia. *Colloquies on the Simples and Drugs of India*. Translated by Clements Markham. London: H. Sotheran, 1913.

Deiwiks, Shu Jyuan, Bernhard Führer, and Therese Geulen, eds. *Europe Meets China, China Meets Europe: The Beginnings of European-Chinese Scientific Exchange in the 17th Century*. Sankt Augustin: Institut Monumenta Serica, 2014.

Delgado, G. C. 'Biopiracy and Intellectual Property as the Basis for Biotechnological Development: The Case of Mexico'. *International Journal of Politics, Culture, and Society* 16, no. 2 (2002): 297–318.

Desmond, Ray. *The European Discovery of the Indian Flora*. Kew: Royal Botanical Gardens; Oxford: Oxford University Press, 1992.

Devika, J. *En-Gendering Individuals: The Language of Re-Forming in Early Twentieth Century Keralam*. New Delhi: Orient Blackswan, 2007.

Drayton, Richard G. *Nature's Government: Science, Imperial Britain and the 'Improvement' of the World*. New Haven: Yale University Press, 2000.

Dutt, Udoy Chand. *The Materia Medica of the Hindus, Compiled from Sanskrit Medical Works*. Calcutta: Thacker, Spink & Co., 1877.

Edmond, Rod. 'Returning Fears: Tropical Disease and the Metropolis'. In *Tropical Visions in an Age of Empire*, edited by Felix Driver and Luciana Martins, 175–96. Chicago: University of Chicago Press, 2005.

Engler, Steven. '"Science" vs. "Religion" in Classical Ayurveda'. *Numen: International Review for the History of Religions* 50, no. 4 (2003): 416–63.

Ernst, Waltraud. *Mad Tales from the Raj: Colonial Psychiatry in South Asia, 1800–58*. Rev. ed. London: Anthem Press, 2010.

Fabian, Johannes. *Time and the Other: How Anthropology Makes its Object*. New York: Columbia University Press, 2014.

Fisher, Michael H. *An Environmental History of Medieval India: From Earliest Times to the Twenty-First Century*. Cambridge: Cambridge University Press, 2018.

Fleck, Ludwik. *Genesis and Development of a Scientific Fact*. Chicago: University of Chicago Press, 1979.

Forbes, Duncan. *A Dictionary, Hindustani and English*. 2nd ed. London: W. H. Allen & Co., 1866.

Foster, William, ed. *The English Factories in India 1646–1650: A Calendar Of Documents In The India Office, Westminster*. Oxford: Clarendon Press, 1914.

Foster, William, ed. *Early Travels in India 1583–1619*. New Delhi: Low Price Publications, 2007.

Foucault, Michel. *The Birth of the Clinic. An Archaeology of Medical Perception*. London: Tavistock, 1973.

Foucault, Michel. 'The Politics of Health in the Eighteenth Century'. In *The Foucault Reader*, edited by Paul Rainbow, 273–89. New York: Pantheon Books, 1984.

Foust, Clifford M. *Rhubarb: The Wondrous Drug*. Princeton: Princeton University Press, 1992.

Francis, Sabil. 'Who Speaks for the Tribe? The Arogyapacha Case in Kerala'. In *Politics of Intellectual Property: Contestation over the Ownership, Use, and Control of Knowledge and Information*, edited by Sebastian Haunss and Kenneth C. Shadlen, 80–106. Cheltenham: Edward Elgar Publishing, 2009.

Fürer-Haimendorf, Christoph von. *Tribes of India: The Struggle for Survival*. Berkeley: University of California Press, 1982.

Gaudillière, J. P. 'An Indian Path to Biocapital? The Indigenous Knowledge Digital Library, Drug Patents and the Reformulation Regime of Contemporary Ayurveda'. *East Asian Science, Technology and Society* 8, no. 4 (2014): 391–415.

Gerard, John. *The Herball or Generall Historie of Plantes*. London: Iohn Norton, 1597.

Gerritsen, Anne and Giorgio Riello, eds. *The Global Lives of Things: The Material Culture of Connections in the Early Modern World*. London: Routledge, 2016.

Gerritsen, Anne, and Giorgio Riello, eds. *Writing Material Culture History*. 2nd ed. London: Bloomsbury Academic, 2021.

Ghosh, Durba. *Gentlemanly Terrorists: Political Violence and the Colonial State in India, 1919–1947*. Cambridge: Cambridge University Press, 2017.

Gilmartin, David and Bruce B. Lawrence, eds. *Beyond Turk and Hindu: Rethinking Religious Identities in Islamicate South Asia*. Gainesville: University Press of Florida, 2000.

Girija, K. P. 'Refiguring of Ayurveda as Classical Tradition'. *Pragmata: Journal of Human Sciences* 3, no. 1 (2016): 43–62.

Girija, K. P. 'Interface with Media and Institutions: The Reordering of Indigenous Medical Practitioners in Twentieth-Century Kerala'. *History and Sociology of South Asia* 11, no. 1 (2017): 1–18.

Goitein, S. D. 'Portrait of a Medieval India Trader: Three Letters from the Cairo Geniza'. *Bulletin of the School of Oriental and African Studies* 48 (1987): 449–64.

Gosden, Chris and Yvonne Marshall. 'The Cultural Biography of Objects'. *World Archaeology* 31, no. 2 (1991): 169–78.

Gowriyamma, Ke Ār. *Aathmakatha*. 3rd ed. Kozhikode: Mathrubhumi Books, 2011.

Grove, Richard. *Green Imperialism: Colonial Expansion, Tropical Island Edens and the Origins of Environmentalism, 1600–1860*. Cambridge: Cambridge University Press, 1995.

Grove, Richard. 'Indigenous Knowledge and the Significance of South-West India for Portuguese and Dutch Constructions of Tropical Nature'. *Modern Asian Studies* 30, no. 1 (1996): 121–43.

Gurukkal, Rajan. *Social Formations of Early South India*. New Delhi: Oxford University Press, 2012.

Gurukkal, Rajan. *Rethinking Classical Indo-Roman Trade; Political Economy of Eastern Mediterranean Exchange Relations*. Oxford: Oxford University Press, 2016.

Gussow, Z. and G. S. Tracy. 'Stigma and the Leprosy Phenomenon: The Social History of a Disease in the Nineteenth and Twentieth Centuries'. *Bulletin of the History of Medicine* 44, no. 5 (1970): 425–49.

Habib, S. Irfan and Dhruv Raina. 'Reinventing Traditional Medicine: Method, Institutional Change and the Manufacture of Drugs and Medication in Late Colonial

India'. In *Asian Medicine and Globalization*, edited by Joseph S. Alter, 67–77. Philadelphia: University of Pennsylvania Press, 2005.

Hacking, Ian. 'Nineteenth Century Cracks in the Concept of Determinism'. *Journal of the History of Ideas* 44, no. 3 (1983): 455–75.

Hacking, Ian. 'Kinds of People: Moving Targets'. *Proceedings of the British Academy* 151 (2007): 285–318.

Haider, Najaf. 'Violence and Defiance of Authority in Mughal India: A Study of the Shoe Sellers' Riot of Shahjahanabad'. *Studies in History* 36, no. 2 (2020): 163–77.

Hanks, William F. 'Text and Textuality'. *Annual Review of Anthropology* 18 (1989): 95–127.

Hardiman, David. 'Healing, Medical Power and the Poor: Contests in Tribal India'. *Economic and Political Weekly* 42, no. 16 (2007): 1404–8.

Hardiman, David. *Missionaries and Their Medicine: A Christian Modernity for Tribal India*. Manchester: Manchester University Press, 2008.

Hardiman, David and Projit Bihari Mukharji, eds. *Medical Marginality in South Asia; Situating Subaltern Therapeutics*. New York and London: Routledge, 2013.

Harilal, M. S. '"Commercialising Traditional Medicine": Ayurvedic Manufacturing in Kerala'. *Economic & Political Weekly* 44, no. 16 (2009): 44–51.

Harley, John, ed. *Royle's Manual of Materia Medica*. 6th ed. London: J. and A. Churchill, 1876.

Harrison, Mark. *Climates and Constitutions: Health, Race, Environment and British Imperialism in India, 1600–1850*. Delhi: Oxford University Press, 1999.

Harrison, Mark. 'Racial Pathologies: Morbid Anatomy in British India, 1770–1850'. In *The Social History of Health and Medicine in Colonial India*, edited by Biswamoy Pati and Mark Harrison, 173–94. Abingdon: Routledge, 2008.

Hasan, Farhat. 'Forms of Civility and Publicness in Pre-British India'. In *Civil Society, Public Sphere, and Citizenship: Dialogues and Perceptions*, edited by Rajeev Bhargava and Helmut Reifeld, 84–105. New Delhi: Sage Publications, 2005.

Hasan, Farhat. *Paper, Performance and the State: Social Change and Political Culture in Mughal India*. Cambridge: Cambridge University Press, 2021.

Hayden, C. *When Nature Goes Public: The Making and Unmaking of Bioprospecting in Mexico*. Princeton: Princeton University Press, 2003.

Haynes, Douglas E., 'Creating the Consumer? Advertising, Capitalism, and the Middle Class in Urban Western India, 1914–1940'. In *Towards a History of Consumption in South Asia*, edited by Douglas E. Haynes, Abigail McGowan, Tirthankar Roy, and Haruka Yanagisawa, 185–223. New Delhi: Oxford University Press, 2010.

Heniger, J. *Hendrik Adriaan Van Reede Tot Drakenstein (1636–1691) and Hortus Malabaricus; A Contribution to the History of Dutch Colonial Botany*. Rotterdam: A. A. Balkema, 1986.

Hofmeester, Karin and Bernd-Stefan Grewe, eds. *Luxury in Global Perspective: Objects and Practices, 1600–2000*. Cambridge: Cambridge University Press, 2017.

Hooper, David. 'Drug Culture in British India'. *Indian Forester* 39, no. 9 (1913): 440–6.

Hurcombe, Laura. *Archaeological Artefacts as Material Culture*. London; New York: Routledge, 2007.

Husain, Ali Akbar. *Scent in the Islamic Garden: A Study of Deccani Urdu Literary Sources*. Karachi: Oxford University Press, 2000.

Hussain, Nasser. 'Hyperlegality'. *New Criminal Review* 10, no. 4 (2007): 514–31.

Ingold, Tim. 'Materials Against Materiality'. *Archaeological Dialogues* 14, no. 1 (2007): 1–16.

Isla, Ana. 'An Ecofeminist Perspective on Biopiracy in Latin America'. *Signs* 32, no. 2 (2007): 323–32.

Jardine, Nicholas and Emma Spary. 'Introduction: Worlds of Natural History'. In *Worlds of Natural History*, edited by Helen A. Curry, Nicholas Jardine, James A. Secord and Emma Spary, 3–16. Cambridge: Cambridge University Press, 2018.

Jensen, Niklas T. 'The Medical Skills of the Malabar Doctors in Tranquebar, India, as Recorded by Surgeon T. L. F. Folly, 1798'. *Medical History* 49, no. 4 (2005): 489–515.

Kaicker, Abhishek. *The King and the People: Sovereignty and Popular Politics in Mughal India*. New York: Oxford University Press, 2020.

Karanjia, B. K. *Godrej: A Hundred Years (1897–1997)*. New Delhi: Penguin Books, 1997.

Kaur, Harminder. 'Of Soaps and Scents: Corporeal Cleanliness in Urban Colonial India'. In *Towards a History of Consumption in South Asia*, edited by Douglas E Haynes, Abigail McGowan, Tirthankar Roy, and Haruka Yanagisawa, 246–67. New Delhi: Oxford University Press, 2010.

Khan, Dargah Quli. *Muraqqa e Dehli: The Mughal Capital In Muhammad Shah's Time*. Translated by Chander Shekhar and Shama Mitra Chenoy. New Delhi: Deputy Publication, 1989.

Khân, Muḥammad Sharîf. *The Taleef Shereef, or Indian Materia Medica*. Translated by George Playfair. Calcutta: Baptist Mission Press, 1833.

Khan, Sumbul Halim. *Art and Craft Workshop Under the Mughals: A Study of Jaipur Karkhanas*. New Delhi: Primus Books, 2015.

Kingsbury, Benjamin. *The Dark Island: Leprosy in New Zealand and the Quail Island Colony*. Christchurch: Bridget Williams Books, 2019.

Kirtikar, Kanhoba Ranchoddas and Baman Das Basu. *Indian Medicinal Plants*, Vol. 2. Bahadurganj: Sudhindra Nath Basu, Pâninî Office, 1918.

Knight, Leah. *Of Books and Botany in Early Modern England; Sixteenth Century Plants and Print Culture*. Burlington: Ashgate, 2009.

Ko, Dorothy. 'Itineraries of Inkstones in Early Modern China'. In *Entangled Itineraries: Materials, Practices, and Knowledges Across Eurasia*, edited by Pamela H. Smith, 202–23. Pittsburgh: University of Pittsburgh Press, 2019.

Krishnankutty, Gita. *A Life of Healing: A Biography of Vaidyaratnam P. S. Varier*. New Delhi: Viking, 2001.
Kumar, Deepak, ed. *Disease and Medicine in India: A Historical Overview*. New Delhi: Tulika, 2001.
Kumar, Suresh, Jitpal Kamboj, Suman, and Sunil Sharma. 'Overview for Various Aspects of the Health Benefits of *Piper Longum* Linn. Fruit'. *Journal of Acupuncture and Meridian Studies* 4, no. 2 (2011): 134–40.
Kumar, T. P. Bharath, M. T. Lakshminarayan and A. T. Krishnamurthy. 'Extraction of Medicinal Plants by Tribals in Kerala'. *Journal of Pharmacognosy and Phytochemistry* 7, SP 3 (2018): 242–5.
Kumar, Udaya. 'Self, Body and Inner Sense: Some Reflections on Sree Narayana Guru and Kumaran Asan'. *Studies in History* 13, no. 2 (1997): 247–70.
Lach, Donald P. *Asia in the Making of Europe, Volume I: The Century of Discovery*. London: Chicago University Press, 2008.
Lai, Fang, Yan Zhang, Dong-ping Xie, Shu-tao Mai, Yan-na Weng, Jiong-dong Du, Guang-ping Wu, Jing-xia Zheng, and Yun Han. 'A Systematic Review of Rhubarb (a Traditional Chinese Medicine) Used for the Treatment of Experimental Sepsis'. *Evidence-Based Complementary and Alternative Medicine* (2015): 1–12.
Lambourn, Elizabeth A. *Abraham's Luggage: A Social Life of Things in the Medieval Indian Ocean World*. Cambridge: Cambridge University Press, 2018.
Latour, Bruno. 'The Berlin Key or How to Do Words with Things'. In *Matter, Materiality and Modern Culture*, edited by P. Graves-Brown, 10–21. London: Routledge, 2000.
Laufer, Berthold. *Sino-Iranica: Chinese Contributions to the History of Civilization in Ancient Iran, with Special Reference to the History of Cultivated Plants and Products*. Chicago: Field Museum of Natural History, 1919.
Leslie, Charles. 'The Professionalizing Ideology of Medical Revivalism'. In *Entrepreneurship and Modernisation of Occupational Cultures in South Asia*, edited by Milton Singer, 216–42. Durham: Duke University Press, 1973.
Leslie, Charles. *Asian Medical Systems: A Comparative Study*. Berkeley: University of California Press, 1976.
Leslie, Charles. 'Interpretations of Illness: Syncretism in Modern Ayurveda'. In *Paths to Asian Medical Knowledge*, edited by Charles Leslie and Allan Young, 177–209. London: University of California Press, 1992.
Leung, Angela Ki Che. *Leprosy in China*. New York: Columbia University Press, 2009.
Levi-Strauss, Claude. 'Introduction: History and Anthropology'. In *Structural Anthropology, Volume I, Claude Levi-Strauss*, translated by Claire Jacobson and Brooke Grundfest Schoepf, 1–27. New York: Basic Books, 1963.
Lewis, Brian. *'So Clean': Lord Leverhulme, Soap and Civilisation*. Manchester: Manchester University Press, 2012.
Liu, Xinru. *Ancient India and Ancient China: Trade and Religious Exchanges AD 1–600*. New York: Oxford University Press, 1988.

Livingstone, David N. 'Tropical Climate and Moral Hygiene: The Anatomy of a Victorian Debate'. *The British Journal for the History of Science* 32, no. 1 (1999): 93–110.

Lo, Vivienne and Sylvia Schroer. 'Deviant Airs in "Traditional" Chinese Medicine'. In *Asian Medicine and Globalization*, edited by Joseph S. Alter, 45–67. Philadelphia: University of Philadelphia Press, 2005.

Low, Sidney. *A Vision of India*. 2nd ed. London: Smith, Elder & Co., 1907.

Madhavan, Harilal and Jean-Paul Gaudillière. 'Reformulation and Appropriation of Traditional Knowledge in Industrial Ayurveda: The Trajectory of Jeevani'. *East Asian Science, Technology and Society: An International Journal* 14, no. 4 (2020): 603–21.

Mahone, Sloan and Megan Vaughan, eds. *Psychiatry and Empire*. Basingstoke: Palgrave Macmillan, 2007.

Malekandathil, Pius. *Portuguese Cochin and the Maritime Trade of India; 1500–1663*. New Delhi: Manohar, 2001.

Malekandathil, Pius. 'Introduction'. In *Maritime Trade: Trade, Religion and Polity in the Indian Ocean*. New Delhi: Primus Books, 2013.

Manilal, K. S. *Hortus Malabaricus and Itty Achuden: A Study on the Role of Itty Achuden in the Compilation of Hortus Malabaricus*. Kozhikode: Mentor Books, 1996.

Manilal, K. S. *Hortus Malabaricus and the Socio-Cultural Heritage of India*. Kozhikode: Indian Association of Angiosperm Taxonomy, 2012.

Marshall, John and Shafaat Ahmad Khan. *John Marshall in India: Notes and Observations in Bengal, 1668-1672*. London: Oxford University Press, H. Milford, 1927.

Martin, James Ranald. *The Influence of Tropical Climates on European Constitutions*. London: John Churchill, 1856.

Maturo, Antonio. 'Medicalization: Current Concept and Future Directions in a Bionic Society'. *Mens Sana Monographs* 10, no. 1 (2012): 122–33.

McGowan, Abigail. 'An All-Consuming Subject? Women and Consumption in Late-Nineteenth and Early-Twentieth-Century Western India'. *Journal of Women's History* 18, no. 4 (2006): 31–54.

McLaughlin, Raoul. *Rome and the Distant East: Trade Routes to the Ancient Lands of Arabia, India and China*. London: Bloomsbury Publishing, 2010.

McLaughlin, Raoul. *The Roman Empire and the Indian Ocean; The Ancient World Economy and the Kingdoms of Africa, Arabia and India*. Barnsley: Pen and Sword Books, 2014.

McLeod, Ray. *Nature and Empire: Science and the Colonial Enterprise*. Chicago: University of Chicago Press, 2000.

McNeil, Peter and Giorgio Riello. *Luxury: A Rich History*. Oxford: Oxford University Press, 2016.

Mehta, Uday Singh. *Liberalism and Empire: India in British Liberal Thought*. New Delhi: Oxford University Press, 1999.

Menon, Sreddhara A. *A Survey of Kerala History*. Kottayam: DC Books, 2007.
Menon, Vallathol Narayana. *Arogya Chinthamani*. 3rd ed. Thrissur: Vallathol Press, 1976.
Merson, John. 'Bio-Prospecting or Bio-Piracy: Intellectual Property Rights and Biodiversity in a Colonial and Postcolonial Context'. *Osiris* 15, no. 1 (2000): 282–96.
Meulenbeld, G. J. *Studies in Indian Medical History*. Groningen: Forsten, 1987.
Mills, James H. *Madness, Cannabis and Colonialism: The 'Native-Only' Lunatic Asylums in British India, 1857–1900*. London: Palgrave Macmillan, 2000.
Mohan, Sanal P. *Modernity of Slavery: Struggles Against Caste Inequality in Colonial India*. New Delhi: Oxford University Press, 2015.
Mohanavelu, C. S. *German Tamilology: German Contribution to Tamil Language, Literature and Culture During the Period 1706–1945*. Madras: Saiva Siddhanta, 1993.
Monahan, Erika. 'Locating Rhubarb: Early Modernity's Relevant Obscurity'. In *Early Modern Things: Objects and Their Histories, 1500–1800*, edited by Paula Findlen, 227–51. London: Routledge, 2013.
Morris, Malcolm. 'Arsenic'. In *Dangerous Trades: The Historical, Social, and Legal Aspects of Industrial Occupations as Affecting Health*, edited by Thomas Oliver, 378–81. London: John Murray, 1902.
Mukharji, Projit Bihari. 'Vishalyakarani as Eupatorium Ayapana : Retro-Botanizing, Embedded Traditions, and Multiple Historicities of Plants in Colonial Bengal, 1890–1940'. *The Journal of Asian Studies* 73, no. 1 (2014): 65–87.
Mukherjee, Rila. 'Introduction: Bengal and the Northern Bay of Bengal'. In *Pelagic Passageways: The Northern Bay of Bengal Before Colonialism*, edited by Rila Mukherjee, 1–260. Delhi: Primus Books, 2011.
Mukherjee, Rila, ed. *Vanguards of Globalization: Port-Cities from the Classical to the Modern*. Delhi: Primus Books, 2014.
Mukherjee, Tilottama. 'The Co-Ordinating State and the Economy: The Nizamat in Eighteenth-Century Bengal'. *Modern Asian Studies* 43, no. 2 (2009): 389–436.
Mukherjee, Tilottama. *Political Culture and Economy in Eighteenth-century Bengal: Networks of Exchange, Consumption and Communication*. New Delhi: Orient Blackswan, 2013.
Mulligan, S. and P. Stoett. 'A Global Bioprospecting Regime: Partnership or Piracy?'. *International Journal* 55, no. 2 (2000): 224–46.
Nadkarni, K. M. *Indian Plants and Drugs with Their Medical Properties and Uses*. Madras: Norton, 1908.
Nadri, Ghulam A. *The Political Economy of Indigo in India, 1580–1930: A Global Perspective*. Leiden: Brill, 2016.
Nair, Aparna. 'Magic Lanterns, Mother-Craft and School Medical Inspections: Fashioning Modern Bodies and Identities in Travancore'. *Tapasam* 8, no. 1–4 (2013): 62–87.
Nair, Preetha. *Raja Serfoji II: Science, Medicine and Enlightenment in Tanjore*. New Delhi: Routledge India, 2014.

Naraindas, Harish. 'Poisons, Putrescence and the Weather: A Genealogy of the Advent of Tropical Medicine'. *Contributions to Indian Sociology* 30, no. 1 (1996): 1–35.

Naraindas, Harish. 'Care, Welfare, and Treason: The Advent of Vaccination in the 19th Century'. *Contributions to Indian Sociology* 32, no. 1 (1998): 67–96.

Naraindas, Harish. 'Nosopolitics, Epistemic Mangling and the Creolization of Contemporary Ayurveda'. In *Medical Pluralism and Homeopathy in India and Germany (1810–2010)*, edited by M. Dinges, 105–36. Stuttgart: Franz Steiner Verlag, 2014.

Naraindas, Harish. 'Of Shastric 'Yogams' and Polyherbals: Exogenous Logics and the Creolisation of the Contemporary Ayurvedic Formulary'. *Asian Medicine* 9, no. 1–2 (2014): 12–48.

Naraindas, Harish. 'Psychedelic Therapy: Diplomatic Re-compositions of Life/Non-life, the Living and the Dead'. In *The Movement for Global Mental Health: Critical Views from South and Southeast Asia*, edited by William Sax and Claudia Lang, 165–209. Amsterdam: Amsterdam University Press, 2021.

Naraindas, Harish, Johannes Quack, and William Sax, eds. *Asymmetrical Conversations: Contestations, Circumventions, and the Blurring of Therapeutic Boundaries*. New York: Berghahn Books, 2014.

Needham, Joseph. *The Grand Titration: Science and Society in East and West*. London: George Allen & Unwin, 1969.

Nichter, Mark. 'Negotiation of the Illness Experience: Ayurvedic Therapy and the Psychosocial Dimension of Illness'. *Culture, Medicine, Psychiatry* 5, no. 1 (1981): 5–24.

Nigh, Ronald. 'Maya Medicine in the Biological Gaze: Bioprospecting Research as Herbal Fetishism'. *Current Anthropology* 43, no. 3 (2002): 451–77.

O'Hanlon, Rosalind. 'Kingdom, Household and Body History, Gender and Imperial Service Under Akbar'. *Modern Asian Studies* 41, no. 5 (2007): 889–923.

Olsen, Carsten Smith and Finn Helles. 'Medicinal Plants, Markets, and Margins in the Nepal Himalaya: Trouble in Paradise'. *Mountain Research and Development* 17, no. 4 (1997): 363–74.

Padmnabhan, D. 'From Distress to Disease: A Critique of the Medicalisation of Possession in DSM-5'. *Anthropology and Medicine* 24, no. 3 (2017): 261–75.

Pandian, M. S. S. 'One Step Outside Modernity: Caste, Identity Politics and Public Sphere'. *Economic & Political Weekly* 37, no. 18 (2002): 1735–41.

Panikkar, K. M. *Asia and Western Dominance: A Survey of the Vasco Da Gama Epoch of Asian History, 1498–1945*. London: George Allen and Unwin, 1959.

Panikkar, K. N. *Culture, Ideology, Hegemony: Intellectuals and Social Consciousness in Colonial India*. New Delhi: Tulika, 1995.

Panikkar, K. N. *Colonialism, Culture, and Resistance*. New Delhi: Oxford University Press, 2007.

Parascandola, John. 'Chaulmoogra Oil and the Treatment of Leprosy'. *Pharmacy in History* 45, no. 2 (2003): 47–9.

Pearson, Michael. *The Portuguese in India*. Cambridge: Cambridge University Press, 2006.
Pearson, Michael. *The Indian Ocean*. London; New York: Routledge, 2003.
Pearson, Michael. 'Medical Connections and Exchanges in the Early Modern World'. *PORTAL* 8, no. 2 (2011): 1–15.
Pelner, Louis. 'Garcia de Orta: Pioneer in Tropical Medicine and Botany'. *Journal of the American Medical Association* 197, no. 12 (1966): 996–8.
Peterson, Indira V. 'The Cabinet of King Serfoji of Tanjore: A European Collection in Early Nineteenth-Century India'. *Journal of the History of Collections* 11, no. 1 (1999): 71–93.
Pierce, Steven and Anupama Rao, eds. *Discipline and the Other Body: Correction, Corporeality, Colonialism*. Durham: Duke University Press, 2006.
Polo, Marco. *The Travels of Marco Polo*. Translated by R. E. Latham. Harmondsworth, Middlesex: Penguin Books, 1958.
Pomata, Gianna and Nancy Siraisi, eds. *Historia: Empiricism and Erudition in Early Modern Europe*. Cambridge, MA: MIT Press, 2005.
Ponder, C. F. and D. Hooper. *An Introduction to Materia Medica for India*. Calcutta: Thacker, Spink & Co., 1901.
Pordié, L. 'The Politics of Therapeutic Evaluation in Asian Medicine'. *Economic and Political Weekly* 45, no. 18 (2010): 57–64.
Pordié, L. and J. P. Gaudillière. 'The Reformulation Regime in Drug Discovery: Revisiting Polyherbals and Property Rights in the Ayurvedic Industry'. *East Asian Science, Technology and Society* 8, no. 1 (2014): 57–79.
Porter, Roy and Dorothy Porter. 'The Rise of the English Drugs Industry: The Role of Thomas Corbyn'. *Medical History* 33, no. 3 (1989): 277–95.
Poskett, James. *Materials of the Mind: Phrenology, Race, and the Global History of Science, 1815–1920*. Chicago: University of Chicago Press, 2019.
Povinelli, Elizabeth. *Geontologies: A Requiem to Late Liberalism*. London: Duke University Press, 2016.
Prakash, Gyan. *Another Reason: Science and the Imagination of Modern India*. Princeton: Princeton University Press, 1999.
Pushpangadan, Palpu, L. S. Amma, C. R. Jawahar, N. Lakshmi, V. V. Nair, S. Rajasekharan, and P. K. Ratheshkumar. '"Arogyappacha" (Trichopus Zeylanicus Gaerin), the "Ginseng" of Kani Tribes of Agasthyar Hills (Kerala) for Ever Green Health and Vitality'. *Ancient Science of Life* 8, no. 1 (1988): 13–16.
Quack, Johannes. *Disenchanting India: Organized Rationalism and Criticism of Religion in India*. Oxford: Oxford University Press, 2011.
Raj, Kapil. *Relocating Modern Science: Circulation and the Construction of Knowledge in South Asia and Europe, 1650–1900*. Basingstoke: Palgrave Macmillan, 2007.
Ramezany, Farid and Mohammad Reza Shams Ardakani. 'Ali Ibn Hosein Ansari (1330–1404): A Persian Pharmacist and His Pharmacopoeia, Ekhtiyarat i Badi i'. *Journal of Medical Biography* 19, no. 2 (2011): 80–3.

Rangan, Haripriva, Judith Carney, and Tim Denham. 'Environmental History of Botanical Exchanges in the Indian Ocean World'. *Environment and History* 18, no. 3 (2012): 311–42.

Reddy, Sita. 'Making Heritage Legible: Who Owns Indigenous Medical Knowledge?'. *International Journal of Cultural Property* 13, no. 2 (2006): 161–88.

Reveal, James L. and James S. Pringle. 'Taxonomic Botany and Floristics'. In *Flora of North America North of Mexico. Volume I: Introduction*, edited by the Flora of North America Editorial Committee, 157–92. New York: Oxford University Press, 1993.

Riddle, John M. *Dioscorides on Pharmacy and Medicine*. Austin: University of Texas Press, 1985.

Rohel, Jaclyn. 'Empire and the Reordering of Edibility: Deconstructing Betel Quid Through Metropolitan Discourses of Intoxication'. *Global Food History* 3, no. 2 (2017): 150–70.

Romaniello, Matthew P. 'True Rhubarb? Trading Eurasian Botanical and Medical Knowledge in the Eighteenth Century'. *Journal of Global History* 11, no. 1 (2016): 3–23.

Rosenberg, Charles E. 'Erwin H. Ackerknecht, Social Medicine, and the History of Medicine'. *Bulletin of the History of Medicine* 81, no. 3 (2007): 511–32.

Roy, Rohan Deb. 'Mal-Areas of Health: Dispersed Histories of a Diagnostic Category'. *Economic and Political Weekly* 42, no. 2 (2007): 122–9.

Sarkar, Aditya. *Trouble at the Mill: Factory Law and the Emergence of the Labour Question in Nineteenth-Century Bombay*. Delhi: Oxford University Press, 2018.

Schaffer, Simon, Lissa Roberts, Kapil Raj, and James Delbourgo, eds. *The Brokered World: Go-Betweens and Global Intelligence, 1770–1820*. Sagamore Beach, MA: Watson Publishing International, 2009.

Schiebinger, Londa. *Plants and Empire: Colonial Bioprospecting in the Atlantic World*. Cambridge, MA: Harvard University Press, 2004.

Schiebinger, Londa and Claudia Swan, eds. *Colonial Botany; Science, Commerce, and Politics in the Early Modern World*. Pennsylvania: University of Pennsylvania Press, 2005.

Sen, Colleen Taylor. *Feasts and Fasts: A History of Food in India*. London: Reaktion Books, 2014.

Sen, Satadru. 'On the Beach in the Andaman Islands: Post Mortem of a Failed Colony'. In *Disciplined Natives: Race, Freedom and Confinement in Colonial India*, edited by Satadru Sen, 274–94. Delhi: Primus, 2012.

Sen, Satadru. 'Rationing Sex: Female Convicts in the Andaman Islands'. In *Disciplined Natives, Race, Freedom and Confinement in Colonial India*, edited by Satadru Sen, 243–73. Delhi: Primus, 2012.

Shaffer, Lynda. 'Southernization'. *Journal of World History* 5, no. 1 (1994): 1–21.

Sherratt, Andrew. 'Introduction: Peculiar Substances'. In *Consuming Habits: Drugs in History and Anthropology*, edited by Jordan Goodman, Paul E. Lovejoy and Andrew Sherratt, 1–10. London: Routledge, 1995.

Shiva, Vandana. 'Bioprospecting as Sophisticated Biopiracy'. *Signs* 32, no. 2 (2007): 307–13.
Sinclair Stevenson, Margaret. *Rites of the Twice-Born*. London: Oxford University Press, 1920.
Singha, Radhika. *A Despotism of Law: Crime and Justice in Early Colonial India*. Delhi: Oxford University Press, 1998.
Singha, Radhika. 'Punished by Surveillance: Policing Dangerousness in Colonial India, 1872–1918'. *Modern Asian Studies* 49, no. 2 (2015): 241–69.
Sinha-Kerkhoff, Kathinka. *Colonising Plants in Bihar (1760–1950): Tobacco Betwixt Indigo and Sugarcane*. India: Partridge Publishing, 2014.
Sivaramakrishnan, Kavita. *Old Potions, New Bottles: Recasting Indigenous Medicine in Colonial Punjab (1850–1945)*. New Delhi: Orient Longman, 2006.
Smith, Frederick. *The Self Possessed: Deity and Spirit Possession in South Asian Literature and Civilization*. Columbia: Columbia University Press, 2006.
Smith, Pamela H. 'Nodes of Convergence, Material Complexes, and Entangled Itineraries'. In *Entangled Itineraries: Materials, Practices, and Knowledges Across Eurasia*, edited by Pamela H. Smith, 5–24. Pittsburgh: University of Pittsburgh Press, 2019.
Snelders, Stephen, Leo van Bergen, and Frank Huisman. 'Leprosy and the Colonial Gaze: Comparing the Dutch West and East Indies, 1750–1950'. *Social History of Medicine* 34, no. 2 (2021): 611–31.
Sood, Gagan D. S. 'Circulation and the Exchange in Islamicate Eurasia: A Regional Approach to the Early Modern World'. *Past & Present* 212, no. 1 (2011): 113–62.
Sreejith, K. 'Negotiating Tradition and Modernity: Middle-Class Dilemmas in Colonial Malabar'. *Social Scientist* 41, no. 3–4 (2013): 35–48.
Steinberg, Philip E. 'Of Other Seas: Metaphors and Materialities in Maritime Regions'. *Atlantic Studies* 10, no. 2 (2013): 156–69.
Stella, Mary Sr. *Makogai: Image of Hope*. Christchurch: Lepers Trust Board, 1978.
Subrahmanyam, Sanjay, ed. *Merchants, Markets and the State in Early Modern India*. New Delhi: Oxford University Press, 1990.
Subrahmanyam, Sanjay. *Penumbral Visions: Making Polities in Early Modern South India*. Ann Arbour: University of Michigan Press, 2002.
Swaminathan, Padmini. 'Prison as Factory: A Study of Jail Manufactures in the Madras Presidency'. *Studies in History* 11, no. 1 (1995): 77–100.
Thapar, Romila. 'Perceiving the Forest: Early India'. *Studies in History* 17, no. 1 (2001): 1–16.
Thappa, D. M. 'History of Dermatology, Venereology and Leprology in India'. *Journal of Postgraduate Medicine* 48, no. 2 (2002): 160–5.
Tharakan, P. K. Michael. 'A Note on Sree Narayana Guru's Teachings and Health in Rural Kerala'. *Review of Agrarian Studies* 8, no. 1 (2018): 109–15.
Thomas, Keith. *Religion and the Decline of Magic: Studies in Popular Beliefs in Sixteenth and Seventeenth Century England*. London: Weidenfeld and Nicolson, 1971.
Torri, Maria-Costanza. 'Bioprospecting and Commercialisation of Biological Resources by Indigenous Communities in India: Moving Towards a New Paradigm?'. *Science, Technology and Society* 16, no. 2 (2011): 123–46.

Uberoi, J. P. Singh. *Science and Culture*. Delhi: Oxford University Press, 1978.
Vaidyar, C. R. Kesavan. *Gurucharanangalil*, 2nd edn. Kottayam: Current Books, 1993.
Vaidyar, C. R. Kesavan. *Vichara Darppanam*. Iringalakkuda: Vivekodayam Printing & Publishing Company, 1976.
Varier, N. V. Krishnankutty. *Ayurveda Charitram*. Kottakkal: Arya Vaidya Sala, 1980.
Varma, S. K., D. K. Sriwastawa, and A. K. Pandey. *Ethnobotany of Santhal Pargana*. Delhi: Narenda, 1999.
Veblen, Thorstein. *The Theory Of Leisure Class*. London: Transaction Publishers, 1929.
Vianello, Andrea, ed. *Exotica in the Prehistoric Mediterranean*. Oxford: Oxbow Books, 2011.
Waldram, J. B. 'The Efficacy of Traditional Medicine: Current Theoretical and Methodological Issues'. *Medical Anthropology Quarterly* 14, no. 4 (2000): 603–25.
Wallace, Robert. *India in 1887*. Edinburgh: Oliver and Boyd, 1888.
Waring, Edward John. *Pharmacopaoeia of India*. London: W. H. Allen & Co., 1868.
Whitmer, Kelly Joan. 'What's in a Name? Place, Peoples and Plants in the Danish-Halle Mission, c. 1710–1740'. *Annals of Science* 70, no. 3 (2013): 337–56.
Winterbottom, Anna. *Hybrid Knowledge in the Early East India Company World*. Basingstoke: Palgrave Macmillan, 2016.
Winterbottom, Anna and Facil Tesfaye, eds. *Histories of Medicine and Healing in the Indian Ocean World*. 2 vols, Basingstoke: Palgrave Macmillan, 2016.
Wise, T. A. *Commentary on the Hindu System of Medicine*. London: Smith, Elder & Co., 1845.
Wood, Frances. *The Silk Road: Two Thousand Years in the Heart of Asia*. Berkeley: University of California Press, 2002.
Wujastyk, Dominik. *The Roots of Ayurveda: Selections from Sanskrit Medical Writings*. New Delhi: Penguin Books, 1998.
Xavier, Ângela Barreto and Ines G. Županov. *Catholic Orientalism: Portuguese Empire, Indian Knowledge (16th-18th Centuries)*. New Delhi: Oxford University Press, 2015.
Xaxa, Virginius. 'Tribes as Indigenous People of India'. *Economic and Political Weekly* 34, no. 51 (1999): 3589–95.
Yang, Anand. 'Indian Convict Workers in South-East Asia in Late Eighteenth and Early Nineteenth Centuries'. *Journal of World History* 14, no. 2 (2003): 179–208.
Yang, Shouzhong. *The Divine Farmer's Materia Medica: A Translation of the Shennong Bencaojing*. Boulder: Blue Poppy Press, 1998.
Zerner, C. and Kelly Kennedy. 'Equity Issues in Bioprospecting'. In *The Life Industry: Biodiversity, People and Profits*, edited by M. Baumann, J. Bell, M. Pimbert and Florianne Koechlin, 96–109. London: Intermediate Technology Publications, 1996.
Zimmermann, Francis. *The Jungle and the Aroma of Meats: An Ecological Theme in Hindu Medicine*. Berkley: University of California Press, 1987.
Zohar, Amar and Efraim Lev. 'Trends in the Use of Perfumes and Incense in the Near East After the Muslim Conquests'. *Journal of the Royal Asiatic Society* 23, no. 1 (2013): 11–30.

Index

Achuden, Itti 46–8, 60
adivasi 129, 213
advertising 4, 148, 164, 233
aetiology 116, 239, 270, 273, 274, 278
Agasthya 214, 215, 219, 221, 223, 226–8
agency 5–7, 17, 22, 82, 87, 102, 131, 140, 152, 223, 225, 232, 242, 261, 263
agnotology 10, 23
Akbar 89, 91, 96, 101–3, 105, 107
Alipore 194, 196, 198–201, 203, 204
America 9, 14, 26, 32, 36, 38, 60, 77, 142, 177, 183, 186, 243, 247, 249, 274
Andamans 23, 210, 223–30, 232–40, 243
anthropologist 5, 77, 169, 243, 256, 266
aphrodisiac 98, 129, 133, 134, 140, 213, 218, 219
apothecaries 19, 130
Arabs 9, 49
archaeology 4, 22, 81, 101, 107, 277
areca 1–3, 21
arogyapacha 16, 17, 20, 211–28, 244, 247
aromatic 17, 87–9, 92–6, 99–101
arsenic 18, 128, 132–40, 142, 143, 175
arthritis 157
Aryavaidyasala 19, 111, 116, 118, 121, 122, 126
ashramam 157
ashtangahridhaya 114, 116, 224, 272
Asian 8, 9, 12, 20, 32, 36, 41, 44, 47, 52, 53, 56–9, 65, 74, 81, 85, 96, 101, 103, 104, 108, 109, 125, 141, 171, 172, 189, 208, 220, 247–50, 256, 257, 275, 276, 279
asymmetrical 20, 21, 41, 45, 56, 235, 241, 247, 249, 253, 258, 273, 275, 280
Atlantic 8, 23, 36, 42, 50, 52, 57, 127, 189, 243
Avicenna 44, 49, 68, 75, 82
Ayurveda 10, 13, 14, 24, 41, 42, 48, 51, 53–5, 61, 62, 82, 111–22, 124–6, 129, 130, 133, 157, 169, 172, 174, 187, 212, 213, 216–18, 225–8, 233, 238, 241, 242, 245–50, 253–7, 262, 269, 270, 273, 275, 276
AYUSH 233, 240, 245, 246, 250

Bailey, E. C. 203
barbarism 50
bazaar 96, 98, 107, 108, 115, 136, 154
Bengal 49, 68, 76–8, 94, 95, 99, 105–9, 142, 163, 173, 176, 180, 188, 193, 199, 207, 226
Bhavaprakasha 10, 61, 278
Bible 15
biomedicine 20, 21, 129, 212, 236, 238, 249, 256–8, 260, 264, 271, 273–6
bioprospecting 9, 20, 23, 41, 43, 44, 56, 57, 59, 231–40, 242–5, 247–9, 251
blood 54, 61, 64, 67, 88, 115, 118, 122–4, 132, 136, 228
botany 31–4, 38, 40, 41, 43–5, 47, 52, 56, 59, 60, 64, 75, 89, 94, 141, 143, 226, 236, 243, 248
British 1, 2, 10–16, 23, 27, 30–3, 36, 66, 74–6, 78–80, 82, 84, 101–3, 105–8, 111–13, 117, 124, 125, 127, 130, 132–5, 140, 142–4, 147, 162, 163, 167, 169–76, 178–80, 184, 185, 187–9, 192, 193, 206, 207, 209, 227, 243, 263, 277
Buddhist 16, 171, 228, 263

Calcutta Medical College 12
Calcutta 73, 129, 133, 136–8, 141, 144, 176, 184
Cambay 49, 94, 95
camphor 61, 92–5, 104, 183
Catholic 26, 30, 37, 39, 57, 58, 266, 267
ceramic 3, 22, 23
Chandrika 157, 165
chaulmoogra 16–18, 171–90
chemist 1, 5, 130, 131, 140, 149, 153, 165, 189, 228, 232, 248

China 8, 16, 42, 44, 56, 57, 61, 66, 68, 71, 73–6, 78–83, 85, 93, 94, 134, 172, 182, 183, 186, 187, 257, 276
Chinamen 182, 183
Chinese 8, 9, 16, 22, 23, 42, 57, 63, 67–70, 73–7, 79–85, 107, 171, 172, 182, 185, 257, 276, 279
cholera 115, 121, 128
Christian 12, 15, 24, 28, 30, 33, 37, 38, 50, 59, 118, 126, 155, 158, 162, 164, 279
Cingalese 2
circulation 4, 9, 13, 17, 23, 37, 41, 50, 52, 57, 60, 87, 92–6, 100, 105, 111, 118, 128, 142, 191, 193, 195, 197, 199, 201, 203, 205, 207, 209
civet 93, 94
clerk 112
clinic 19, 20, 111, 115–17, 136, 157, 207, 208, 233, 234, 238, 240, 244, 250, 253, 256, 257, 260, 268–70, 272, 277, 279
Cochin 46, 47, 57, 131, 147–50, 155, 157, 159, 162, 163, 166, 184, 190, 227
colloquies 48, 49, 59–61, 71, 83, 93, 94, 105
colonialism 10–15, 23, 56, 105, 111–14, 119, 124, 125, 142, 162, 206, 207, 209, 231, 233, 235, 237, 239, 241–3, 245, 247, 249, 251
commercial 8–11, 15, 17, 21, 31, 32, 34, 36, 49, 66, 73, 74, 78–81, 85, 95, 98–100, 108, 112, 124, 129, 131, 157, 169, 177, 179, 180, 183–6, 211–13, 220, 221, 223–5, 231, 232, 245, 251, 276
constitution 12, 16, 20, 41, 112, 129, 143, 166, 167, 192, 198, 207, 244, 272
consumption 8, 10, 12–16, 54, 87–92, 96, 99, 108, 112, 115, 117, 119, 121–3, 128, 145–9, 151–4, 158, 161, 164, 166–8, 220
convicts 18, 191–204
Coromandel 8, 27–30, 32, 36, 39
Creolisation 249, 272, 275
Criminal Tribes Act 130
crops 14, 15, 66, 89, 112, 182
culture 1, 4–6, 8–10, 13, 16, 17, 21–3, 25, 27, 28, 34–7, 41, 43, 52, 59, 65, 80–2, 87, 89, 91, 96, 97, 99–101, 107, 108, 125, 127, 130, 131, 134, 137, 142, 143, 150, 152, 154, 158, 161, 163, 171–3, 175, 177, 185, 187, 188, 203, 207, 218, 220, 223, 234, 247, 256, 257, 261, 273–5, 278, 279

dalit 158–62, 169, 257
Danish 27–9, 32, 33, 35, 37, 38
Da Orta, Garcia 9, 44, 48, 49, 52, 58, 60, 61, 71, 83
Davies, H. N. 195, 203
dietary 10, 12–14, 20, 43, 61, 119, 120, 122, 173
Dioscorides 44, 52, 64, 68–70, 72, 74, 81
disciplinary 5, 11, 65, 187, 206, 209, 227, 275
disease 10, 12–15, 18, 20, 23, 24, 28, 38, 42, 43, 50, 51, 54, 56, 58, 61, 63, 64, 68, 69, 88, 111–13, 115–25, 127, 136, 141, 157, 172–5, 177–81, 183–8, 194, 196–8, 200–2, 205, 207, 218, 228, 234, 237, 238, 246, 249, 258–60, 262–4, 270–2, 274, 275, 277, 278, 280
diversity 193, 212, 213, 219, 226, 227, 229, 231, 232, 240, 241, 243, 244, 248
diwan 98, 120
drugs 13–15, 20, 26–9, 31, 32, 39, 44, 45, 49, 51, 58, 60, 75, 83, 84, 111, 115–17, 119–22, 125, 128–34, 136, 139, 141, 142, 177, 217, 231–5, 237–41, 243, 245–7, 249–51, 259, 260, 270, 271, 273, 274, 277
Dutch 8, 9, 14, 23, 29–31, 35, 37, 38, 42, 45, 46, 50, 57, 59, 60, 90, 94, 95, 107, 174, 184, 186–8, 195

endemic 172, 174, 175, 211, 212, 215
ethnographers 9–12, 130, 243
Eucharist 20, 265, 266
Eurocentric 5
Europe 1, 5, 8–13, 15, 16, 18, 19, 22, 23, 25–45, 48–50, 52, 54–7, 59–61, 66, 68, 72, 73, 77, 80, 82, 94, 95, 103, 114, 120, 127, 130, 131, 133, 140, 142, 143, 154, 155, 158, 162, 167, 168, 172–7, 179, 192, 205, 231, 236, 239–41, 266, 269, 275
exotic 9, 25, 26, 30–2, 34, 35, 52, 65, 66, 74, 77, 91, 96, 152
Ezhava 13, 46, 48, 53, 59, 61, 123, 157, 158, 160, 162, 163, 169

fetish 261
fever 64, 68, 89, 116, 182, 194, 201, 264, 265
Fiji 16, 171, 174, 178–81, 185, 186, 188–90
folk 21, 42, 52, 57, 59, 175, 185, 245, 273
forest 55, 57, 63, 112, 129–33, 141, 142, 171–9, 185–7, 193, 213–15, 217, 220–5, 227, 229, 232, 237, 244, 272
French 8, 29, 33, 50, 100, 107, 131, 171, 174, 277

Gandhi, M. K. 159, 160, 170
geographical 25, 35, 43, 79, 93, 94, 105, 112, 113, 123, 134, 141, 149, 193, 211, 213, 221–3, 225, 226, 236
geographies 16, 18, 113, 122
German 27, 29, 32, 33, 37, 38, 77, 132, 158, 169, 195, 213, 249, 258, 267, 275
Ginseng 212, 215, 218, 219, 227, 229
Goa 44, 58, 94, 95, 106, 179, 227
governor 19, 33, 45, 190, 191
Gowda Saraswath Brahmins 46
Gowriyamma, K. R. 145, 162
Grose, John Henry 1, 21

healthy 11, 12, 15, 124, 192–4, 196–8, 200, 202
Hendley, H. 205
Hendrik Adriaan Van Rheede tot Drakenstein 9, 23, 43, 57, 59
herb 25, 28, 31, 32, 39, 44–9, 51, 52, 56, 61, 67, 117, 152, 157, 166, 211–13, 215–21, 223, 225, 226, 228, 232, 233, 245, 246, 263, 271, 273, 274
hide 134, 135
Himalaya 22, 75–80, 84, 93, 129, 143, 233, 237, 247
Hindu 29, 37, 42, 48, 62, 67, 75, 76, 78, 82, 99, 101, 102, 104, 114, 135, 141, 148, 155, 160, 161, 164, 174, 187, 231, 243, 245, 246, 250, 251, 263, 277
homeopathy 233, 245, 246, 249, 275, 278
Honolulu 181, 183
Hortus Indicus Malabaricus 19, 23
hospital 11, 32, 39, 79, 115, 120, 125, 136, 171, 174, 176–9, 181–4, 196, 242, 253, 259, 277
hydnocarpus 176, 177, 179, 186

hygiene 1, 2, 4, 12, 15, 16, 18, 145, 154–6, 158–60, 162, 168, 170, 190, 207

illness 118, 122, 124, 146, 174, 177, 182, 249, 274–6
imperial 8, 16, 19, 21, 37, 41, 42, 56–60, 67, 82, 87, 92, 98, 99, 103, 131, 132, 164, 173, 174, 178, 191, 192, 194, 207, 236
imperialism 58, 59, 207, 236
Indian Medical service 205, 209
Indology 274
industrial 6, 12, 121, 128, 131, 133, 134, 136, 140, 142, 143, 146, 149, 161, 163, 165, 167, 179, 225, 226, 231, 248, 250, 260, 271–3, 275
infection 228, 237, 238, 260, 262, 264
Intellectual Property Rights 211, 219

Jeevani 211, 212, 216, 219–21, 224–6, 229, 230, 244
JNTBGRI 211, 212, 215–17, 219–21, 223–5, 227–9, 244

Kani 17, 212–16, 218–25, 227–30, 242, 244
karkhana 93, 96, 107, 188
kashayam 116, 129, 131, 271
Kerala 1, 13, 17, 19, 20, 43, 46, 47, 57–9, 61, 111–18, 123–6, 145–51, 153–66, 168–70, 211–15, 218, 219, 221–3, 225–30, 237, 247, 248, 272, 276
kerosene 18, 128, 137–40
KIRTADS 211, 214, 223, 224
Konkani 46, 48, 49, 59
Kottakkal 19, 111, 116, 118–22, 126, 228

laboratory 2, 135, 149, 163, 179, 183, 211, 215, 216, 276
laxative 64, 68, 96, 98, 132
leather 98, 134, 135, 164
leper 174, 178–81, 183, 187, 189, 198, 199, 201
leprosy 16, 17, 48, 157, 171–5, 177–85
lethal 133, 139
linguistics 16, 75–7, 82, 113, 114, 117, 155, 170, 222, 223, 229, 234, 249, 276
Linschoten, Jan Huygen van 19

Lord Minto 191
Lukis, C. P. 200, 205
Luther 27, 29, 30, 32, 33, 35, 38, 266, 267, 279

Madagascar 1, 21
Madras 12, 27, 31–4, 37–9, 120, 125, 129–31, 141, 142, 147, 149, 162–7, 206, 207, 228, 232, 253, 268
Makogai 174, 178–85, 188, 189
Malabar 8, 9, 23, 28, 29, 31, 32, 34, 35, 38, 39, 42–7, 49, 50, 53, 57, 61, 81, 83, 147, 148, 150, 153, 156–9, 162–4, 166, 167, 169, 227
Malacca 71, 94, 95, 106
malaria 111, 112, 115–17, 134, 138, 193, 194, 201, 205, 228, 232, 264
Malay 44, 49, 107, 120, 215
Malayalam 45, 46, 48, 49, 113, 117, 125, 130, 150, 151, 153, 157, 160, 162, 168–70, 221, 239
Malayali 46, 48, 146–8, 151, 152, 155, 156, 160, 161, 168, 222
Manipravalam 50, 61
market 8–10, 13–15, 22, 32, 65, 66, 70, 71, 74, 80, 84, 94–6, 98–100, 108, 117, 131, 146–8, 150, 153, 163, 175, 176, 179, 213, 219, 220, 223, 224, 226, 233, 237, 241, 276
marketing 4, 18, 149, 150, 224, 240, 241, 246
materia medica 19, 20, 25–8, 30–3, 36, 39, 41, 44, 50–2, 54, 55, 60, 67, 68, 75, 81, 82, 129, 130, 132, 141–3, 176, 185, 259, 260, 274, 275, 278
Menon, Karat Achyutha 121, 151, 152, 155, 162–4, 166–8, 170
mercantile 49, 57, 95, 96, 98, 99, 184, 190
mercantilism 19, 42, 99
mercury 48, 61, 175
metropole 19, 131
miasmatic 14, 194
micro-organism 231
microscope 135
mimesis 275
missionaries 12, 15, 24, 26–36, 38, 52, 118, 126, 158, 169
Mughals 87, 89–92, 94, 96–103, 107, 108

muscles 9
museum 2, 3, 36, 40, 77, 84, 103, 105, 106, 108, 189, 223
Muslim 64, 72, 106, 108, 131, 134, 162, 164, 272, 277

Nair 118, 120, 152, 153, 160, 162, 163, 167, 168, 170, 188, 227
Namboothiri 151–3, 160, 162, 167, 170
Narayana 13, 123, 126, 158, 162–4, 166–8, 170, 278
nattuvaidya 149, 157, 158, 165, 167
natural history 25, 26, 29, 30, 32, 34–7, 40, 75, 79, 84, 143, 188, 189
naturalist 25, 27, 30–4, 36, 75–7
naturopathy 233, 244, 245
Nellore 129, 130, 132, 140
network 5–7, 9, 12, 15, 17–19, 22, 34–6, 41, 42, 48–50, 53, 56, 57, 60, 87, 92–4, 96, 100, 108, 114, 117, 118, 127, 140, 146, 149–51, 171–4, 176, 178–81, 184, 186, 212, 214
Niuean 184
noxious 194
nutmeg 9, 94

oriental 2, 3, 21, 26, 31, 37, 39, 45, 52, 57, 58, 106
Orissa 121, 204
orpiment 134
oushadha 146, 149, 155–8, 161

Paludanus, Bernardus 9
Parsi 131, 134
Patanjali 233, 241, 245, 246
patent 132, 212–14, 216, 217, 219, 225, 230, 231, 240, 241, 243, 244, 247, 248, 250
pathyam 269, 270
penal 191–203, 206, 209
pepper 9, 44, 216, 241
perfumes 17, 87–93, 95–101, 109, 147, 150, 168
Persian 44, 49, 68, 71, 72, 75–8, 82, 83, 87–9, 96, 99, 102, 107, 134, 172
pharmacognosy 228, 248
pharmacology 44, 131, 133, 218, 228, 229
pharmacopoeia 51, 54, 55, 79, 80, 83, 85, 114, 117, 130, 132, 133, 137, 140, 142,

144, 172, 175, 239, 240, 246, 262, 270, 271, 273, 274, 278
Phirangi   10
physician   1, 25, 28, 29, 31, 35, 44–7, 53, 54, 56, 59, 61, 64, 67–9, 76, 82, 83, 88, 91, 101, 112–17, 119, 121, 125, 130–3, 135, 143, 181, 245, 254, 255, 263, 264
plantation   17, 19, 112, 125, 178–80, 186, 193, 199
planters   181
Pliny   44
pluralism   249, 253, 258, 273, 275
polyherbal   211, 214, 224, 249, 250, 271, 275, 278, 280
Port Blair   192–202, 204, 205, 207–10
Portuguese   8–10, 14, 26, 30, 31, 37, 39, 42, 44, 46, 49, 50, 57, 59, 61, 70, 83, 94, 104, 107
potato   10, 15
practitioner   13, 28, 40, 51, 53, 61, 68, 111, 114, 117, 119, 123, 130, 131
princely   15, 115, 147, 149, 127, 154, 162
proselytization   15
psychiatry   125, 208, 274, 275
psychoanalysis   274
psychological   273
psychosis   262, 264
putrid   18, 123, 193

Quail   178, 180–3, 185, 189

religion   8, 21, 27, 28, 30, 35–8, 41, 42, 111, 114, 125, 187, 243, 256, 257, 266, 273, 274, 277, 279
renaissance   44, 45, 59
rhubarb   16, 18, 63–71
Roman   43–6, 49, 52, 58
Roxburgh, William   31, 32, 34–6, 40, 176, 177

Sahara   8
sailors   11, 13, 24, 31, 42, 45–51, 55, 61, 67, 82, 88, 111, 113–15, 117, 122, 125, 141, 175, 217, 196, 218, 262
Samhita   114, 116, 172, 217, 226, 245
sandalwood   92–5, 101, 102, 104, 109
Sanskrit   11, 13, 24, 30, 42, 45–51, 55, 61, 67, 82, 88, 111, 113–15, 117, 122, 125, 151, 175, 217, 218, 262

savage   50
sensual   90–2, 124
shastric   121, 249, 271, 272, 275, 278, 280
Shillong   22, 33, 35, 94, 105, 112, 121
shudham   154, 155, 168
siddha   55, 157, 169, 213, 216, 217, 225, 226, 228, 233, 240, 245, 250, 256
sin   12, 15, 118
sinology   274
Sloane, Hans   19, 37
soap   15–18, 129, 145–70
sodium   181, 182
southeast   1, 8, 16, 104, 171, 280
Sowa Rigpa   213, 225, 233, 245, 246
stomach   1, 64, 67, 68, 73, 116, 118, 228
strychnine   131, 132, 139, 152, 184
Sundarbans   193
superintendent   31, 85, 165, 181, 194, 197, 200, 204, 205, 209
Surat   94, 95
surgeon   11, 27, 32, 33, 39, 75, 125, 197
Swadeshi   147–9, 153, 163, 167, 245, 246
syphilis   10, 54, 61

tallow   146, 148, 149, 155, 163, 164
taxonomy   43, 60, 190, 236
technology   4, 6, 8, 57, 60, 85, 143, 172, 219, 226, 228, 232, 239, 243–5, 248, 250
textuality   7, 22
thechukuli   151, 152, 155, 166
therapeutic   11, 12, 16, 18, 20, 21, 27, 29, 30, 32, 33, 35, 38, 41, 42, 47, 51, 54–6, 61, 69, 75, 80, 83, 87–90, 112–16, 119, 120, 124, 127–9, 131, 132, 134, 136, 137, 139, 140, 146, 155, 156, 158–60, 171–81, 183–6, 211, 212, 216, 232, 236, 238, 239, 241, 243, 253, 254, 257, 259–62, 264, 268, 269, 272–5
Tibet   78, 79, 84, 94, 232, 238, 247, 276
tobacco   1, 9, 10, 23, 31, 54, 55, 61, 112, 122, 131
tonic   68, 73, 116, 129, 130, 132, 134–6, 140, 165, 218, 270
toothpaste   1–3
toxic   67, 127–37, 139–43, 169, 247
trade   1, 3–5, 7–9, 13, 15–17, 19, 21–3, 25, 27, 31, 32, 41, 43, 46, 50, 57–60, 65, 66, 70, 73, 75, 78, 79, 92–6, 98–100, 104, 127, 129–31, 133–5, 139, 141, 143,

146, 163, 164, 171–4, 177, 178, 183, 184, 186, 190, 207, 216, 224, 225, 231, 239, 240, 259, 261, 273
trade mark   183, 184, 225, 240
traders   8, 17, 25, 27, 75, 130, 135, 140, 164, 171, 224
Tranquebar   27–30, 32–5, 37–40, 188
Travancore   15, 24, 32, 69, 115, 125, 129, 132, 147–50, 152, 153, 157, 159, 162, 163, 165, 166, 168–70, 215, 227, 229
tribal   24, 42, 55, 57, 129–31, 141, 187, 198, 211–25, 227, 229–34, 236–8, 241–5, 248, 251
tropical   1, 37, 51, 53, 54, 131, 137, 145, 200, 202–4, 209, 210, 225, 248, 249
tropics   1, 9, 14, 44, 59, 114, 124, 175, 193

Unani   17, 55, 68, 69, 75, 82, 88, 129, 141, 213, 225, 233, 240, 245, 250, 256, 276

vaidyan   47, 111–17, 119, 123, 125, 126, 157, 159, 169, 213, 218–21, 223–5, 228, 233, 244, 275, 280
Varier, M. R. Raghava   59
Varier, N. V. Krishnankutty   228
Varier, Panayinpalli Shankunni   116–19, 121, 122, 126
Viceroy   191
vishachikitsa   114
Vishavaidyam   157, 179
vomica   18, 128–34, 137, 139–42
voyage   1, 21, 71, 106, 128, 131

Yanadis   129, 130, 132, 140
Yohannan, Poikayil   159, 160
Yule, Henry   72, 83, 105

Ziegenbalg, Bartholomäus   28, 33, 36–8, 40

www.ingramcontent.com/pod-product-compliance
Lightning Source LLC
Chambersburg PA
CBHW070750020526
44115CB00032B/1607